Disorders and Interventions

Disorders and Interventions

Norma Whittaker

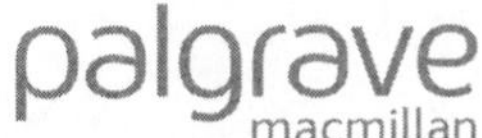

First published 2004 by
PALGRAVE MACMILLAN
Houndmills, Basingstoke, Hampshire RG21 6XS and
175 Fifth Avenue, New York, N.Y. 10010
Companies and representatives throughout the world

PALGRAVE MACMILLAN is the global academic imprint of the Palgrave Macmillan division of St. Martin's Press, LLC and of Palgrave Macmillan Ltd. Macmillan® is a registered trademark in the United States, United Kingdom and other countries. Palgrave is a registered trademark in the European Union and other countries.

ISBN-13: 978-0-333-92263-7 paperback
ISBN-10: 0-333-92263-8 paperback

This book is printed on paper suitable for recycling and made from fully managed and sustained forest sources.

A catalogue record for this book is available from the British Library.

10 9 8 7 6 5 4 3 2
13 12 11 10 09 08 07 06 05

Printed and bound in Great Britain by
Creative Print & Design (Wales), Ebbw Vale

Contents

List of Tables

List of Figures

Acknowledgements

Many thanks to my husband Terry for his technical expertise and invaluable help in editing the chapters and proofreading the manuscript, without which the book would not have come to fruition. Also, to Philippe Marie, who had the original idea for this book.

NORMA WHITTAKER

Notes on Contributors

Norma Whittaker, MA, BA(Hons), RGN, RNT, Dip. N., Dip. H.S., CMB Part1 Cert., Cert. Ed.
Senior Lecturer (Adult Nursing), School of Nursing and Midwifery, De Montfort University.

Philippe Marie, MA, BA, RGN, RNT, RCNT, Dip. N., Cert. Ed.
Senior Lecturer (Adult Nursing), School of Nursing and Midwifery, De Montfort University.

Sandra Johnson, MSc, BSc, RMN, RGN, RNT, Dip. N., Cert. Ed.
Senior Lecturer (Adult Nursing), School of Nursing and Midwifery, De Montfort University.

Introduction

Norma Whittaker, Philippe Marie and
Sandra Johnson

The aim of this book is to present an overview of a selection of common disorders, with consideration of the potential for nursing interventions of a general nature rather than detailed care. This detailed information may be readily acquired from other appropriate nursing texts. The need for a holistic approach to care that incorporates such issues as socio-environmental issues, ethnicity and aspects relevant to the care of relatives is an integral part of nursing care and is accordingly acknowledged by the inclusion of specific chapters. The disorders included in the book can affect clients in any branch of nursing and therefore the information presented in this text may be a useful resource for nurses in any clinical setting.

The rationale for the inclusion of a chapter on sociological issues is to emphasize that nursing interventions should take account of external factors if holistic care is to be practised. Health resources are useless if individuals cannot access them. The chapter explores a number of issues that have potential bearing upon the health experience of individuals and the implications for nursing practice. These include factors such as social class and differences in the social patterning of health and mortality, the latter highlighting regional variations and differences in the distribution of diseases among different groups. The ways in which individuals' attitudes to health and illness are examined and the potential effects upon health of unemployment, poverty and the environment are discussed. All these factors are potentially pertinent considerations when planning nursing interventions but also have a wider political agenda of which nurses should be aware.

Illness can affect other people than the sick person. In discussing any disorder the effects upon other family members can be an important consideration that must be taken into account by nurses. The chapter on family-centred care seeks to increase the reader's awareness of the significant roles of the family in health related matters and the potential need to care for family members when illness occurs within the family. The chapter outlines the influence that the family has upon individual family members, in most cases from childhood and continuing throughout life's spectrum. It seeks to emphasize the important roles that families play in the development of health related and help-seeking behaviour. Such knowledge is vital if nurses are to understand how families may influence healthcare. Understanding how relatives can have positive and negative influences, for example, in adherence to treatment regimens is a significant consideration when planning care of the ill person. The chapter also highlights the detrimental effects upon relatives' physical and psychological health and well-being that can occur as a result of a family member becoming sick. The shift of care from institutions to the community has, in many cases, placed the burden of care on carers. The need to care for the carers has, therefore, never been greater than it is at the present time, in this climate of community-based care. This care of the carers can be facilitated within the framework of family-centred care. In essence, the ethos of family-centred care is the focus, by nurses, on potential and actual problems experienced by relatives and the planning and implementation of nursing care to meet the needs of relatives, and this can take place in any area of practice.

Healthcare provision may be available but may not be accessible to all people and it is important for nurses to be aware of this. Therefore the chapter on ethnicity sets out to highlight the potential barriers to access that some individuals from ethnic minority groups may experience. It focuses upon a number of issues for the reader to consider in relation to the experience of health and healthcare of individuals from ethnic minority groups. The plight of individuals seeking political asylum is also given consideration with regard to health care needs. The chapter also identifies disorders that occur more frequently among certain groups, highlighting the need for specific targeting of health promotion and resources. It seeks to identify how some of the barriers can be removed and to promote an approach to nursing interventions that values individuals, no matter what their colour, race or religion.

The financial cost of nosocomial infection today is considerable, both to the government, to tax payers and to patients. Hospital admissions are increased, so 'hotel' costs are often substantially increased, in addition to the extra funding required to treat with drugs, dressings and more nursing time. There is also a cost to the individual in terms of discomfort, major inconvenience and distress; there is also a 'knock-on' effect in terms of increased waiting time for elective procedures. The need for effective control measures includes having informed nurse practitioners. The chapter on infectious diseases seeks to address this by giving the reader an overview of such things as the chain of infection, microorganisms, body defence mechanisms and insight into the potential for the transmission of infection that is of concern to all healthcare workers with regard to nosocomial infections. The chapter on infectious diseases also provides a basis for better understanding of the issues relevant to the chapter on tuberculosis.

In choosing the disorders to be included a number of factors were taken into consideration, for example epidemiological issues such as the increasing incidence and prevalence of the disorders and the average ages of those affected. (See chapters on tuberculosis, chronic obstructive pulmonary disease and chronic inflammatory bowel disease and women's and men's cancers.) Epilepsy was chosen as this is considered to be the most common serious neurological disorder in the United Kingdom (UK). It can affect individuals of any age and crosses the boundaries of all branches of nursing. For example, there is a higher prevalence of epilepsy among individuals with a learning disability. Epilepsy poses a challenge for nurses to provide support that takes account of the chronic nature of the disorder and thus the need for ongoing support and also highlights the potential role of the specialist practitioner. The contributions of such practitioners appear to be increasingly valued by patients, relatives and other members of the multidisciplinary team.

Multiple sclerosis is a chronic degenerative disease that can have profound affects upon not only the individual, but also the family. The age of onset of multiple sclerosis is 20 to 40 years, a time when many of those affected are likely to be rearing children. This has implications for nursing practice with regard to the need for family-centred care. Multiple sclerosis represents a significant healthcare problem that accounts for a great deal of expenditure on healthcare related costs in the UK. This disorder was chosen to highlight the variable demands for care and resources that the disease gives rise to, and the implications for family members in relation to long-term care.

The choice of tuberculosis reflects the increasing concern, both globally and nationally, at the present upsurge of this disease. Tuberculosis was declared a global emergency in 1993. Not only has tuberculosis re-emerged in developed countries but also there are concerns about the increased incidence of multidrug resistant strains of tuberculosis in the UK. Nurses have an important role to play in preventing the spread of tuberculosis and in encouraging adherence to drug treatments. There is also the need for nurses to be aware of the potential risk to themselves, following exposure to a patient with undiagnosed tuberculosis infection when infection control measures are not in place. The chapter on tuberculosis also explores the contribution that nurses make in relation to primary, secondary and tertiary health promotion.

The rationale for including chronic obstructive pulmonary disease is that the UK has the world's highest prevalence of chronic obstructive pulmonary disease and it is also the largest single cause of absence from work in the UK. It is a major cause of both morbidity and mortality and the rate of increase in the prevalence among women continues to rise. It affects people at the height of their productive years, placing a heavy burden on society, industry and the health services. Chronic obstructive pulmonary disease is more prevalent among people who smoke cigarettes and there is therefore a significant role for nurses to play in health education and primary health promotion.

Chronic inflammatory bowel disease is included to highlight the increasing incidence of these disorders, particularly Crohn's disease, amongst a lowering age group. All aspects of an individual's life can be disrupted and the consequences of these disorders can be costly, not only in terms of personal suffering, but also in primary and secondary healthcare settings. Nurses, particularly the clinical specialist nurse can have an invaluable role in providing educational, emotional and physical support influencing the quality of care offered to those affected by chronic inflammatory bowel disease.

The reason for selecting disorders such as coronary heart disease, stroke and hypertension is that they are the major causes of death in this country as well as in the world. They are very closely related and interrelate with devastating consequences. Coronary artery disease accounts for up to 28 per cent of deaths in the UK; in England heart disease is very much on the increase. Stroke is the third biggest cause of death in the UK. Every year about 100 000 people are said to experience a stroke for the first time. Hypertension is intricately linked with the above disorders and diabetes and can cause significant damage to vital organs. While great strides have been made regarding treatment, it is thought that many people with hypertension remain undiagnosed. Diabetes is included because it is not only a world-wide problem in its own right, with millions of cases remaining undiagnosed, but also a very major risk factor for all the three major disorders mentioned above. While it is not always possible to prevent disease, health education can play a vital role in reducing the incidence of the above disorders and nurses are well placed to provide the information on which informed decisions can be made. It therefore makes sense that nurses should have a sound understanding of its effects on the individual, family and society at large. The above chapters seek to highlight for the reader the significant role that nurses may have with regard to primary health promotion and education as well as support of patients once disease is established.

Most people know of, or have known, friends, relatives or acquaintances for whom cancer has been a significant health problem. It is estimated that one in three people will develop malignant disease at some stage during their life. Many myths and misunderstandings have persisted over the centuries and an overview of cancer aims to enlighten the reader regarding the epidemiology and pathophysiology of cancer, in order to reduce some of the common misconceptions still held today. It is likely that any nurse will be consulted about investigations, diagnostic procedures and treatments, together with the likely outcome. A reasonable understanding should be held of the carcinogenic process, common methods of determining the presence of the disease and its extent. This is essential in order that a degree of professional support can be offered or, at least, knowledge of where a person suffering from cancer may seek such help.

An overview of the disease process is offered in the first of the three oncology chapters together with an indication of the epidemiological situation and trends world-wide. This is followed by a chapter on women's cancers covering breast and cervix cancer, two of the commonest and feared diseases. Whilst there is cause for concern relating to other female cancers that are reported to be rising in incidence, for example, ovarian cancer, there are limitations as to how many of these can be included in a book of this nature.

The third oncology chapter explores prostatic and testicular cancer, both frequently encountered, and with rising numbers of men being affected in this country. These two cancers are usually curable or controllable, thus the intention is to leave the reader with a 'positive' approach to the disorder. In all chapters there is reference to the nurse's role in prevention, by health promotion, and in assisting the patient through the treatment regime both physically and psychologically.

In writing this book, our aim is mainly to give a good grounding to student nurses as well as qualified nurses about the disorders, in terms of their effects on the individual and his or her family. It is also our intention to explore the nurse's contribution in the overall management of these conditions; we have therefore chosen to examine the possible contributions of nurses, in terms of prevention, containment, and eventually in the general interventions once the patient has contracted the disorder. In that sense, we do not deal with nursing care or care-planning specifically. Inevitably there are constraints as to the number of disorders to be included but we believe that the contents of our book highlight the enormous contribution that nurses can play in terms of health promotion and general support of individuals and their families in times of illness and specifically in relation to a number of common disorders.

Social and Environmental Effects on Health and Well-being

1

NORMA WHITTAKER

Health and illness cannot be seen in a vacuum; social and environmental factors have a profound effect upon the occurrence of illness as well as how individuals react to being ill. Nurses should take account of the fact that people's experience of health and access to healthcare is due to a variety of causes. External factors such as an individual's attitude to health and illness and the financial implications of accessing healthcare are significant issues that nurses should be aware of, if holistic care is to be accomplished. This chapter sets out to explore a number of issues; ways in which individuals may be affected and the potential implications for nursing practice.

Contents

- Social class
- Social patterning of health and mortality including
  - regional variations
  - high risk groups
  - differences in morbidity and mortality
- Attitudes to health and illness
- Unemployment
- Poverty and health
- Environmental effects on health

Learning Objectives

By the end of the chapter you should be able to demonstrate knowledge of:

- The potential effects that social class; attitudes to health; unemployment; poverty and environmental factors may have upon an individual's well-being and healthcare experience.

- The need for health promotion to reflect the specific needs of the target group.
- Ways in which nursing care should take account of the individual's social background.

Changes in work conditions, housing, sanitation and diet brought about changes in the pattern of diseases during the twentieth century. At the turn of the nineteenth century, diseases reflected the poor and unsanitary conditions that prevailed; as the century progressed, there was a growth in the diseases of affluence but as we begin the twenty-first century the former disease pattern can be found in the deprived areas of many of our cities. Communicable diseases, respiratory problems and hypothermia are prevalent among those living in overcrowded and impoverished conditions. Life expectancy and the chances of contracting cancer and coronary heart disease are strongly influenced by social characteristics (Giddens, 1993). The more affluent the individual's background the more likely he or she is to make full use of healthcare services and be proactive in health promoting activities (Ham, 1985). A study by Evandrou *et al.* (1992) found no consistent impact of economic circumstances on the use of primary health care. Such figures, however, do not account for differences in the health of the different social groups. The groups most likely to be poor are the elderly; the unemployed; single parent families; the sick and disabled; low-wage earners and those with large families and low incomes (Trowler, 1989). It is important if nurses are to practise holistic care that the social history of patients is taken into account. Nurses must be aware that social backgrounds can profoundly affect the experience of health, attitudes to health and illness and the ability to access healthcare.

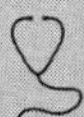

Nursing action points

Social background influences the patterns of disease

- Be aware of the significance of social history when admitting a patient.
- Consider the type of housing your patient lives in, for example could the current disease be associated with overcrowding?
- Take into account the person's current or past occupation. Could the current illness be associated with the individual's employment and/or lifestyle? Consider the potential impact of unemployment upon an individual and their family.
- Note that ethnic origin is related to social class in that most immigrants find themselves in the lower part of the class structure (Trowler, 1989). (See the sections on Social Class and Poverty and Health that follow later.)

Connections

- Chapter 10 (Infectious Diseases) considers ways in which infectious diseases can be transmitted.
- Chapter 4 (Hypertension), Chapter 5 (Coronary Heart Disease) and Chapter 6 (Stroke) discuss how an individual's lifestyle can increase his or her risk of developing these disorders.
- Chapter 9 (Chronic Obstructive Pulmonary Disease) links the development of respiratory problems to environmental pollutants.

Healthcare provision is useless if people are unable to access it. Social class differences in health and the uptake of healthcare have been shown to exist. If nurses are unaware that, or fail to understand that, such differences exist, false assumptions may be made about the way that people are expected to respond to illness and compliance with health promotion and/or treatment. Taking account of the individual's social background enables nurses to deliver individualized care. For example, two people may be admitted to a hospital ward for the same treatment for the same disorder. Their social backgrounds may, however, differ considerably. One may have a good salaried job, no problems with regard to taking time off work on full pay and no dependants; whereas the second person may have recently acquired a low-paid job, have very little income during the period of treatment and convalescence, a young family to support and worries that he or she will not be able to return to that job after discharge. These differences could influence the individual's response to the disorder and the recovery from treatment.

Social Class

The Black Report (1980) highlighted the inequalities in health and healthcare that existed between the social classes (Department of Health and Social Security [DHSS], 1980). An update of that report called 'The Health Divide' was published in 1987 (Whitehead, 1988). Explanations for the inequalities in health were put forward as follows:

- The structural/material explanation
  This suggests that the poorer health of working class people stems from such things as poor housing; low finance; hazardous jobs; severe life events; stress and related use of cigarette smoking and alcohol; operation of the Tudor Hart's 'inverse care law'. This states that the availability of good medical care tends to vary inversely with the need for it. Lack of services available may be

linked to:

- □ The geographical area: areas most heavily populated by working-class people tend to be provided with the fewest and worst health facilities.
- □ Inequalities in knowledge: middle-class people are more likely to demonstrate knowledge of the nature of illness, pregnancy and birth control than people from the working classes. Patients in the professional class may be more likely to ask questions, while those in the unskilled manual group more often wait to be told. Middle-class people are more likely to be critical of services and more demanding of them and to be proactive in relation to health rather than reactive (Trowler, 1989).
- □ Differential treatment by healthcare professionals: doctors and other healthcare professionals may deal differently with patients from different social groups. Referrals to specialist care have been found to be highest among patients in social class I and lowest in social class V, despite the inverse relationship between social class and mortality (Blaxter, 1984). Middle-class patients have also been shown to have longer consultations with general practitioners (GPs) and to receive more information about their condition than working-class patients, even when attending the same practice. The main reason for this appears to be the readiness of middle-class patients to ask questions (Cartwright and O'Brien, 1976). Evidence in 1994 from the Office of Home Economics was that underprivileged social groups were getting the least information about their health during consultations with their doctors (Marsh and McKay, 1994). While black patients have been found to talk more to psychiatrists from the same ethnic background, white psychiatrists appear more likely to classify black people as mentally disturbed than white people. As most doctors are drawn from the ranks of the white middle class they may find it difficult to empathize with other social groups (Trowler, 1989).

- ■ The social selection explanation
This argues that people in poor health tend to move to or stay at the bottom of the employment scale or are unemployed as a direct result of ill health. It is therefore poor health that determines low social class rather than vice versa.
- ■ Genetic differences explanation
This argues that the lower social class groups are more prone to certain diseases and less resistant to others in comparison with higher social groups.
- ■ The artefact explanation
This explanation says that the statistics are misleading, as they are artificial and inaccurate therefore any conclusions are invalidated (Whitehead, 1988).
- ■ The behavioural/cultural explanation
This explanation blames ill health upon individuals for not looking after themselves. The cause lies in unhealthy behaviour such as cigarette smoking, unhealthy eating, lack of exercise and in failing to take advantage of the facilities provided, such as health screening programmes, family planning and well-person checkups at GP surgeries. Respiratory disease in children has been linked to parents' smoking. The risk of infection increases with the size

of the family and poor parental supervision explains the higher fatal accident rate amongst children from the lower social classes. This explanation points out that it takes money to smoke and drink whereas exercise is free, so people from social class V are not forced into bad behaviour as a result of structural/materialistic circumstances.

Changing Behaviour and Influencing Social Factors

Health education is part of the nurse's role; the aim of this is to provide the clients with sufficient information for them to make an informed choice with regard to health related behaviour. This often involves making changes to current lifestyle and certain activities such as smoking, alcohol intake and eating habits. Health education must, however, take account of the fact that poverty often restricts the individual's choice with regard to diet (see the section that follows on Poverty and Health). Changing behaviour is not easy, for example, smoking is not a series of random individual acts but a group phenomenon, a cultural norm rather than a personal habit. Smoking is known to be implicated in a number of common disorders.

Connections

- Chapter 9 (Chronic Obstructive Pulmonary Disease) provides details of smoking related diseases.
- Chapter 4 (Hypertension), Chapter 5 (Coronary Heart Disease), Chapter 6 (Stroke) and Chapter 13 (Diabetes) highlight the link between cigarette smoking, excessive alcohol intake and diet with the increased risk of developing one or more of the above disorders.

Failure of health education to make an impact may be because smoking remains closely interwoven with the culture of everyday life. The prevalence of smoking in England is increasing among children and young teenage girls in particular. A third of girls and over a quarter of boys were regular smokers by the age of 15 years (Office for National Statistics [ONS], 1999). Smoking among the young has long been a significant symbol of growing up and the increase in smoking among women testifies to its continuing importance as a symbol of independence and adulthood. Giving up therefore involves more than overcoming an addiction; it also requires a cultural redefinition of the behaviour. As smoking becomes unfashionable among middle-class groups, those who persist will encounter peer-group pressure to stop, whereas in manual groups, continued high consumption positively reinforces and perpetuates the habit (Hart, 1985). The indications are that smoking has halved among the better-off families in Britain but those on low income have continued to smoke at the same high levels as in the 1970s (Marsh and McKay, 1994).

Connection

Chapter 4 (Hypertension) outlines ways in which individuals can be supported when advised to stop smoking.

Manual workers tend to make the transition from school to work earlier and so have more need of external symbols of their change in status. The transition is usually more gradual for those in the middle classes, where there is a tendency towards a continuing development involving further education or training and occupational career developments. The symbolic value of smoking is therefore often less. If an individual's reluctance to take health warnings seriously stems from the narcotic value of cigarettes as a means of reducing the sheer physical stress of manual work, then the problem is one of material deprivation and not cultural deprivation (Hart, 1985). The implications are that health promotion, to be effective, must aim at changing society's view of smoking and not only the individual's. The societal change approach requires health to be put on the political agenda. The nurse's role is to educate patients of health hazards to enable them to make an informed choice. Nurses who smoke can still act as role models by not smoking in front of patients. Wider measures include no smoking policies, making the sale of cigarettes less accessible to children and limiting tobacco advertising and sponsorship of sports (Ewles and Simnett, 1992).

It is easy to blame individuals for lack of exercise and the media highlight the growing trend of the rich and famous to employ personal trainers. Sessions in leisure centre gymnasiums or swimming pools cost money and their use may therefore be restricted for those on very low income who cannot afford the membership/admission fees. It also costs money to take time off from work to attend health checkups and for the unemployed there is the potential cost of travelling to a hospital or health centre. The decision as to whether or not to take up health surveillance or treatment may therefore be a rational decision based upon the potential consequences of attending.

Government policies such as 'Saving Lives: Our Healthier Nation' (Department of Health [DOH], 1999a) identified certain diseases with a high incidence and prevalence. The aim of such policies is to target resources, health promotion and health education appropriately in order that the incidence and prevalence of such diseases is reduced. Statistical evidence highlights many variations in the social patterning of health and mortality. Geographical variations occur and certain groups of the population are at a higher risk than others in

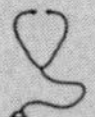 *Nursing action points*

Inequalities in health according to social class

- Recognize that people's experience of health and illness varies according to their social class. This is essential if holistic and individualized care is to be practised. Whatever the explanation, inequalities in health do exist.
- Consider the implications for nurses working in densely populated and deprived inner city areas. How might the lack of resources affect nursing services and patient care?
- Examine the way that you relate to your patients, do you show any bias towards people from your own social class/ethnic group?
- Consider the fact that some patients may wait for you to give them information and so be proactive in keeping them informed. Just because they do not ask does not mean that they are not interested in knowing about their illness and treatment.
- Remember that giving information allows people to make an informed choice.
- Target groups where behaviour detrimental to health is more prevalent and where there is a need to educate people of the risks to health that such behaviour incurs.
- Consider that inviting all new patients for health checks may result in poor targeting and could in fact widen the inequalities in health (Griffiths *et al.*, 1994).
- Aim to be a good role model when promoting healthy behaviour.

relation to certain diseases. If health promotion, health education and nursing care are to be effective, nurses must have knowledge of the types of diseases that are common in the geographical area and among high risk groups in the locality of their work. They should also take account of the predominant social grouping of the local population and the potential implications for health and well-being associated with social-class groups.

Social Patterning of Health and Mortality

The good news is that a number of diseases have been virtually eradicated. These are the diseases that are amenable to treatment by immunization programmes. Pregnancy and childbirth are relatively safe and while the infant mortality rate has dropped, life expectancy has increased. The bad news is that certain diseases have increased. These include cancers; there has been an almost ten-fold increase in the number of deaths from cancer in the United Kingdom

(UK) since the middle of the nineteenth century. Mental disorder, diabetes, cardiovascular disease, degenerative disease and diseases associated with AIDS have all increased (Trowler, 1989).

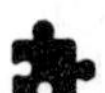

Connection

Chapter 5 (Coronary Heart Disease), Chapter 13 (Diabetes), Chapter 15 (Women's Cancers) and Chapter 16 (Men's Cancers) provide further details of the epidemiology of these disorders.

Life expectancy is a widely used indicator of the nation's health. Since the beginning of the century there has been a steady increase in life expectancy so that the expectation of life at birth in the UK in 1997 was over 74 years for males and over 79 years for females (ONS, 1999). Life expectancy has increased for all social classes since 1972 but this disguises increasing inequality, it also tells us little about the health of the living. For men the difference in life expectancy at birth between social classes I and V has risen from 5.5 years in 1972 to 9.5 years by 1996. For women the difference has risen from 5.3 years to 6.4 years. Women were showing decreasing class inequalities until 1991 but more recently these inequalities are rising. Most gains for men occur in older age groups whilst women in social classes IV and V continue to gain more years of life at a younger age (Hattersley, 1999).

Although life expectancy for men and women in all classes is increasing the likelihood of surviving to older ages shows a definite class gradient. Studies of mortality and social class have shown that although there has been a fall in the death rates for both men and women of working age (35–64), deaths from ischaemic heart disease, cancers, respiratory diseases and indeed all causes are showing a widening manual/non-manual divide (Harding *et al.*, 1999). Recent work examining the effect on men of adverse childhood conditions on adult mortality suggests that certain causes of death, for example stroke and stomach cancer, are related to deprived socio-economic conditions operating in childhood only. Diseases such as coronary heart disease and respiratory disease are related to childhood deprivation plus adult circumstances. Others such as lung cancer are associated with social circumstances and adulthood risk factors (Davey Smith *et al.*, 1998). The key findings of an ONS longitudinal study were that childhood and adulthood circumstances were both important predictors of long-term illness in adulthood and premature mortality. The current socio-economic position was the strongest association, and accidents and injuries accounted for most of the deaths. Persisting disadvantage over the course of life was significantly associated with worse health and survival (Harding *et al.*, 1997). A study by Bosma *et al.* concluded that unhealthy psychological attributes (personality factors and coping styles) are more common in individuals who reported low childhood social class (Bosma *et al.*, 1999).

One factor that has contributed to the increase in life expectancy is the continuing reduction in the infant mortality rate (IMR). This has almost halved since 1981 from 11.2 deaths per thousand live births to 5.9 deaths per thousand live births in 1997. Despite the overall improvement in IMR, social class differences remain. In 1996, for babies born in marriage the IMR was more than twice as high for those babies whose fathers were unskilled as for those whose fathers were in the professional social class. Low birthweight has a particularly strong association with infant mortality and the average birthweight for babies born in marriage and whose fathers were in the professional social class was 115 grams heavier than for those babies whose fathers were in the unskilled social class (ONS, 1999).

Regional Variations

During the latter half of the nineteenth century, analyses of death certificates by the Registrar General highlighted consistently higher death rates in the northern and western regions of England and Wales than in the south and east. The decline in mortality during the twentieth century has not eliminated the disparity between regions and social class. Higher mortality rates in the north occur primarily in middle age, though for men higher rates in the north and west have been found at every age up to the 75 plus group (Blaxter and Prevost, 1993) (see Table 1.1). Regional variations are found in the prevalence of a range of common and important diseases such as coronary heart disease, peptic ulcer, gallstones and diabetes. They are also seen in diseases of children, for example anencephaly and Perthe's disease of the hip. Infant mortality rates are twice as high in poor areas such as Glasgow and Manchester compared with the wealthy Home Counties. During the last decade of the twentieth century recent data suggest that premature death rates for all children and adults under the age of 65 have soared as much as 2.6 times as quickly in areas such as Glasgow, Liverpool and Newcastle upon Tyne as in places such as south Suffolk, Wokingham and Berkshire, which have the lowest death rates in Britain (Brindle, 1999). Socio-economic influences, in terms of income and population density are to some extent implicated in the regional variation in mortality and morbidity; as also to a lesser extent are the adverse effects of urban life, occupational factors and possibly genetic factors. The discovery of modifiable influences in the environment, which adversely affects the health of people living in certain regions, remains a major challenge to preventative medicine (Barker *et al.*, 1998).

The government's annual statistics survey of regional trends in 1995 showed that the north/south divide is increasing. Figures show that redundancy rates were highest in the north and that men in the southeast worked the shortest

Table 1.1 Regional variations in mortality rate in England and Wales in 1985

Region	***Standardized mortality rate***	
	Men	***Women***
North	113	112
North-west	112	111
Wales	105	103
Yorks and Humberside	106	103
West Midlands	105	103
East Midlands	100	100
South-west	89	92
South-east	93	94
East Anglia	90	94
England and Wales	100	100

Note: All-cause mortality is expressed as standardized mortality ratios. These ratios are calculated so that the overall ratio for England and Wales is 100. Regions with ratios above 100 have therefore above average mortality rates, after allowance for the age structure of their population (Barker *et al.*, 1998).

Source: Barker *et al.*, 1998.

hours with the highest pay. People in the north remained the biggest spenders on alcohol and tobacco. Nearly half the elderly people in the northwest had a limiting long standing illness, a higher proportion than any other region (Nursing Standard, 1995).

High Risk Groups

Differences are found in the distribution of disease among different ethnic groups. For example, the incidence of non-insulin-dependent diabetes and coronary heart disease is high among Asian populations, and the incidence of hypertension is high among Afro-Caribbean people (Nazroo, 1997). Death from hypertension and stroke is very high among African and Caribbean immigrants while more Asians die of coronary heart disease than their white counterparts. Psychiatric illness appears to be more common among Afro-Caribbeans living in Britain than among the population as a whole. The perinatal mortality rate of babies born in Britain to mothers from the West Indies, India, Bangladesh and (particularly) Pakistan is higher than the national average for all babies (Trowler, 1989).

 **Connection**

Chapter 4 (Hypertension) and Chapter 6 (Stroke) provide further details of the incidence and prevalence of these disorders among ethnic minority groups.

Tuberculosis has virtually disappeared among well-housed white people but there is a high prevalence among immigrants, especially those from Asia (Barker *et al.*, 1998).

Connection

Chapter 11 (Tuberculosis) discusses the prevalence of tuberculosis among certain populations.

Differences in Morbidity

Accurate statistics on morbidity are difficult to find. There is evidence from a variety of sources, however, that in men and women there is an increasing gradient of various disease categories across the social classes with the highest figures in social class V. Children of poor families have more bad teeth and bad lungs than those children in affluent families. Children in social classes IV and V are between five and seven times more likely to die from accidental death by fire, falling down stairs, drowning or a road traffic accident than are children from social class I. Coronary heart disease, strokes and peptic ulcers, the so-called 'executive diseases' are now more common among the working class than social classes I and II (Trowler, 1989).

Causes of Death

All the major killing diseases are now associated with a low socio-economic level and this is reflected in the all-causes mortality gradient (see Table 1.2). All-causes mortality in unskilled labourers and their wives is almost twice as high as among professional families at the present time. Classification by profession therefore identifies a group with special risk for most major diseases, including cardiovascular disease, bronchitis, peptic ulcer, cirrhosis and a number of cancers (Barker *et al.*, 1998). In the UK the most common cause of death for women below the age of 65 is breast cancer, which has recently overtaken coronary heart disease, while for men of this age coronary heart disease is the leading cause of death (ONS, 1999).

Connections

- Chapter 9 (Chronic Obstructive Pulmonary Disease) addresses bronchitis.
- Chapter 15 (Women's Cancers) addresses breast cancer.

Table 1.2 Examples of conditions for which mortality rates have risen (England and Wales)

Cause of death	*Percentage increase 1975–85*	
	Men	*Women*
Diabetes mellitus	55	38
Cirrhosis of the liver	50	31
Prostate cancer	47	
Oesophageal cancer	42	22
Skin cancers	36	16
Osteomyelitis	33	46
Multiple sclerosis	17	20
Lung cancer	(−2)	42

Source: Barker *et al.*, 1998.

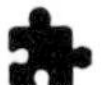

Connection

Chapter 7 (Multiple Sclerosis) explores the long-term effects of the disorder that may reduce life expectancy.

Differences in Mortality Relative to Social Class

Parallel trends in mortality were highlighted in a survey of rates, by percentage of mortality over seven years by age in 1984/85. The differences between non-manual and manual, was unsurprisingly the greatest, especially for men, in late middle age. Though patterns for specific age groups were more irregular, remarkably smooth gradients in all-age mortality in accordance with social class were shown (Blaxter and Prevost, 1993).

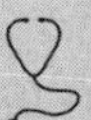

Nursing action points

Social patterning of health and mortality

- Be aware that the need for resources will vary according to the local population and this must be taken into account by nurse managers.
- Identify regional high risk groups in order to ensure that health promotion is appropriately targeted.
- Identify the needs of ethnic groups in order to ensure that health promotion is appropriate and acceptable to their specific needs.

Connection

Chapter 3 (Health Issues Related to Ethnic Minority Groups) discusses the potential difficulties in accessing healthcare experienced by people from ethnic minority groups.

People's attitudes to health and illness also vary considerably and this factor may enhance or impede the care that nurses set out to provide. Individuals who have a positive and proactive approach to health may respond more readily to health-related advice and seek help more readily than those individuals who do not accept responsibility for their own well-being or whose perceptions of good and bad health differ from those of health care professionals. Health education and promotion must take account of people's attitudes and perceptions of being well or being ill and be tailored accordingly.

Attitudes to Health and Illness

The World Health Organization (WHO) (1984) defines health rather vaguely as: "Not the mere absence of disease, but the total physical, mental and social well-being."

This has been criticized on the grounds that it is unrealistic and idealistic, as it is not often that individuals claim to be in a state of total well-being and also it implies a static state, whereas little about life is static. Ewles and Simnett (1992) suggest that the idea of health means having the ability to adapt to constantly changing demands, expectations and stimuli. In practice the medical profession and the general population tend to define health negatively as 'the condition in which there is absence of disease', but this raises the problem of how to distinguish between illness and disease. Illness refers to a subjective feeling of being unwell; the more subjective term disease refers to the medically diagnosed condition, which has given rise to the signs and symptoms in a patient. In order for a disease to be identified the individual must first go through a process of recognizing bodily events as symptoms of disease. The next step is of defining the symptoms as serious enough to consult a doctor and thirdly to act upon them by seeking help from a doctor (Trowler, 1989). Everyone does not share the very concept of illness as involving physical malfunction of the body. Sickness and even death are thought of in some cultures as produced by evil spells, not by treatable physical causes (Giddens, 1993). It is also possible to have no illness and yet to have a disease, as is the case with asymptomatic hypertension (Trowler, 1989).

Variations in defining illnesses are one of the principal problems concerned with morbidity statistics. For some people a common cold or backache represents 'illness' and justifies them seeking medical help or taking absence from work and this 'illness' may be recorded in a data system. On the other hand other people with symptoms that doctors would view as indicative of a major disease would tolerate the symptoms as an inconvenience until recovery takes place. Such illnesses would not appear in any morbidity statistics because the individuals concerned did not seek medical help nor allow the symptoms to interfere with their lifestyle (Farmer *et al.*, 1986). There are also strongly defined social rules about how individuals are expected to behave when they become ill.

Parsons (1951) presented the socially prescribed role of the sick person as follows:

1. The sick person is allowed exemption from the performance of normal social role obligations.
2. The sick person is allowed exemption from responsibility for his or her own state.
3. The sick person must be motivated to get well as soon as possible.
4. The sick person should seek technically competent help and cooperate with medical experts.

The sick person cannot voluntarily recover or be held responsible for his or her condition (Smith, 1985). In essence a person who is ill is excused from many of the duties of everyday life; however, the sickness must be acknowledged as serious enough to claim such benefits without criticism. An individual whose illness has not been legitimized by a distinct diagnosis or whose symptoms are considered by others to be giving rise to a mild form of infirmity are likely to be labelled as malingerers, with no right to escape their daily responsibilities.

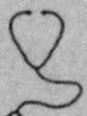

Nursing action points

Individuals may perceive health and illness differently

- Consider how individuals' perceptions of health and illness can influence both their health seeking behaviour and help seeking behaviour.
- Consider how such knowledge might enhance nursing practice in relation to health promotion/education activities?
- Be aware that patients' symptoms may not always fall into recognizable categories or be easily verified.
- Remember that nurses must be non-judgemental; examine your own beliefs and values to identify any negative feelings towards your patients.

The implications of unemployment for health are considerable. Medical opinion increasingly relates cancer, suicide, mental illness and other ailments to the effects of unemployment. Nurses cannot solve the problem of unemployment but are well placed to recognize in their clients the potential physical, psychological and social effects that unemployment can bring about, not only in the affected individuals but also in their families.

Unemployment

A powerful correlation has been found between the rates of unemployment and the number of admissions to mental hospitals of those under the age of 65 (Kammerling and O'Connor, 1993). The link between suicide and unemployment is the strongest link so far established (Laurance, 1986). Unemployed people on low incomes are likely to have an inadequate diet, often missing meals because they cannot afford to eat (Lang *et al.*, 1984). Unemployed men are more likely to smoke more, drink more alcohol and to binge than employed men according to the General Household Survey 1982 (Office of Population Censuses and Surveys [OPCS], 1984). An increase in drug misuse, particularly among the young has also been correlated with unemployment (Plant *et al.*, 1984). All these have implications for the physical health of individuals and this is supported by the findings of the OPCS report of 1987, which found high levels of lung cancer, suicide and heart disease among the unemployed (Homer, 1994). Individuals in social class V and those who are long-term unemployed are likely to have higher blood pressure and tend to be fatter than their counterparts in class I. They are also more likely to suffer from haemorrhoids, angina, respiratory problems and deafness (Trowler, 1989).

The unemployed role does not have the same exemptions from social commitments as the sick role; individuals are expected to continue to fulfil their social obligations despite financial or emotional problems. They are expected to be able to recover and are held responsible if unable to find work. The unemployed must regard unemployment as undesirable and temporary and must accept work of any type and at any wage. Failure to find work labels the individual as lazy or incompetent; permanent status is granted only if there is evidence of unemployability, chronic disease, total abandonment or demoralization (Smith, 1985).

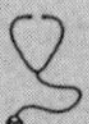

Nursing action points

The potential effects of unemployment

- Consider the potential effects of unemployment on the physical/mental health of your patient and his or her family.
- Consider whether the period of sickness has any implications for the individual in terms of employment status.
- Decide whether a referral to a social worker would be appropriate and/or helpful to the patient?
- Have knowledge of local initiatives to help the unemployed, which would be useful to pass on to patients.

Studies consistently show that worse off families risk significantly higher rates of mortality and morbidity. Factors such as poor housing, poor nutrition, lack of heating and unemployment are linked to poor physical and mental health. Again nurses cannot solve the problem of poverty but in recognizing the limitations placed upon families living 'on the bread line', health education and promotion can be realistically tailored to meet the resources available to the individuals concerned. Health visitors and school nurses working among 'at risk groups' are particularly well placed to monitor the development of children and to assess the potential effects of poverty upon them. There is the potential for nurses to act as advocates on behalf of their clients and to refer to other agencies if appropriate. An essential requisite for holistic care is to 'know' the population being cared for.

Poverty and Health

The poorer areas are said to have 4.2 times as many children living in poverty as the more affluent areas, 3.6 times as much unemployment and 1.5 times as many GCSE failures (Brindle, 1999). The inability to purchase fuel consistent with an individual's needs rose by a quarter and fuel debt by a half in the 1980s (Linehan, 1994). Poverty is dragging the UK back into the nineteenth century according to a Health Visitors Association survey in 1996. The survey found widespread child malnutrition and families in overcrowded accommodation struggling with fuel debt and utility disconnections. It also highlighted the re-emergence of diseases of poverty, such as tuberculosis and rickets (Nursing Standard, 1996). There have also been reported increases in the incidence of dysentery; an infection often associated with poor environmental conditions of overcrowding and squalor. The number of cases of hepatitis has also increased; this disease is associated with overcrowding and faecal contamination of food and water (Linehan, 1994).

 **Connection**

Chapter 10 (Infectious Diseases) details ways in which infectious diseases are transmitted.

Low income can act as a key health hazard and set off a domino effect involving hazards such as poor housing, pollution, the lack of safe play areas and poor social support systems (Blackburn, 1994). Household income shapes health behaviour. Choices of food for example are governed by available income after other fixed costs have been met. The Poverty and Nutrition Survey found that one in five adults and one in ten children in low-income households had gone without food in the previous month because there was not enough money to buy food. There was no evidence to suggest that parents were ignorant about what constitutes a healthy diet (National Children's Home, 1991).

The task for health professionals in relation to health promotion is immense. Clients living in situations of social and economic deprivation may have lost interest in their own health (Linehan, 1994). Paradoxically, health promotion strategies that ignore the socio-economic status of clients may increase health inequalities by improving the health of the more affluent groups while doing nothing to improve the health of the poor (Blackburn, 1994).

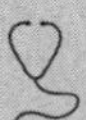

Nursing action points

The effects of poverty on health

- Identify the needs of vulnerable groups, such as the young, the old and those on low incomes.
- Consider the potential for and limitations of client advocacy.
- Ensure that health promotion strategies take account of the socio-economic background of the client groups.
- Be aware of the broader agenda of health policies and social security policies.
- Refer patients to a social worker, if appropriate, for advice on benefits.

Occupational Health Nurses have a specific role to play with regard to monitoring the health of people within a given working environment. However, a person's occupation, whether current or past, may have a bearing on the presenting symptoms and is therefore a relevant part of the nursing history at home or in hospital. Health Visitors, School Nurses, Community Nurses and hospital-based nurses are all well placed to offer appropriate health education with regard to common environmental hazards and their potential effects upon health. This does require the practitioner, however, to be knowledgeable about these issues. There is a great opportunity for nurse-led health education campaigns that can serve to highlight such things as the links of parents smoking to childhood asthma.

Environmental Effects on Health

While many diseases have a genetic component, in many cases environmental and behavioural factors are also part of the aetiological equation. What we eat and drink can be health promoting or detrimental to health. The long-term effect of eating genetically modified foods is of current concern and the subject of ongoing research. Pesticides have been linked to cancer in those who use them or eat food contaminated by them. The excess consumption of alcohol can lead to cancer and to cirrhosis of the liver, and can be responsible for loss of earnings and lead to physical abuse in some families. Even chemicals added to water may be potentially hazardous; fluoride may be damaging to health in large concentrations (Fish, 1997). Changes in behaviour related to an upsurge in the use of mobile phones have been linked with brain cancers.

Environmental pollutants have long been associated with respiratory disorders. Many people died as a result of the infamous 'smogs' during the early part of the twentieth century. The increasing incidence of asthma in young children has been linked to pollution from car exhausts and to adults smoking cigarettes within the family home. The fact that modern homes are centrally heated and carpets are mechanically cleaned rather than taken outside and beaten may add to the problem of limiting house dust mites and animal fleas, both of which can exacerbate the problem of asthma and allergy. Cigarette smoking is also linked to emphysema, bronchitis and vascular diseases such as coronary heart disease, strokes and peripheral vascular disease. Various types of cancer are also associated with cigarette smoking including cancer of the lungs, mouth, pharynx, oesophagus, bladder, pancreas, cervix and kidney.

Connections

- Chapter 4 (Hypertension) discusses the links between cigarette smoking, hypertension, coronary heart disease and strokes.
- Chapter 9 (Chronic Obstructive Pulmonary Disease) discusses the links of environmental pollutants and cigarette smoking with the development of chronic bronchitis and pulmonary emphysema.
- Chapter 14 (Overview of Cancer) discusses the pathogenesis of malignant changes.

Parental smoking is also considered to be a contributing factor in sudden infant death syndrome (Chandler, 1996). Smoking during pregnancy carries a risk of the baby being of low birth weight and the consumption of large amounts of alcohol, particularly at the time of conception can be detrimental to the developing embryo. There may be an association between mothers living near to toxic waste sites and a range of congenital abnormalities (Dolk *et al.*, 1998; Elliott *et al.*, 2001).

Occupational exposure to coal dust, leading to pneumoconiosis; exposure to asbestos, leading to pulmonary asbestosis and mesothelioma of the pleura and exposure to radiation, leading to leukaemia are well-known industrial diseases but there are many other substances linked with industrial activities that have the potential to cause diseases. For example, arsenic and lead, which are often found in the paint used in old houses. Pollutants may be carried home on the clothes and shoes of workers if safe working practices are not followed.

Industrial accidents have been responsible for local populations being exposed to potentially lethal toxins and lethal doses of radiation. Organophosphates in some sheep dips, head lice lotions and pet flea preparations have been blamed for symptoms such as anxiety, restlessness, insomnia, convulsions, slurred speech and depressed respiratory and circulatory centre. Individuals may also be adversely affected by airborne allergens and infectious agents, such as bacteria ingested when swimming in sewage polluted seawater and legionnaires' disease contracted via showers or other water outlets (Sinclair, 1999).

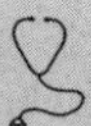

Nursing action points

Environmental effects on health

- Note the occupational history when taking a patient's admission history.
- Be aware that industrial pollutants can affect all members of a family.
- Advise clients about the potential effects of the environment upon health.
- Have knowledge of the local industries in order to recognize potential work related health issues.

Conclusion

Factors that harm people's health such as air pollution, unemployment, low wages and poor housing are beyond the control of any single individual. The government White Paper 'Saving Lives: Our Healthier Nation' reaffirms the government's clear responsibility to address the fundamental problems. To tackle health and health inequality, a new three way partnership comprising individuals, communities and government is outlined. People need to take responsibility for their own health by what they do and what actions they take. Better health information is the basis on which improvements to health will be made but, as discussed earlier in this chapter, better health opportunities and decisions are not available to everyone due to financial constraints. NHS Direct is a nurse-led telephone helpline and Internet service the aim of which is to empower people in relation to health, by providing rapid access to professional advice and information (DOH, 1999a).

Working in partnership through local organizations is seen by the government as the best means of delivering information, better services and better community wide programmes, which will lead to better health. The roles of the NHS and of local authorities are viewed as crucial. They must become organizations for health improvement, as well as healthcare and service provision. The Health Act (1999) underlines the joint responsibilities by establishing the new duty of partnership. All aspects of the way the NHS works with other bodies will be geared not only to treatment of illness but to the prevention and early detection of ill health.

Care Trusts were announced in the NHS plan in July 2000; they offer a pragmatic way forward as important vehicles for modernizing both social and healthcare and for helping to ensure integrated services that are focused on the needs of patients and users. They will be established on a voluntary basis and in partnership where there is a joint agreement at local level that this model will offer the best way to deliver better health and social care services (DOH, 2002). The White Paper also outlined a number of toughened targets, for example with regard to cancers and coronary heart disease with targets by 2010. The target is to reduce the death rate due to cancer in people under 75 by at least a fifth, saving 100 000 lives and to reduce deaths from coronary heart disease and stroke in people under 75 by at least two-fifths, saving 200 000 lives (DOH, 1999a).

An independent review by Derek Wanless, the first evidence-based assessment of the long-term resource requirements for the NHS, concluded that in order to meet people's expectations and to deliver the highest quality care over future years, the UK will need to devote more resources to health care and this must be matched to needs to ensure that these resources are used effectively (Wanless, 2002).

Holistic care encompasses the whole person and this must take account of all aspects of a person's life. This chapter has outlined how socio-economic factors can influence individuals' health experience and life expectancy, and also how changes can occur, over time, in social conditions, which are then reflected in the pattern of diseases and the subsequent demands upon medical and nursing services. Nursing services must develop in line with such changes in order to continue to meet the dynamic health needs of the population. Recognizing that the health experience of individuals may vary according to their economic status is essential if individualized nursing is to be practised. It is incumbent upon nurses within the scope of their professional practice that there is equity of care for all individuals. All the factors discussed in this chapter have important implications for nursing practice. Understanding and taking account of the potential effects of socio-economic and environmental factors can only serve to promote and enhance holistic nursing care. In the reality of increased need derived from social inequality and poverty, with limited resources to meet the needs of such underprivileged and vulnerable groups, nurses face a considerable challenge. In order to meet the challenge, nurses must be well informed of the current evidence identifying those who are vulnerable, whether services are currently meeting their needs, the changing face of services and the shifting professional role boundaries within such services.

Ultimately, tackling underlying social, economic and environmental conditions is vital. Those factors operate independently and through specific lifestyle factors. Health inequality can only be reduced by giving more people better education; creating employment so that people can escape poverty; building social capital by increasing social cohesion and reducing social stress by regenerating neighbourhoods and communities; and tackling aspects of the workplace that are damaging to health (DOH, 1999b).

References

Barker, D. J. P., Cooper, C. and Rose, G. 1998, *Epidemiology in Medical Practice*, 5th edn, Edinburgh, Churchill Livingstone.

Blackburn, C. 1994, 'Low income, inequality and health promotion', *Nursing Times*, 90(39), 42–3.

Blaxter, M. 1984, 'Equity consultation rates in general practice.' *British Medical Journal*, 288, 1963–70.

Blaxter, M. and Prevost, A. T. 1993, in Cox, B. D., Huppert, F. A., and Whichelow, M. J. (eds), *Health and Lifestyle Survey 1993*. Aldershot, Dartmouth Publishing Company Limited.

Bosma, H. H., Dike van de Mheen, D. and Mackenbach, J. P. 1999, 'Social class in childhood and general health in adulthood: questionnaire study of contribution of psychological attributes'. *British Medical Journal*, 318, 18–22.

Brindle, D. 1999, 'Ministers fail to tackle biggest health gap.' *The Guardian*, Tuesday, 2 December 1999, 6.

Cartwright, A. and O'Brien, M. 1976, 'Social class variations in health care and in general practitioner consultations', in Stacey, M., *The Sociology of the NHS, Sociological Review Monograph. No. 22*. Keele. University of Keele.

Chandler, S. 1996, 'Sudden infant death: an update', *Update*, 91(9), 115–21.

Davey Smith, G., Hart, C., Blane, D. and Hole, D. 1998, 'Adverse socio-economic conditions in childhood and cause specific adult mortality: prospective observational study', *British Medical Journal*, 316, 1631–5.

Department of Health and Social Security (DHSS), 1980, *Report on the Working Group on Inequalities in Health*. London. DHSS.

Department of Health (DOH) 1999a, *Saving Lives: Our Healthier Nation*. London. The Stationery Office.

Department of Health (DOH) 1999b, 'Saving Lives: Our Healthier Nation.' http://www.archive.official-documents.co.uk/document/cm43/4386/4386-06.htm

Department of Health (DOH) 2002, 'Care Trusts'. http://www.doh.gov.uk/caretrusts/index.htm

Dolk, H., Vrijheid, M., Armstrong, B., Abramsky, L., Bianchi, F., Nelen, V., Scott, J. E., Stone, D. and Tenconi, R. 1998, 'Risk of congenital anomalies near hazardous waste landfill sites in Europe: the EUROHAZCON study'. *Lancet*, 352, 423–7.

Elliott, P., Briggs, D., Morris, S., De Hoogh, C., Hurt., C., Jensen, T. K., Maitland, I., Richardson, S., Wakefield, J. and Jarup, L. 2001, 'Risk of adverse birth outcomes in populations living near landfill sites.' *British Medical Journal*, 323(7309), 363–8.

Evandrou, M., Falkingham, J., Le Grand, J. and Winter, D. 1992, 'Equity in health and social care.' *Journal of Social Policy*, 21(4), 489–523.

Ewles, L. and Simnett, I. 1992, *Promoting Health. A Practical Guide*. 2nd edn. Harrow, Middlesex. Scutari Press.

Farmer, R., Miller, P. and Lawrenson, R. 1986, *Lecture Notes on Epidemiology and Public Health Medicine*. 4th edn. Oxford. Blackwell Science Ltd.

Fish, H. 1997, 'Freshwaters' in Harrison, R. M. (ed.), *An Introduction to Environmental Chemistry and Pollution*. 2nd edn. Cambridge. Royal Society of Chemistry.

Giddens, A. 1993, *Sociology*. 2nd edn. Cambridge. Blackwell Publishers.

Griffiths, C., Cooke, S. and Toon, P. 1994, 'Registration health checks: inverse care law in the Inner City'. *British Journal of General Practice*, 44(382), 201–493.

Ham, C. 1985, *Health Policy in Britain*. 2nd edn. London. Macmillan Education Ltd.

Harding, S., Bethune, A., Maxwell, R. and Brown, J. 1997, 'Mortality trends using the Longitudinal Study' in Drever, F. and Whitehead, M. (eds), *Health Inequalities*. Series DS15. London. The Stationery Office.

Harding, S., Rosato, M., Brown, J. and Smith, J. 1999, Social patterning of health and mortality: children aged 6–15 years, followed up for 25 years in the ONS Longitudinal Study. *Health Statistics Quarterly*, 03 Autumn 1999. London. The Stationery Office.

Hart, N. 1985, *The Sociology of Health and Medicine*. Ormskirk, Lancashire. Causeway Press Ltd.

Hattersley, L. 1999, Trends in life expectancy by social class – an update. *Health Statistics Quarterly*, 02(1999). London. The Stationery Office.

Health Act, 1999, http://www.legislation.hmso.gov.uk/acts/acts1999/99008--a.htm

Homer, M. 1994, 'Links between unemployment and mental health problems'. *Nursing Times*, 90(30), 42–4.

Kammerling, R. M. and O'Connor, S. 1993, 'Unemployment as a predictor of Rate of Psychiatric admission'. *British Medical Journal*, 307(6918), 1536–9.

Lang, T., Andrews, H., Bedale, C. and Hannaon, E. 1984, *Jam Tomorrow?* Manchester. Food Policy Unit.

Laurance, J. 1986, 'Unemployment health hazards.' *New Society*. 21 March 1986, 492–3.

Linehan, T. 1994, 'Poverty and health: the problem in perspective'. *Healthiness*, July/August 1994, 14–16.

Marsh, A. and McKay, S. 1994, *Poor Smokers*. London. Policy Studies Institute.

National Children's Home 1991, *Poverty and Nutrition Survey*. London. National Children's Home.

Nazroo, J. Y. 1997, *The Health of Britain's Ethnic Minorities*. London. Policy Studies Institute.

Nursing Standard 1995, 'Statistics show an increase in the North South divide'. *Nursing Standard*, 9(40), 6.

Nursing Standard 1996, 'Poverty drags UK into 1800s'. *Nursing Standard*, 11, 10.

Office of Population Censuses and Surveys (OPCS) 1984, *General Household Survey 1982*. London. HMSO.

Office for National Statistics (ONS) 1999, *Social Trends, 29*. London. The Stationery Office.

Parsons, T. 1951, *The Social System*. London. Routledge and Kegan Paul.

Plant, M. A., Brocke, E. M. and Freeman-Browne, D. 1984, *Alcohol, Drugs and School Leavers*. London. Tavistock.

Sinclair, J. 1999, 'Environmental effects on health'. *Nursing Standard*, 13(26), 42–6.

Smith, R. 1985, 'Occupationless Health'. *British Medical Journal*, 291, 1626–9.

Trowler, P. 1989, *Investigating Health Welfare and Poverty*. London. Unwin Hyman Ltd.

Wanless, D. 2002, 'Securing our future health: taking a long term view'. HM Treasury. http://www.hm-treasury.gov.uk/Consultations_and_Legislation/wanless/consult_wanl

Whitehead, M. 1988, *Inequalities in Health. The Health Divide.* Harmondsworth. Penguin Books Ltd.

World Health Organization (WHO) 1984, 'Health promotion: a WHO discussion document on the concepts and principles'. Reprinted in *Journal of the Institute of Health Education*, 23(1), 1985.

Family-centred Care

2

NORMA WHITTAKER

The concept of family-centred care is not new; perhaps what is new is the concept of formalizing the role that nurses and midwives have in caring for both the patient and his or her relatives. Recent changes in the way that the chronically sick, the old and the disabled are cared for have shifted care away from institutions and into the community, the burden of care falling to relatives. Family-centred care acknowledges the burden that this places upon carers but it also acknowledges the important roles that families play in terms of the health and well-being of family members and the potential effects that the illness of one person in a family may have upon others in the family.

Contents

Learning Objectives

By the end of the chapter you should be able to demonstrate knowledge of the following:

- The roles and functions of families in health related issues.
- The potential ways in which an illness in one family member can affect other family members.
- The need for nurses to recognize the potential health risks to relatives particularly relatives undertaking long-term care of the sick.
- Models for family-centred care.

Family-centred care is a multidimensional approach to care. In order for nurses to be effective practitioners in family-centred care there is a need to first understand a number of factors.

Points for consideration

1. What is a family?
2. How might the family influence individual family members in relation to health?
3. How might family members be affected by the illness of another family member?
4. What can nurses do to support and meet the needs of family members?

Definition of a Family

The word family is used confidently in everyday speech with the assumption that everyone knows exactly what it means. Defining the family, however, is not as straightforward as was the case in the past. Traditional definitions of the family have focused upon describing a nuclear family, that is, parents and their offspring, and the extended family, which included grandparents, aunts, uncles and cousins. A much broader definition is, however, more relevant given the diversity of family grouping in today's society. Re-ordered families, which are where parents no longer live together, are now fairly commonplace. Parents make new relationships so that a family may include children from the new as well as previous relationships. There are also many different family groups that may include several generations living together, homosexual families, single parent families or groups of people that have no blood ties and yet function in all ways as a family. Such families share a number of characteristics in relation to the roles that various family members undertake and the functions that the families carry out (Whittaker, 1998).

Identifying who is the family is a central component of family-centred care but can be problematic according to a study by Philip Darbyshire. The study focused upon the experiences of resident parents and paediatric nurses. In the study it is argued that nurses' perceptions of 'family' were often constituted through their understandings of both social relationships and parents' perceived moral adequacy. Family, therefore, became a moral as well as a kinship issue, in that some parents (for example, fathers and young single mothers) were marginalized, while others were welcomed (Darbyshire, 1995). There are potential difficulties in dealing with complex, delicate or acrimonious visitation problems related to parents who may have separated or remarried. However, the most important factor for nurses to recognize is that the family is central in a child's life and should be central in a child's plan of care. The same can be true in relation to patients in any branch of nursing or midwifery. Their families may be central to their lives and should be considered central in any planned care. Family-centred care embraces diversity in family structures, cultural backgrounds, choices, strengths and needs (Ahmann, 1994).

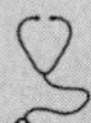

Nursing action point

The family group

- Understand and accept the diversity of family structures.

Family Influences upon the Health and Well-being of Family Members

Idealistically the family provides individuals with food, shelter and warmth and the materialistic things in life that are necessary for survival. The family also provides a loving, caring, supportive network and environment in which its young may learn and grow emotionally and physically, until they are ready to take their place as adults in society. Unfortunately this idealistic picture of the family is not true for all. Children whose families undergo a series of disruptions are more likely to suffer health problems than children whose families remain intact. A report by the Joseph Rowntree Foundation based on an analysis of 200 British research studies on the impact of divorce on children, concedes that such children are twice as likely to experience psychological, economic and social problems in adolescence and adulthood. Poor outcomes for these children are not inevitable, however, if there is better professional support during and after divorce for parents and children (Frean, 1998).

In some cases poverty prevents families from providing the basic necessities of life, which has implications for the health of family members. The problems of poverty and unemployment can lead to family stresses and domestic violence (Chappel, 1982). Studies of abuse have frequently noted that women and children are more at risk of physical and sexual abuse behind their own front doors than outside them (Wright, 1994). Family life has never been more problematic according to Slipman (1994). She argues that if young people are to build successful families, adults need to show them the way and offer positive guidance. Women's aspirations have changed but these have not been matched by changes in male patterns of parenting. Women are expected to work, but their partners do not expect to be active homebuilders or child carers. Where men are no longer the breadwinners they have not found a role as joint carers. These are the messages parents are giving to adolescents who therefore have none of the traditional routes into adulthood.

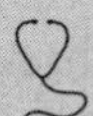

Nursing action points

The following are important considerations for nurses when assessing the needs of patients and families

- Assess whether the family structure provides a supportive network.
- Remember that poverty prevents some families from providing the basic essentials of food, clothing, shelter and warmth.
- Remember that family homes are not always places of safety for individuals.
- Remember that family roles may not conform to traditional patterns.

The ways in which families function, their socio-economic status and the individual roles adopted within the family structure, influence the nursing interventions required.

Family Influences on Health-Related Behaviour

Learned Behaviour from Within the Family (Whittaker, 1998)

Positive behaviour	*Negative behaviour*
■ Proactive in terms of health promotion and health education ■ Early diagnosis and help-seeking behaviour ■ Treatment adherence	■ Little or no interest in health promotion or health education ■ Poor or late diagnosis and help-seeking behaviour ■ Little or no adherence to prescribed treatment

The family influences the lifestyles, health and non-health behaviours of its members. As a basic unit of health care management the family assumes responsibility for at least 75 per cent of all health care provided for its members. This includes health promotion, disease prevention, early intervention and rehabilitation (Duffy, 1988).

Children are influenced by the beliefs, values and behaviour of older family members, so that the family can shape the future lifestyles and behaviour of its young in positive health-seeking ways and in negative ways that pose a risk to health. Children as young as four years old can understand and practice health behaviours (Danielson *et al.*, 1993). A study by Mechanic (1964) found that young adults who reported fewer symptoms of illness recalled an emphasis on self-care and healthy practices during their childhood.

Most people discuss their symptoms with someone else, usually a relative, before seeking help (Scambler *et al.*, 1981). The family acts as a lay referral system that will influence an individual's help-seeking behaviour, positively or negatively. A well-informed family is more likely to initiate early referral to professional agencies. Decisions about health may be weighed against family and work needs as finances and other social needs may compete with healthcare needs. Culture is also a significant factor inasmuch as some cultures rely more upon folk medicine and family care than upon modern medicine. Some problems may be viewed as serious in some cultures whereas doctors would not share this view. Conversely, some problems that doctors consider serious would not be viewed as such by the individuals concerned (Mechanic, 1978). The family can also influence how well or otherwise a patient complies with prescribed treatment regimes. Compliance with the treatment prescribed for children may be linked to parents' satisfaction of consultations with doctors (Korsch and Negrete, 1972).

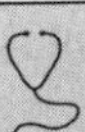

Nursing action points

Family influences on health related behaviour

Nurses have an important role to play in educating and promoting the health of families.

- Establish who within the family group is influential in matters relating to health.
- Maximize opportunities to pass on relevant health promotion and health education information to the person who is most likely to influence the family's behaviour.
- Offer advice, to correct misconceptions about healthy and unhealthy behaviours.
- Remember that early referral and help-seeking behaviour are influenced by the family.
- Recognize differences in the ways that different cultures interpret illnesses, in order to ensure that the appropriate action is taken.
- Gain the trust and confidence of relatives and convince them of the benefits of the prescribed treatment. The chances of the patients adhering to treatments may then be increased.

The Effects of Illness upon Relatives

Illness in one member of a family can produce a crisis that affects the whole family system. Roles and responsibilities of the sick person may have to be delegated to others and the anxiety generated by the illness is compounded by the extra responsibilities. The impact of the illness is determined by factors such as the nature and length of the illness, any residual effects, the financial impact and whether or not the future family functioning can be restored (Kozier and Glenora, 1988).

Relatives may initially experience a number of emotions when a sick person becomes ill and requires admission to hospital. Anxiety, fear of the outcome of the illness and guilt may be experienced. Estrangement from the patient may require an adjustment by relatives to a loss that can be temporary or permanent. It may well be that relatives will experience the five stages of loss as described by Kubler-Ross (1969) before the final adjustment to the loss. These stages are used as a means of coping. The concept of loss may also include the relative who is confronted with the future care of a sick family member and so suffer a social loss (Brown, 1987). This would explain the reaction of relatives who appear unable to accept a diagnosis and whose consequent anger nurses encounter sometimes when they are dealing with relatives. It is easier perhaps to understand and support such relatives if nurses are able to recognize the stages of denial, anger, guilt, and resentment that relatives are experiencing and finally in terminal illness the preparatory grief, the final stage of adjustment.

The way in which the family adapts to an individual's illness can affect the patient and the outcome of his or her illness. If relatives cannot determine the progress of the patient, it is incumbent upon nurses to recognize stressed relatives, to identify the cause of the stress and to implement action to reduce or alleviate it. Relatives who constantly seek information or attempt to do so and relatives who avoid contact with nursing staff may be experiencing stress (Gibbon, 1988). Giving information may reduce anxiety; relatives most frequently seek information about the patient's diagnosis, treatment and prognosis (Gibbon, 1988). The involvement of relatives in care and in giving information is normally with the consent of the patient; the patient's right to confidentiality will always be respected. There is much anecdotal and research evidence however, to suggest that relatives are frequently dissatisfied with the level of information they have received from healthcare practitioners (Whittaker, 1998). Relatives may be intimidated by nurses and apprehensive about approaching busy staff. They may find it difficult to articulate the questions or are afraid that they will not understand the answers. If nurses respond using jargon this will reinforce such feelings. The onus should be upon nurses actively to seek out relatives and not the other way around (Gibbon, 1988). Nurses can do much to meet the needs of relatives by the simple act of good communication.

It is easy for nurses to forget how difficult it can be for relatives when professionals usurp their caring role and the relatives are left on the 'sidelines', feeling helpless and frightened and in some cases having only limited access to their relative. Relatives need to be with the ill person and restricted visiting has been questioned on the basis of the following points:

- Physically ill patients need emotional support from their close relatives and friends.
- There is evidence that family interactions are less stressful than staff–patient interactions.

- There have been marked changes in paediatric visiting that have resulted in marked psychological benefits for patients.
- Patients and relatives have a right to see each other which nurses cannot ethically prevent (Pottle, 1990).

Admission to high dependency units causes great fear in relatives who are likely to be experiencing denial and shock and may have difficulty in understanding what is going on. To exclude them can only make the situation worse for them. The stress that relatives experience can be reduced if they are regarded as a valuable contributor to the patient's care. Involving relatives allows them to feel that they are doing something positive and strengthens the valuable role that relatives play in the patient's recovery (Gibbon, 1988).

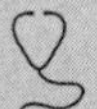

Nursing action points

The potential effects of illness upon relatives

Relatives may be under a great deal of stress as a result of the illness, admission to hospital and change in roles.

- Identify signs and symptoms of stress in relatives.
- Take account of the fact that stress may be manifested in different ways.
- Determine the cause of stress and plan interventions to reduce the stress.
- Ensure that relatives are kept informed.
- Invite them to participate in care if they and the patient so wish it.
- Allow relatives reasonable access to the patient.
- Foster a good relationship with relatives. They know the patient best and can be a great asset.

The Experience of Caring

There are estimated to be 6.8 million unpaid carers in Britain and 25 per cent of these people spend more than 20 hours a week caring for someone (General Household Survey, 1990). Carers save the health service costs in the region of 24 billion pounds if the care had to be provided by statutory services (Bibbings, 1997). The work of caregiving is often accompanied by considerable physical, emotional and material stresses (Mudge, 1995). Caregiving is taken on in addition to prior responsibilities, resulting in drastic lifestyle changes that leave caregivers feeling trapped. Taking on the responsibility of caregiving for a loved one at home occurs in the absence of any alternative. The context is one of uncertainty and unpredictability about the consequences of the decision, overpowered by a sense of moral duty (Wilson, 1989).

Caring for a chronically sick, disabled or elderly relative can be exhausting, physically taxing, emotionally draining and socially limiting. Relatives may have little respite from their caring role. In many cases relatives are faced with 24-hour care that includes washing, dressing, feeding and toileting the sick person. Caregivers often report a decline in physical health, but evidence from several studies is inconclusive. However, a few studies do indicate that caregivers have more chronic illness than controls (Neundorfer, 1991).

Burnout Syndrome

Burnout has been described as a syndrome of physical and emotional exhaustion involving a negative self-concept and attitude, a loss of concern for others and a loss of focus upon one's own life (Pines and Maslach, 1978). The carer's close contact with a chronically sick or disabled person, hour after hour, day after day and year after year may lead to burnout (Ekberg *et al.*, 1986). The findings of a study of people caring for demented elderly relatives suggest that caregivers with initially high levels of poor health, limited social life and a negative outlook on the caregiving situation appear more likely to suffer from burnout. Older wives caring for their husbands followed by daughters caring for parents are most likely to experience a high burden and burnout (Almberg *et al.*, 1997).

It has been long established that caring for a family member with dementia is often very stressful. Caring for the mentally impaired causes more problems than caring for the physically infirm elderly (Gilhooly, 1984). Caregivers who care for a mentally impaired elderly person for an extended time and have low social support are at high risk of suffering psychological stress or depression (Baillie *et al.*, 1988).

Socially the lifestyles of carers can be severely restricted in a number of ways. The primary caregiver may be forced to give up his or her work; this has financial implications and can also leave the carer isolated. Social meetings and holidays may depend upon arranging for someone to stay with the dependent person. It may be difficult to invite friends to the house, particularly if there has been a need to turn a downstairs room into a bedroom. Materially, the carer can be faced with extra laundry and soiled furnishings if the dependant is incontinent. There are also the problems faced when the dependent person is confused and forgetful (Whittaker, 1998). Sadly for many caregivers the stresses and resentment can be overwhelming at times and knowing that the end of their burden of care can only end with the death of someone they love can lead to feelings of remorse and guilt.

Young Carers

Sometimes the roles in families are turned upside down when a child has to care for a parent. Estimates of young carers vary from 40 000 (Watson, 1999) to more than 51 000 youngsters under the age of 18 years caring for a family member (Magnus, 1997). In some cases the child may be the only carer for a disabled or mentally sick parent. The plight of young carers is in many ways a hidden one due in part to the fear of separation, by either the adult or the child being removed from the family. In addition there are sexual taboos that make it socially unacceptable for children to carry out intimate tasks on a parent of the opposite sex. Families, because of guilt and pride often do not seek outside help, which inevitably means that young carers go unsupported. The effects of caring upon the child are complex. Children's psychological development can be impaired by the effects of caring upon education, friendships and socializing, which can be severely affected by the demands and restrictions that caring places upon them. Health problems can be caused to children by lifting adults but to train children to lift adults is to condone and legitimize the activity (Dearden *et al.*, 1995).

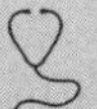

Nursing action points

Caring for carers

- Do not underestimate the impact of care upon relatives; the burden of care can be considerable.
- Identify those carers at high risk of burnout syndrome.

Addressing the needs of carers is a neglected area of nursing practice. Failure to adequately conceptualize the needs of carers has in the past resulted in interventions being inappropriate, irrelevant or unavailable (Nolan and Grant, 1989). The Carers (Recognition and Services) Act 1995 gives carers a right in law to have an assessment made of their needs (Watson, 1999).

- Respond to the needs of carers in order to avoid carers themselves suffering from ill health.
- Refer to a medical social worker for social support. Regular periods of respite from caregiving are needed. This can reduce the risk of burnout.
- Recognize and support young carers. This would improve their health and well-being and promote good nursing practice (Dearden *et al.*, 1995). School and community nurses may be well placed to identify children who are undertaking care of an adult relative.
- Do not assume that where other adults are living in the same house that the child is not the primary carer.
- Remember that young carers are often reluctant to complain about their situation or to complain therefore gaining their trust is vital (Godfrey, 1995).
- Take account of the fact that if the person being cared for has a mental illness or an HIV/AIDS related illness, there may be considerable social stigma associated with caring for them. This may make many carers reluctant to seek help and so remain 'invisible' to the health-related agencies.

Supporting and Meeting the Needs of Carers

Family-centred Care

Family-centred care suggests a global concept of nursing care that embraces the whole family, with a multifaceted approach to care aimed at promoting the well-being of the family throughout the course of the illness. Family-centred care can be practised on a number of levels and in all branches of nursing and midwifery.

Various authors have described the concept of family-centred care; two examples are included below.

Family Nursing

Wright and Leahey (1990) describe family nursing and suggest that it can be conceptualized in two ways. First, it is the focus on the individual in context of the family. Alternatively, the focus is the family with the individual as context. For example, the nurse focusing upon the individual suffering from a disorder would direct questions to assess the individual's understanding of the disorder, its potential effects on the person's life and how they cope with the condition within the family. Other family members may be similarly questioned about their understanding of the disorder and its potential effects upon the individual concerned. In situations where the focus is upon the family the nurse will be interested in exploring how the illness of one family member is affecting others, emotionally and practically, for example, in caregiving. Family systems nursing on the other hand can be conceptualized as focusing on the whole family as the unit of care. The nurse focuses upon the individual and the family simultaneously and centres upon interaction between family members. The nurse will focus upon relationships or connections between family members' behaviours, beliefs or effects.

Family Systems Nursing

Friedemann (1989) suggests a system-based conceptualization of family nursing (see Figure 2.1). She suggests that the concept of family nursing encompasses three levels of the family system:

- Nursing of the system of individuals.
- Nursing the system of groups of two, three or more members of a family (interpersonal level).
- The entire family system.

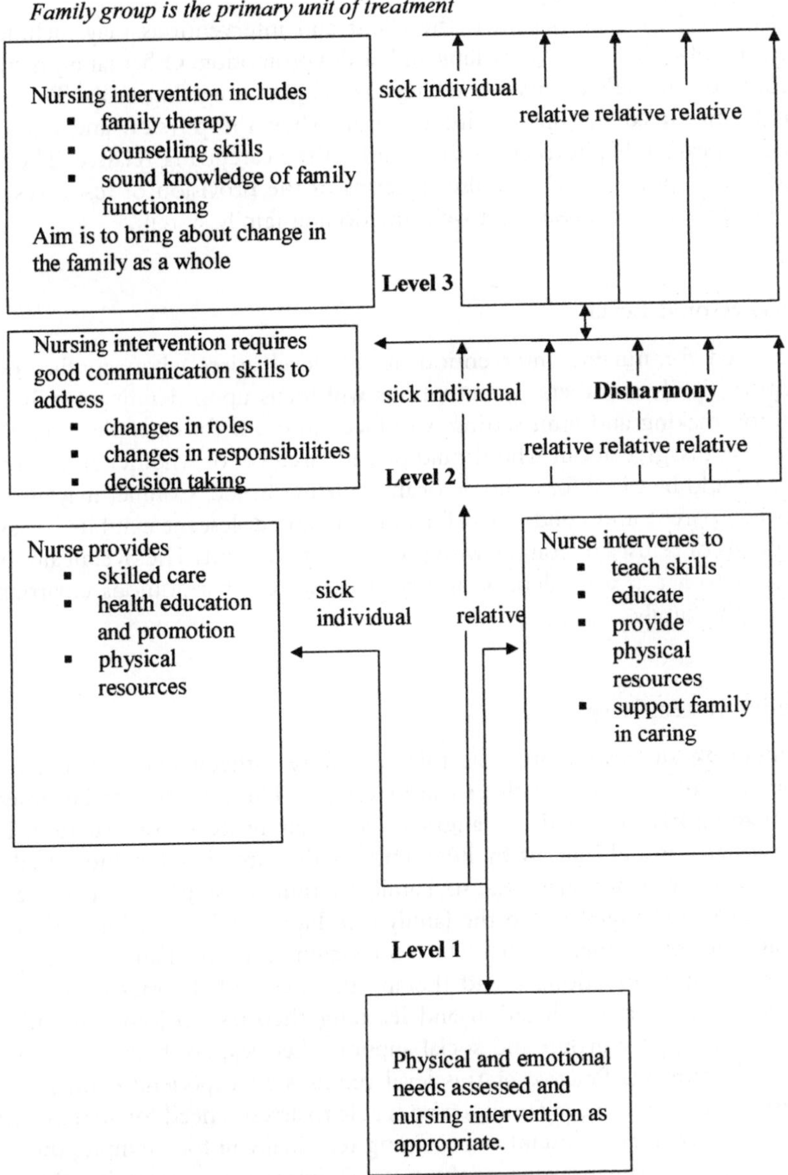

Figure 2.1 Family nursing schema (based on Friedemann's (1989) concept of family nursing)

Source: Whittaker (1998).

Individual Level

At this level the sick person is the client and interventions may include the provision of skilled care, counselling and health promotion. Other family members become the nurse's clients when they are taught caregiving skills. There may also be the need for nursing intervention when the physical and emotional effects of caring begin to affect the health of the caregiving relative. The nurse acts in a supportive role and also in terms of the provision of resources. This level of intervention assumes a well-functioning family system.

Interpersonal Level

The need for nursing intervention at this level arises when conflict occurs between family members. Interventions will focus upon defining family roles, decision making and limit setting. Conflict can occur for example when family members disagree about who should be the caregiver or whether an elderly relative should be cared for at home or in a nursing home. Conflict may also arise between parent and child when for example an adolescent exhibits behaviour problems or refuses to comply with prescribed treatment. The overall aim of the nurse is to act as a moderator and try to restore a harmonious environment within the family.

Family System Level

Friedemann suggests that while this is a more difficult concept to envisage experts of all nursing disciplines can practise it. The total system becomes the client and goals are aimed at changes in the system processes or structure. These changes are brought about by interventions that are aimed at individuals and the family's interactional system. Family system nursing plans personal and interpersonal changes within the family (see Figure 2.2). Nursing actions may involve the environment within which the system interacts. Family development theories, family functioning and therapy theories and theories related to the environment such as education and learning theories, sociological and work environment, peer group and social support theories, are helpful at this level of family nursing. Practice at this level requires an experienced nurse with a holistic understanding of families who is able to assess a need for system change. In the case of a family member becoming terminally ill for example, there may be a need for reorganization of the system's internal resources. Teaching procedures will be at the individual level whereas negotiating responsibilities will be at the interpersonal level. The anticipated goal of all interventions, however, is a system change.

Family System Nursing Using an Alcoholic Family Member as an Example

Assessment

Includes interpersonal and family system interaction with the environment.

Information is obtained by

- Direct questioning of family members
- Observation of interpersonal dynamics, support systems
- Spatial arrangements
- Physical surroundings
- Use of family time

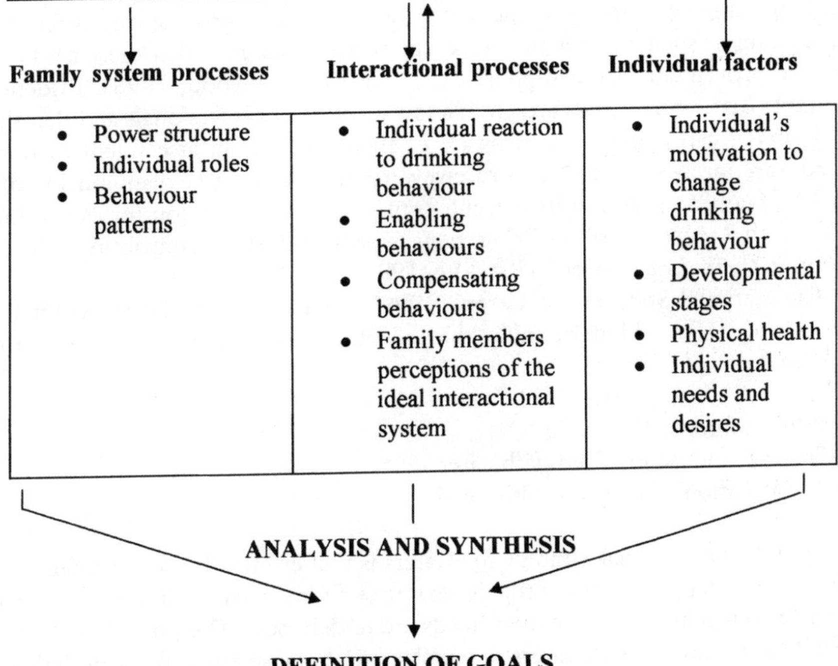

Figure 2.2 Schema based on Friedemann's (1989) concept of family system nursing

Caring for the Carers

The number of older people requiring support to stay in their own homes is increasing. The response of nearly all developed countries has been to introduce a community care policy. A key aim of such a policy is to maintain older people in their own homes at a minimal cost to the state. In order to achieve this attention has been paid to the support needed by carers, the implicit motivation of which is to maintain carers in their roles. The policy focus on carers led to the Carers (Recognition and Services) Act 1995. In principle, the Act provides carers with a statutory right to have their needs assessed and was intended to take account of the carers' perspectives, their ability and willingness to care (Nolan and Lundh, 1999). The Carers Act has been criticized for the over-emphasis within the Act and in guidance notes for social service departments upon tasks and under-emphasis on the psychological effects of caring. Ratcliffe (1998) suggests that rather than rewarding carers it weakens the position of carers by enshrining in statute the previously implicit assumption that the primary responsibility for caring lies with relatives and not with the State. Ratcliffe also points out that the word 'need' does not appear in the Act. In fact, the Carers Act places a duty on local authorities to assess the ability of the carer to provide care when the carer requests such an assessment. Recent evidence suggests that there has been little improvement in the support carers receive (Henwood, 1998). Evidence suggests that carers' needs are given a low priority by professionals and that the majority of carers may not be aware of their right to an assessment of their needs, are rarely consulted and receive very little training (Nolan and Lundh, 1999). The Carers Act in its present form provides recognition for carers, but not in the sense of recognizing their worth and their contribution made through their choice to care (Ratcliffe, 1998).

The National Strategy for Carers (1999) was intended to ensure equitable provision of care. Underpinning the recommended approach to care is the need to

- Provide information
- Support and be involved with carers
- Pay attention to carers' health needs.

An aim of the National Strategy for Carers is that eventually all carers feel prepared and equipped to care if that is what they choose to do, that they feel cared for themselves and feel that their needs are understood. The purpose of therapeutic intervention with carers is problematic because there is an underlying aim to maintain them in the caring role (Twigg and Atkin, 1994).

The change of emphasis needs to be reflected in both pre-registration and post-registration training.

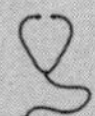

Nursing action points

- Work in close partnership with carers, recognizing their expertise or lack of it, as the basis for therapeutic intervention.
- Adopt a holistic approach to care that identifies and addresses the difficulties and the rewards of caring and carers' strengths and coping strategies.
- Develop skills in psychological interventions in order to maximize carer satisfaction and coping, while minimizing difficulties and burden.

(Nolan and Lundh, 1999)

Conclusion

The structure of family groups in today's society can be very diverse, but generally such groups will share a number of characteristics and, for good or bad, can influence the health and well-being of family members. In order to practise holistic care nurses must acknowledge this potential influence and adopt health promotion strategy accordingly. In times of illness nurses must recognize that relatives can do much to impede or enhance recovery and should value the positive contribution that relatives can make. At the same time it is necessary to recognize the potential effects of illness on other family members and the physical, emotional and social consequences of caring for a chronically sick relative. Family-centred care is a systematic approach to care that enables nurses to assess the needs of families and to plan appropriate interventions to meet those needs. As community care develops, the gap between intention and resources is widening, often leaving carers to take on an increasing load of caring tasks (Whyte and Donaldson, 1999). Nursing must move forward in partnership with those individuals who are undertaking the burden of care, failure to do so may mean that carers will in time become the cared for. Family-centred care can be practised in all settings and with all client groups; ultimately adopting a family-centred nursing philosophy will make nursing care more effective and will, in the long term, be cost effective.

References

Ahmann, E. 1994, 'Family-centred care: shifting orientation'. *Paediatric Nurse*, 20 (2), 113–17.

Almberg, B., Grafstrom, M. and Winblad, B. 1997, 'Caring for a demented elderly person – burden and burnout among caregiving relatives'. *Journal of Advanced Nursing*, 25 (1), 109–16.

Baillie, V., Norbeck, J. S. and Barnes, L. E. A. 1988, 'Stress, social support, and psychological distress of family caregivers of the elderly'. *Nursing Research*, 37 (4), 217–22.

Bibbings, J. 1997, 'Carers', in Leathard, A. (ed.). *Going Interprofessional.* London. Routledge.

Biley, F. 1988, 'Open all hours?' *Nursing Times*, 84 (44), 60–1.

Brown, E. G. A. 1987, 'Meeting the needs of relatives part 2: The nurse and the family'. *Care of the Critically Ill*, 3 (6), 195–6.

Chappel, H. 1982, 'The family life of the unemployed'. *New Society*, 62 (1039), 76–7.

Danielson, C. B., Hamel-Bissell, B. and Winstead-Fry, P. 1993, *Families, Health and Illness: Perspectives on Coping and Intervention.* St. Louis. Mosby.

Darbyshire, P. 1995, 'Family-centred care within contemporary British paediatric nursing'. *British Journal of Nursing*, 4 (1), 31–3.

Dearden, C., Becker, S. and Aldridge, J. 1995, 'Children who care: a case for nursing intervention?' *British Journal of Nursing*, 4 (12), 698–701.

Duffy, M. E. 1988, 'Health promotion in the family: current findings and directives for nursing research'. *Journal of Advanced Nursing*, 13, 109–17.

Ekberg, J. Y., Griffith, N. and Foxall, M. J. 1986, 'Spouse burnout syndrome'. *Journal of Advanced Nursing*, 11, 161–5.

Frean, A. 1998, 'Divorce may offer children of warring parents best future'. *The Times*, Wednesday, 24 June 1998.

Friedemann, M-L. 1989, 'The concept of family nursing'. *Journal of Advanced Nursing*, 14, 211–16.

General Household Survey 1990, London. The Office of Population, Censuses and Surveys. The Stationery Office.

Gibbon, B. 1988, 'Stress in relatives'. *Nursing*, 3 (28), 1026–8.

Gilhooly, M. L. M. 1984, 'The impact of care-giving on care-givers: factors associated with the psychological well-being of people supporting a dementing relative in the community'. *British Journal of Medical Psychology*, 57, 35–44.

Godfrey, K. 1995, 'Children who care too much'. *Community Nurse*, 1 (3), 18–19.

Henwood, M. 1998, *Ignored and Invisible? Carers' Experience of the NHS.*

Report of a UK survey commissioned by Carers National Association. London.

Korsch, B. M. and Negrete, V. F. 1972, 'Doctor–patient communication'. *Scientific American*, 227, 66–74.

Kozier, B. and Glenora, E. 1988, *Concepts and Issues in Nursing Practice.* California. Addison-Wesley Publishing Company.

Kubler-Ross, E. 1969, *On Death and Dying.* New York. Macmillan.

Magnus, S. M. 1997, 'A time to care'. *The Guardian*, 4 June 1997.

Mechanic, D. 1964, 'The influence of mothers on their children's health attitudes and behaviours'. *Paediatrics*, 33, 444–53.

Mechanic, D. 1978, *Medical Sociology.* 2nd edn. New York. Macmillan Press.

Mudge, K. 1995, 'Considering the needs of carers; a survey of their views on services'. *Nursing Standard*, 9 (30), 29–31.

National Strategy for Carers. 1999, *Caring about Carers.* London. The Stationery Office.

Neundorfer, M., M. 1991, 'Coping and health outcomes in spouse caregivers of persons with dementia'. *Nursing Research*, 40 (5), 260–5.

Nolan, M. and Lundh, U. 1999, 'Satisfactions and coping strategies of family carers'. *British Journal of Community Nursing*, 4 (9), 470–5.

Nolan, M. R. and Grant, G. 1989, 'Addressing the needs of informal carers: a neglected area of nursing practice'. *Journal of Advanced Nursing*, 14, 950–61.

Pines, A and Maslach, C. 1978, 'Characteristics of staff burnout in mental health settings'. *Hospital and Community Psychiatry*, 29, 233–7.

Pottle, A. 1990, 'To visit – or not to visit'. *Nursing Practice*, 3 (2), 7–11.

Ratcliffe, P. 1998, 'Not really caring for the carers?' *Journal of Community Nursing*, 12 (4), 18–20.

Scambler, A., Scambler, G. and Craig D. 1981, 'Kinship and friendship networks and women's demands for primary care'. *Journal of the Royal College of General Practitioners*, 26, 746–50.

Slipman, S. 1994, 'The changing family: young people now'. *United Nations International Year of the Family 1994*, 10–11.

Twigg, J. and Atkin, K. 1994, *Carers Perceived: Policy and Practice in Informed Care.* Buckingham. Open University Press.

Watson, S. 1999, 'Meeting the needs of young carers'. *Nursing Standard*, 13 (31), 37–40.

Whittaker, N. A. 1998, 'Family-centred care', in Hinchliff, S., Norman, S. and Schober, J. (eds). *Nursing Practice and Health Care.* 3rd edn. London. Arnold, 434–77.

Whyte, D. and Donaldson, J. 1999, 'All in the family'. *Nursing Times*, 95 (32), 47–8.

Wilson, H. S. 1989, 'Family caregiving for a relative with Alzheimer's dementia: coping with negative choices'. *Nursing Research*, 38 (2), 94–8.

Wright, J. 1994, 'Women and family – a mythical ideal'. *Nursing Standard*, 9, 12–4, 27–30.

Wright, L. M. and Leahey, M. 1990, 'Trends in nursing of families'. *Journal of Advanced Nursing*, 15, 148–54.

Health Issues Related to the Ethnic Minority Groups

3

NORMA WHITTAKER

The National Health Service (NHS) was introduced in 1948 with the aim of providing a high standard of comprehensive care for people from a fairly homogeneous culture and background. The nature of Britain today is multiracial and multicultural and yet NHS provision and training are still based largely on the needs of a homogeneous population. This can affect the care that black and ethnic minority people receive, making care less accessible or less appropriate to their needs in comparison with the care available and received by their white fellow citizens (Henley, 1991). However good the technical facilities available, without access they are useless. The Patient's Charter describes the patient's right to be given detailed information on local health services and to have access to a health service that has respect for privacy and dignity and religious and cultural beliefs (Department of Health [DOH], 1992).

Contents

- Epidemiology
- Potential barriers to access to healthcare including:
  - □ language barriers
  - □ lack of knowledge
  - □ unacceptable services
  - □ lack of specific services
- Potential difficulties faced by asylum seekers and refugees in relation to healthcare

Learning Objectives

By the end of the chapter you should be able to demonstrate knowledge of the following:

- The potential barriers to access to care for black and ethnic minority groups and those seeking political asylum.
- Specific needs of such groups.
- The need for nursing practice to reflect a multiracial and multicultural society.
- Potential ways in which nurses can meet the needs of such clients.

Epidemiology

The number of people describing themselves as belonging to an ethnic minority group increased from 5.8 per cent of the population in Great Britain in 1992 to 6.4 per cent (3.6 million people) in 1998. Just less than half of the ethnic minority population was born in the United Kingdom (UK). Three groups from the Indian subcontinent account for almost half of the ethnic minority population, and nearly half of the population of ethnic minority groups lives in Greater London. All of the ethnic minority groups have a younger age profile than the white population (Schuman, 1999). There will be a tenfold increase in the numbers of black and ethnic minority older people in 30–40 years. Due to the unbalanced age structures of ethnic minorities, the numbers of their elderly will rise dramatically. In all ethnic groups, poor health increases with age, but the rise is sharper and arrives at an earlier age in the minority populations. In all ethnic groups women outnumber men by 2 : 1. This demographic information is important for nurses with responsibility for commissioning or providing services, and for those caring for older people from ethnic minority groups (Royal College of Nursing [RCN], 1998).

Potential Barriers to Access to Health Care

Access to, and ease of use of, health services is an important potential source of inequality in the health experience of different ethnic minority groups. Variations in health may be partly attributable to or amplified by differences in health service use. Differences in the use of health services may be the result of differences in demand rather than inequality of access. Such differences in demand may also result from the inability of health services to address the needs and expectations of different ethnic groups (Nazroo, 1997). In addition to levels of health, usage will depend upon health beliefs and knowledge; attitudes to health services; distribution of resources; sensitivity to the different needs of groups; and variations in the quality of care (Smaje, 1995).

Most studies that have attempted to explore possible variations in health service usage have found that ethnic minority groups make greater use of the health service than the white majority. Such studies do, however, have a number of drawbacks. Differences in use do not necessarily reflect differences in need. It may well be that differences in use disappear or even reverse when differences in need are taken into account. The few studies that have considered use of services by ethnic groups have not directly accounted for differences in need (Nazroo, 1997). The greater use of primary health services by ethnic minority patients may be the result of more frequent consultations for illnesses that have a greater prevalence among various ethnic groups (McCormick and Rosenbaum, 1990). This suggests a greater prevalence of ill health. Also assessments of frequency of use give no indication as to the quality of the services received (Nazroo, 1997). For black and ethnic minority older people, barriers to access exist at many points within services. Most older Asian people, for example, are registered with a general practitioner (GP), yet a considerable proportion receives no treatment for known health problems (RCN, 1998).

Physical accessibility of the services concerns all potential users from whatever background and includes such things as evening clinics and adequate car parking or public transport facilities. Many ethnic minorities are found in the lower socio-economic groups and may find physical access to services difficult. This is particularly so for the elderly ethnic groups. Most live in the poorest housing and most have low income and pension rights. Black elders tend not to be economically active, so they are not free to move. The result will be a concentration of elderly ethnic groups in certain areas and this has implications for community nursing services (Mehta, 1993). The isolation and economic vulnerability of elderly black and ethnic minorities is an example of how racial stereotyping fails to meet their health and social services needs; the assumption being that they are cared for by their families. Bahl (1993) suggests that this is not the case for all people.

Stereotypical attitudes to Asian communities can lead social workers to believe that Asian families prefer to care for their own, leaving young carers without support. It is not unusual for young Asian carers to receive little help from social services (Shah and Hatton, 1999). Stereotypical assumptions that the extended family will help as well as the expectations from the Asian community and the young carers themselves that they have a duty to look after their own, may account for the lack of support to young Asian carers. The myth of the extended family support continues to be perpetuated because the idea of the extended family is a basic racist assumption. The extended family may live locally but may not necessarily provide support. A thorough community care assessment of the cared for person should profile all family members' responsibilities, so that young carers are assessed themselves, as they are entitled to be by the Carers Act. If this does not happen, it means that social workers are putting together a picture based upon their own stereotypes, which is racist. Young carers of every race have it tough but those from Asian communities also face discrimination. It is imperative that all concerned ensure that young Asian carers are not excluded from the services on offer (Valios, 1999).

Carers need a break. It might be someone going into a home to take over care from time to time or admission of the cared for person into a hospital or care home for a short stay. The provision of respite services tends to be extremely inconsistent and for people from ethnic minorities the picture tends to be even worse. Part of the problem relative to poor uptake may be to do with language and a lack of awareness among people from ethnic minority groups about what services are available. The biggest problem, however, is that in many parts of the country the services that are on offer are not culturally sensitive and so people do not feel comfortable about using them (Wellard, 1999). Several reasons have been suggested to account for poor uptake of services (Fletcher, 1997; Redmond, 1993; Rawaf, 1993):

- Language barriers
- Lack of knowledge
- Unacceptable services
- Lack of specific services.

Language Barriers

Many Asian people entered the UK as elderly people and had no opportunity to learn English. Elderly black and ethnic minority people find it difficult to gain access to health services because of lack of interpreters, link workers and advocates. The provision of translated materials is of no use if the person is illiterate (Bahl, 1993). According to Alderman (1993) even where there are good interpreting services available, health professionals lack the skill to use them efficiently and there may be resistance to using them. Difficulties with language can make an individual feel stupid and humiliated. It is important for nurses to recognize that where communication problems exist it is the nurse's responsibility to overcome them; the onus should not be upon the patient.

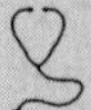

Nursing action points

Using interpreters

- Always check that the interpreter and the patient speak the same language and dialect.
- Ask the patient if he or she prefers an interpreter of the same sex.
- Reassure the patient that everything said will be treated in strictest confidence.
- Allow extra time for the interview.
- Allow the interpreter a few minutes with the patient before the interview takes place.
- Outline the situation to the interviewer.

- Keep your language simple and jargon free.
- Do not marginalize patients from the interaction when using an interpreter.
- Speak directly to the patient, using normal facial expressions and gestures.
- Never leave the interpreter to give clinical advice, the patient is your responsibility.
- Be prepared to support the interpreter if he or she has to give bad news or deal with a difficult situation.
- Encourage the interpreter to find out if the patient has any other problems.
- If the interpreter is a relative or friend, determine his or her command of English and how much you can expect from the translation.
- Find out what the relationship is between the interpreter and the patient as this may affect what you can ask to be translated.
- Be aware that the patient may want to withhold some things from the translator.
- Remember that mistranslation can have serious consequences and cause great personal stress to the patient and family.
- Although you cannot communicate directly, smile a lot and make friendly gestures to show that you want to be helpful.
- Be sensitive to non-verbal signals.

(Henley, 1991)

Lack of Knowledge

To ensure that the patient gets the care that he or she needs it is essential that he or she understands what is happening and can ask the right questions. This is necessary in order for the patient to make informed decisions about care and treatment (Henley, 1991). It is often fear through lack of information that makes people unwilling to use services (Baylow, 1992). Understanding what is happening has also been shown to improve people's tolerance to pain, to reduce stress, aid healing and lower infection rate (Boore, 1978). People are unlikely to use services if they do not know about them. A Birmingham study found that 53 per cent of elderly black people had not heard of district nursing and 72 per cent had not heard of nursing auxiliaries compared with 14 and 32 per cent of white elderly people respectively (Badger *et al.*, 1988). Lack of information about the range and availability of services is a common barrier to service uptake by people from minority ethnic groups (Richardson *et al.*, 1994). A study by Coventry Health Information Forum (1991) found that health information was not getting through to members of ethnic communities. Uptake of cervical and breast screening has been found to be low among some ethnic minority groups mainly because of a lack of awareness of availability rather than a failure of women to attend (Doyle, 1991). Lack of information about services is not, however, the only barrier to appropriate service provision; when information does reach such communities it is often inappropriate in cultural or linguistic terms. Healthcare professionals' lack of knowledge about cultural and religious beliefs creates additional barriers for potential service users (Richardson *et al.*, 1994). In order to practise effectively, healthcare practitioners must be well informed about their client groups. Lack of information about cultural and religious beliefs in terms of diet, religion, language and social customs will impose further barriers to the uptake of care.

Nursing action points

- Be aware that an interpreter can act as the patient's advocate.
- Be aware that improved communication through an advocate can influence the outcomes of clinical practice (Rawaf, 1993).
- Be aware that the use of a patient's advocate helps to redress the imbalance of knowledge and power between healthcare practitioners and patient (Henley, 1991).
- Have knowledge of the local communities and of the various cultural and religious beliefs of ethnic minority groups.
- Ensure that information is appropriate for the client group.

Unacceptable Services

Access to healthcare can be hampered by restricted opportunities or a reliance on services that are inappropriate and insensitive. When providing healthcare many staff may be guilty of racial stereotyping and thus people may be subjected to prejudice and hostility and attitudes that are culture specific. Such discrimination significantly affects the standard of care received and leads to a lack of confidence in the NHS (Fletcher, 1997). Stereotyping can be apparent for example in the lack of available play equipment in hospitals, that reflects the racial and cultural experiences of children from black and ethnic minority families (Alderman, 1993). Racism may be institutional or personal; the latter taking the form of overt racist activities such as verbal abuse, physical attacks and overt discrimination (Bassett, 1993). Racism cannot only affect the health status of people from ethnic minorities, but also the healthcare received. Institutional racism occurs throughout the health service. Racist beliefs are accepted as factual evidence for differences between ethnic groups, and these beliefs become normalized and influence and determine the behaviour of healthcare professionals. This has been clearly identified in the mental health services (Fletcher, 1997). Providing services that are relevant and appropriate to black and ethnic minority groups is not a matter of special treatment or positive discrimination but represents a necessary and reasonable acceptance of the diversity of contemporary multiracial Britain (Connelly, 1988).

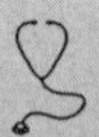

Nursing action points

- Follow the nurses' Code of Professional Conduct (UKCC [now known as the Nursing and Midwifery Council], 1992) which requires nurses to: 'recognize and respect the uniqueness and dignity of each patient and client, and respond to their needs for care, irrespective of their ethnic origin, religious beliefs, personal attributes'.
- Take account of the health consequences of discrimination and harassment on individuals (Chevannes, 1997).
- Understand patients' cultural beliefs, expectations, behaviour and their conceptions of health and illness.
- Recognize that stereotypes and myths about ethnic minority groups must not be relied upon in determining whether nursing interventions are necessary (Henley, 1991)

While services should be acceptable to all users it is essential that services are sensitive to the cultural values and religious beliefs of people from all backgrounds (Rawaf, 1993). When food is a religious issue for patients it is important to ensure that it is prepared and served in an acceptable manner. For Jewish, Hindu, Sikh and Muslim patients who follow food restrictions, the utensils used to prepare their food must be kept separate from those used for food they cannot eat. Many people eat with their fingers and use only their right hands for eating and the left hands for washing and handling dirty things. Fasting has a special value in many religious faiths. For example, Muslims fast during the month of Ramadan, taking nothing to eat or drink between sunrise and sunset (Henley, 1991). This has implications for the administration of medications and health education and promotion.

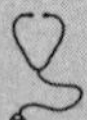

Nursing action points

- Ask each patient whether there are any specific dietary requirements/religious restrictions and ensure that these are met.
- Discuss the local policy/provision, if families wish to bring food into a hospital.
- Ask fasting patients what they need; let the prescribing doctor be aware of this and change medication times or routines if necessary.

- Take periods of fasting and dietary restrictions into account, when advising a patient with diabetes about diet and insulin.
- Ensure that adequate hand washing facilities are made available, if patients usually eat with their hands and ensure that food is served in bite-sized pieces.
- Check when siting intravenous infusions whether the patient needs his or her right hand to eat with.
- Know how to check for signs and symptoms of jaundice, pallor, cyanosis and inflammation in people with dark skins.

(Henley, 1991)

Physical modesty may be a religious as well as a personal issue. Many men and women regard it as morally wrong for a woman to allow any man but her husband to touch her body, especially the genital area. Such women should have the option of consultation and treatment by women doctors and nurses, particularly in the provision of gynaecological and obstetric services (Rawaf, 1993). Women may suffer from long-standing incontinence or gynaecological problems because they are too shy to consult a male doctor (Redmond, 1993). Language barriers and cultural differences isolate Asian women from the facts concerning menopause and hormone replacement therapy (HRT). A study by Sarwar, investigating Asian women's response to HRT concluded that many Asian women were unaware of the acutal medical condition of menopause even though the majority of subjects were experiencing symptoms. The uptake of HRT can be greatly improved as a result of a three-way communication system set up between the client, the health professional and the health educator. It is important that women are aware of the potential side effects of HRT, for example to start bleeding after the menopause may be very frustrating for Muslim women as praying is an important part of their daily chores, which is forbidden if a woman is bleeding (Sarwar, 1998).

Personal preferences and customs should be taken into account in relation to bathing. Sitting in a bath may be distasteful to some people who consider that to be clean the water must be running. Some people may have specific needs in relation to saying prayers and rituals surrounding death. Getting things right for a dying person and their relatives is a way of helping them in their grief. Naming systems may be very different from the British system and this can lead to confusion. For example, in some systems the first name is a religious name and not a personal one. In others the last name is a title that indicates a religion and/or gender and not a family surname and thus of little help in filing records or linking patients and their notes. It is potentially dangerous if notes are mixed up and causes offence and embarrassment by using people's names incorrectly (Henley, 1991).

Nursing action points

- Provide a jug if there are no showers, for those patients who require to bathe in running water.
- Check the significance of religious jewellery, for example an engraved medal or a pouch containing holy writings or objects to give protection; avoid removing if possible, tape and keep dry.
- Ensure that female staff are available as appropriate.
- Respect people's religious beliefs, practices and objects.
- Ask patients if they wish to practice any aspects of their religion while in hospital.
- Be knowledgeable of the various rituals associated with death and dying.
- Be as flexible as possible in allowing access to relatives and religious leaders.
- Seek help and advice from people in different communities, if deemed necessary.
- Find out the patient's full name, how the patient wishes to be addressed and the correct pronunciation.

(Henley, 1991)

Lack of Specific Services

Notwithstanding the socio-economic factors that may predispose certain ethnic groups to particular diseases, there is some epidemiological evidence to suggest that within ethnic minority groups, disease patterns and rates of mortality are different from the white indigenous population (Fletcher, 1997). There is a higher prevalence of coronary heart disease (CHD) among Asian communities (Smaje, 1995; Balarajan and Raleigh, 1993). In contrast men and women born in the Caribbean have lower rates of mortality from CHD than the universal population (Nazroo, 1997). Non-insulin dependent diabetes mellitus has a higher prevalence among minority ethnic populations (Smaje, 1995). Diabetes has an associated mortality three times that of the national level among people from the Indian subcontinent (Simmons *et al.*, 1989). A study by Burden (1998) indicated that Asian patients did not achieve as good diabetic control as their white counterparts; she points out the need to tailor treatment according to the individual's cultural background. Afro-Caribbean people report hypertension more frequently and the risk of dying from a stroke is higher for those born in the Caribbean and South Asia than for those born in Britain (Nazroo, 1997). There is a higher incidence of stomach problems among Bangladeshi people (George, 1995). The mortality rate from tuberculosis (TB) is very considerably raised in all the major migrant groups; this may reflect the endemic nature of TB in the Indian subcontinent and the higher prevalence among newly arrived immigrants and those who make frequent trips back there and also their poor socio-economic conditions in Britain. The prevalence of sickle cell disorders, which are inherited diseases, varies among ethnic groups, but are most common in populations where malaria is endemic. Sickle cell disease is most prevalent among African and Caribbean populations while beta thalassaemia also affects people originating from South Asia, Southern Europe and the Middle East (Smaje, 1995). Women from Indian and Pakistani backgrounds have higher rates of premature labour and low birth weight babies and rates of reported schizophrenia are far greater in black Caribbean people (Steer *et al.*, 1995).

Connection

Chapter 4 (Hypertension), Chapter 5 (Coronary Heart Disease), Chapter 6 (Stroke) and Chapter 11 (Tuberculosis) give further details of the epidemiology of these disorders in relation to people from ethnic minority groups.

The catalogue of misdiagnoses, wrong assessments and inappropriate service delivery that characterizes the way in which mental health care reaches men in black communities is well documented (Wilson, 1995). Differences between ethnic groups and pathways to care and the kind of care received have been highlighted in relation to mental health problems. Caribbean patients are less likely to have had prior contact with a GP and are more likely to be referred by police and compulsorily detained under the 1983 Mental Health Act. They are more likely to be detained in secure units and have major tranquillizers and electro-convulsive therapy in cases where it does not appear to be indicated and are more likely to be seen by junior staff. It is suggested that this may reflect the racism or ethnocentrism of British psychiatry. Most psychiatrists are white and often have a poor understanding of the cultural background of minority ethnic patients and they hold stereotyped views about the behaviour of black people (Raleigh, 1995). Ethnic or cultural differences in the presentation of diseases are such that psychiatrists mistake minor symptoms or delusions for schizophrenia. The existence of genuinely elevated incidence of schizophrenia among Caribbean population in Britain must be regarded as unproven (Smaje, 1995). The medical model of illness in Western society is ill equipped to diagnose and heal people of non-Western cultures. Economic deprivation, unemployment, poor housing and social isolation can contribute to mental illness, and black and minority people are more likely to experience these conditions (Raleigh, 1995). By concentrating on diseases that affect particular groups there is a risk of putting the blame on the individual and their culture and ignoring the experiences associated with ethnicity. It serves to create a misconception that health problems are due to cultural practices and leads to stereotyping, detracting from the underlying socio-economic factors. Rather than observed ethnic variations prompting research into the underlying cause, it becomes the explanation (Donovan, 1984). For example, the high rates of congenital malformation and stillbirth in Pakistani people have been attributed to deviant marriage patterns and other factors such as service provision, environmental and personal factors have received less attention (Fletcher, 1997). These cultures are then seen as deviant or deficient and in need of change, so that health care planners refer to the 'special needs' of ethnic groups rather than devise a health service that responds adequately to our complex population (Hopkins, 1993).

Points for reflection

- The collection and use of ethnic origin data has a key role in establishing epidemiological patterns, aiding purchasers with needs assessment and in providing the most accessible and appropriate services to all patients (Ranger, 1994).
- There is a need for a more balanced representation of health care professionals from black and ethnic minority groups (Carlisle, 1994).
- Those involved in recruiting candidates to posts such as counsellors for sickle cell disease sufferers, should actively seek out applicants from relevant ethnic groups for their community. This can be achieved by advertising posts with relevant organizations and appropriate ethnic minority media (Anionwu, 1996).
- In-service training is needed to enable a wide range of professionals to acquire the skills necessary to work with people from ethnic minority backgrounds in a sensitive and helpful way (Kurtz, 1993).
- Quality support requires knowledge of the language and the specific needs of the client group (Chan, 1994).
- Alliances should be formed with health promotion agencies, Mosques, temples, community centers, Asian radio and other media (Burden, 1998).
- Black groups and community forums are well placed to provide valuable information, knowledge and expertize, which contribute to better links with GPs and other health care professionals and can lead to better services for black communities (Wilson, 1995).
- Health care planning and the provision of care should be tailored to meet the specific needs of the client group taking into account variations in the pattern of diseases among different groups.

Potential Difficulties Faced by Asylum Seekers and Refugees in Relation to Health Care

An asylum seeker is someone who comes to the UK, often fleeing persecution, torture or war, and who applies for refugee status. Individuals remain asylum seekers while their applications to the Home Office are being considered or the appeals on them are continuing (Resource Information Service, 2001). More than 5000 people seek refuge in the UK every month (Hampshire, 2001). While all of the discussion points outlined above can be reflected in the experience of asylum seekers, this group experiences additional problems and hardships. Many asylum seekers have been tortured and have chronic physical and psychological injuries. Some may have been threatened with execution, where they are told that they are going to be killed, hear a gunshot and then realize that they are still alive. Both men and women have been gang raped and many have war wounds such as burns and shrapnel injuries. Individuals so treated can have profound psychological problems, such as post-traumatic stress, and suffer from chronic illnesses including diabetes and kidney failure (Hampshire, 2001). Many have dental problems, including broken teeth and toothache (Leifer, 1999).

Many of the children of asylum seekers will not have had routine health surveillance in the countries of origin. Defects of vision, hearing and speech will have gone undetected and routine immunizations omitted. Children and adults may enter the UK with infections acquired in their country of origin. Asylum seekers from Africa and the Indian subcontinent and some parts of South America may have been exposed to numerous diseases not encountered in the West. Any omissions in routine child health surveillance and immunizations should be rectified. An informed health care professional using a structured history taking and relevant laboratory tests can carry out screening for tropical diseases (Davies *et al.*, 1996).

Common problems encountered by asylum seekers

- Delay in receiving National Asylum Support Service (NASS) vouchers or delay in replacing lost vouchers.
- Need to travel to Immigration or other official interviews.
- Need to travel to see solicitors.
- Unsuitable accommodation provided by NASS.
- Refusal by a GP or dentist to provide care or imposition of additional conditions (for example, time limited appointments).
- Unable to pay health related costs, for example, eye glasses.
- Less favourable treatment by shop staff when using vouchers.
- Changes of circumstances, for example, birth.
- Awaiting a decision on asylum application.
- Completion of Home Office Enquiry form.
- Employment.
- Special or additional needs.
- Getting a positive decision.

(Bateman, 2001)

Asylum seekers also face homelessness and particular difficulties in getting accommodation. Changes in legislation in recent years have restricted their rights to public housing, welfare benefits and employment. Under the Immigration and Asylum Act 1999, asylum seekers lost their entitlement to benefits or support under provisions of the National Assistance Act. Instead the NASS was set up by the Home Office to provide support for asylum seekers outside mainstream UK welfare services. Asylum seekers are being dispersed to cluster areas outside London and the South East to help ease pressure on services (Resource Information Service, 2001).

Government policy to redistribute asylum seekers may however mean that they are placed in the care of people without any specialist knowledge of their problems, including people working in primary care. Although all asylum seekers are eligible for free NHS treatment and have the right to register with a GP, it appears that GPs are often confused about asylum seekers' entitlements. They have been registered on a temporary rather than a permanent basis and thus excluded from a full package of checks. Additionally, various forms of identification are being requested on registration (Dar, 2000). Dentists may not be keen to register asylum seekers as patients because of all the bureaucracy involved. Dental staff may not realize that asylum seekers may be here for years and offering temporary dental repairs is therefore inappropriate (Leifer, 1999). Although entitled to NHS care, the Refugee Council has found that many clients have been turned away by GPs. Clients then appear at accident and emergency departments because they believe that they have nowhere else to go. Refugees also may have no concept of GPs or the NHS and on seeing a big hospital, believe that is where they should go (Hampshire, 2001). Some pregnant asylum seekers and refugees may not seek proper health care because they assume that they would have to pay, as would be the case in their home countries and they have no means of payment (Healy, 2002).

According to Dar (2000), in the absence of national guidelines each health authority should provide guidance for the integration of asylum seekers into general practices. These guidelines should emphasize that additional documents such as immigration and passports are not required as proof of asylum status and that permanent rather than temporary registration should be offered. The presence of asylum seekers undoubtedly presents local authorities with challenges that must be met. GPs have no medical history to refer to and some asylum seekers will have had no medical treatment throughout their lives. Upon their arrival in Glasgow asylum seekers are given a welcome pack, which explains how they can access medical and dental services. The pack contains the name and address of a designated GP who they are asked to register with and who will already have received information. All asylum seekers entering the UK receive free access to general medical, dental and ophthalmic services and free prescriptions. Reimbursement of travel costs to hospital may be available if required (Redpath, 2002).

The Role of the Nurse

Nurses can play a pivotal role. The advantage of having a nursing background is that nurses are taught to look at the whole person. Regardless of the area of nursing practice, looking deeper than what appears on the surface is an essential component of holistic care. The non-verbal skills of nurses, such as listening and observing, have a major impact on the initial assessment and what information is given by the client (Hampshire, 2001). These clients may have suffered appallingly and getting to the crux of their problems requires skill and patience. In understanding the difficulties that asylum seekers face, nurses can act as their advocates in dealing with systems that are cumbersome and often hostile.

Conclusion

Historically, health authorities have failed to identify the needs of ethnic minorities. The NHS has been slow to introduce ethnic monitoring, which is necessary in order to plan systematically health services that are sensitive to the needs of minority groups. While it is now the practice to carry out such monitoring, the information does not relate to socio-economic factors and therefore its value is questionable (Fletcher, 1997).

In terms of meeting the Health of the Nation targets for ethnic minority groups, immigrant mortality suggests that there is still a long way to go (Nazroo, 1997). The ultimate aim of any attempt to address the health needs of a multicultural Britain is to ensure a multicultural consumer-involving NHS. While it is important to acknowledge that certain diseases are more prevalent among certain groups and that distinct patterns of morbidity are sometimes identifiable, it is equally important that the process of identifying and addressing the health needs of black and ethnic minority groups never becomes marginalized, but is wholly integrated into the general process of planning, personnel training and healthcare delivery (Nzegwu, 1993). A philosophy that ensures that the needs, services and rights of every sector of society are clearly defined and that healthcare is available and accessible to everyone, regardless of race, colour or creed is required.

It has been suggested that there has been no real NHS planning for the health needs of asylum seekers and that no thought has been given to their health needs or the social infrastructure around them and it is possible to see the whole process as an abuse of human rights (Carlowe, 2001). The main obstacles to providing appropriate care are the inflexibility of the NHS and the delays and bureaucracy inherent in the arrangements for the support of asylum seekers. Many people arrive with no money at all and it takes time for them to receive vouchers or money. In the meantime babies still need nappies, a menstruating woman needs sanitary protection and it takes three weeks for an exemption certificate to be issued for vital medicines. While solving such problems can be time consuming, GPs should be reassured that asylum seekers are resourceful and their needs are not overwhelming, neither are the language barriers insurmountable (Montgomery and Le Feuvre, 2000).

It is clear that there are still barriers to access to healthcare for many people in Britain today. Whilst some issues need to be addressed by government others are within the remit of every nurse. Recognizing the barriers to access to care is the first step towards removing them. Ensuring that clients are informed of available services, using appropriate aids such as videos and leaflets in different languages, using interpreting services appropriately, tailoring health promotion according to the client group and most importantly finding out as much as possible about patients' and clients' wishes and needs are examples of how difficulties can be addressed. In order to practise holistic care, nurses must be knowledgeable about their patients' culture and religious beliefs. Each person has a right to expect that nurses will respect their individuality and this includes cultural and religious beliefs. Minority groups are not seeking other than equitable care that addresses their specific needs and that is no more and no less than the expectation of every British citizen.

References

Alderman, C. 1993, 'A colour blind health service'. *Nursing Standard*, 7 (26), 18–19.

Anionwu, E. N. 1996, 'Ethnic origin of sickle and thalassaemia counsellors', in Kelleher, D. and Hillier, S. (eds), *Researching Cultural Differences in Health*. London. Routledge.

Badger, F., Cameron, E., Evers, H. and Griffiths, R. 1988, 'Put race on the agenda'. *Health Service Journal*, 98 (5129), 1426–27.

Bahl, V. 1993, 'Access to health care for black and ethnic minority elderly people', in Hopkins, A. and Bahl, V. (eds), *Access to Health Care for People from Black and Ethnic Minorities*. London. Royal College of Physicians.

Balarajan, R. and Raleigh, V. 1993, *Ethnicity and Health*. London. Department of Health.

Bassett, C. 1993, 'Health versus racism'. *Journal of Community Nursing*, 7 (4), 24–6.

Bateman, N. 2001, 'Asylum seekers: A guide to sorting out money and support problems'. http://www.careandhealth.com/arch/article_162.asp

Baylow, A. 1992, 'Equality of access: are we meeting the challenge?'. *Primary Health Care Management*, 2, 7.

Boore, J. R. P. 1978, *Prescription for Recovery*. London. Royal College of Nursing.

Burden, M. 1998, 'Approaches to managing diabetes in Asian people'. *Community Nurse*, 4 (4), 31–4.

Carlisle, D. 1994, 'Facing up to race'. *Nursing Times*, 90 (26), 14–15.

Carlowe, J. 2001, 'The doctor won't see you now ... '. http://www.observer.co.uk/life/story/0,6903,511637,00.html

Chan, Dr. M. 1994, 'Breaking down barriers'. *Healthlines*. November 1994, 10.

Chevannes, M. 1997, 'Nurses caring for families – issues in a multicultural society'. *Journal of Clinical Nursing*, 6, 161–7.

Connelly, N. 1988, *Care in the Multicultural Community.* London. Policy Studies Institute.

Coventry Health Information Forum 1991, *Information Needs of Black and Ethnic Minority Groups in Coventry.* Coventry. CHIF.

Dar, S. 2000, 'General practitioners' knowledge of issues relating to asylum seekers is poor'. *British Medical Journal,* 321, 893.

Davies, E. G., Elliman, A. C., Hart, C. A., Nicoll, A. and Rudd, P. T. 1996, *Manual of Childhood Infections.* London. W. B. Saunders Company Limited.

Department of Health (DOH) 1992. *The Patients' Charter.* London. HMSO.

Donovan, J. 1984, 'Ethnicity and health: a research overview'. *Social Science and Medicine,* 193, 663–70.

Doyle, Y. 1991, 'A survey of the cervical screening in a London district'. *Social Science and Medicine,* 32, 953–7.

Fletcher, M. 1997, 'Equal health services for all'. *Journal of Community Nursing,* 11 (7), 20–4.

George, M. 1995, 'Perceptions of health'. *Nursing Standard,* 9 (28), 18–19.

Hampshire, M. 2001, 'Out of reach'. *Nursing Standard,* 15 (51), 16–17.

Healy, P. 2002, 'Opening doors'. *Nursing Standard,* 8 (16), 13.

Henley, A. 1991, *Caring for Everyone.* The National Extension College Trust Ltd.

Hopkins, A. 1993, 'Envoi', in Hopkins, A. and Bahl, V. (eds), *Access to Health Care for People from Black and Ethnic Minorities.* London. Royal College of Physicians.

Kurtz, Z. 1993, 'Better health for black and ethnic minority children and young people', in Hopkins, A. and Bahl, V. (eds), *Access to Health Care for People from Black and Ethnic Minorities.* London. Royal College of Physicians.

Leifer, D. 1999, 'Giving refuge to those in need'. *Nursing Standard,* 13 (43), 16–17.

McCormick, A. and Rosenbaum, M. 1990, *Morbidity Statistics from General Practice, Third National Survey: Socio-economic Analysis.* London. HMSO.

Mehta, G. 1993, 'The ethnic elderly'. *Journal of Community Nursing,* 6 (12), 16–20.

Montgomery, S. and Le Feuvre, P. 2000, 'Health care for asylum seekers: main obstacles are inflexibility of NHS and bureaucracy of support systems'. *British Medical Journal,* 321, 893.

Nazroo, J. Y. 1997, *The Health of Britain's Ethnic Minorities.* London. Policy Studies Institute.

Nzegwu, F. 1993, *Black People and Health Care in Contemporary Britain.* Reading, Berks. The International Institute For Black Research.

Raleigh, Dr. V. S. 1995, *Mental Health in Black and Minority Ethnic People – The Fundamental Facts.* London. The Mental Health Foundation.

Ranger, C. 1994, 'Kings Evidence'. *Health Service Journal.* April 1993, 22–3.

Rawaf, S. 1993, 'Access to health care for people from ethnic minorities'. *The Health Service.* July, 4.

Redmond, E. 1993, 'Reaching out to the Asian community'. *Community Outlook,* 3 (7), 13–15.

Redpath, K. 2002, 'Health services for asylum seekers'. Greater Glasgow Primary NHS Trust. http://www.show.scot.nhs.uk/ggpct/asylum/services.htm

Resource Information Service 2001, 'Asylum seekers and refugees'. http://www.homelesspages.org.uk/subjects/S0000016.html

Richardson, J., Leisten, R. and Calviou, A. 1994, 'Lost for words'. *Nursing Times.* 90 (26), 18–19.

Royal College of Nursing 1998, Resource Guide. *The Nursing Care of Older Patients from Black and Minority Ethnic Communities.* London. Royal College of Nursing.

Sarwar, Z. 1998, 'Helping Asian women to understand the menopause'. *Community Nurse*, 4 (3), 12–13.

Schuman, J. 1999, 'The ethnic minority populations of Great Britain – latest estimates'. *Population Trends 1996 – Summer 1999.* London. The Stationery Office.

Shah, R. and Hatton, C. 1999, *Caring Alone: Young Carers in South Asian Communities.* London. Barnardo's.

Simmons, D., Williams, D. and Powell, V. 1989, 'Prevalence of diabetes in a predominantly Asian community'. *British Medical Journal*, 298, 18–21.

Smaje, C. 1995, *Health, 'Race' and Ethnicity: Making Sense of the Evidence.* London. Kings Fund Institute.

Steer, P., Alam, M., Wadsworth, J. and Welch, A. 1995, 'Relation between maternal haemoglobin concentration and low birth weight in different ethnic groups'. *British Medical Journal*, 310, 489–91.

UKCC 1992, *Code of Professional Conduct.* 3rd edn. London. United Kingdom Central Council.

Valios, N. 1999, 'Young, alone and marginalised'. *Community Care*, 1300, 26.

Wellard, S. 1999, 'Caring about culture'. *Community Care*, 1297, 26–7.

Wilson, M. 1995, 'Black women and men. Stereotypes, racism and the mental health system', in Harding C. (ed.), *Not Just Black and White.* London. Good Practices in Mental Health Publications.

4

Hypertension

PHILIPPE MARIE AND SANDRA JOHNSON

Hypertension, or raised blood pressure, is a major disorder common throughout the world. There is much evidence that accurate detection, diagnosis, investigation and treatment of patients with hypertension is highly effective in promoting well-being and preventing life-threatening medical conditions, such as heart disease and stroke, to which it makes a significant contribution (Izzo and Black, 1999).

While there is much evidence to confirm the benefits of early detection and management of high blood pressure, the 'Rule of Halves' (O'Brien *et al.*, 1995) suggests that fewer than 13 per cent of hypertensive people in the United Kingdom (UK) receive adequate intervention to control this problem, unless a comprehensive set of guidelines is followed. According to O'Brien *et al.* (1995), of 100 people with hypertension, only 50 will be diagnosed, of that 50, only 25 will be treated and, of the 25 treated, half will be poorly controlled and half will be well controlled. A similar situation exists in the United States of America (USA) where, according to Burt *et al.* (1995), more than 70 per cent of known hypertensive patients are improperly managed. Calhoun and Oparil (1999), however, reported that only an alarming 6 per cent of British people treated for the disorder were effectively managed.

Contents

Learning Objectives

By the end of this chapter, you should be able to demonstrate knowledge of:

- Blood pressure and the mechanisms by which it is normally controlled.
- Factors that contribute to raised blood pressure.
- How hypertension and its sequelae may be detected and controlled.
- The role of the nurse in assisting with blood pressure management.

Definitions

Blood Pressure

Blood pressure may be defined as the force exerted on arterial walls by the blood circulating through them. It occurs cyclically, peaking as the cardiac ventricles contract (the reading being designated systolic) and at its lowest when the cardiac ventricles relax (the reading being designated diastolic). Blood pressure measurement is expressed as the ratio of the systolic pressure (peak) over the diastolic pressure (resting). There are wide variations within the individual during 24 hours, between age ranges and cultural groups, but 'normal' values range from 100/60 millimetres of mercury (mmHg) to 140/85 mmHg with an 'average' blood pressure usually projected as 120/80 mmHg.

The difference between the two readings, usually around 40 mmHg, is known as the pulse pressure, and reflects stroke volume, ejection velocity from the heart and systemic resistance by the peripheral blood vessels. It may assist as an indication of the patient's ability to maintain cardiac output and further assessment of the patient's cardiovascular status may be judicious if the pulse pressure falls below 30 mmHg.

Marieb (2001) formulated blood pressure as cardiac output multiplied by peripheral resistance. Cardiac output is the amount of blood ejected from the left ventricle of the heart in one minute, or stroke volume (in millilitres) multiplied by heart rate (beats per minute) and a general rule of thumb is stroke volume of 70 ml multiplied by a heart rate of 70 beats per minute is equal to 4900 millilitres of blood per minute (roughly the total blood volume in circulation). Blood pressure is this figure multiplied by peripheral resistance.

Classification of Hypertension

Hypertension is defined as a sustained increase in blood pressure. Since a number of factors induce a change in blood pressure, for example, suddenly being confronted by an anxiety-provoking situation where the sympathetic nervous system increases heart rate and constricts peripheral arterioles in preparation for the 'fight or flight' phenomenon, a single measurement of blood pressure indicating an elevated reading would not normally be of great significance. If readings remained raised several hours later, however, and in the absence of known cardiovascular stimulation, then further investigation would be appropriate. During the measurement of blood pressure, if only the systolic reading is raised, and there is widening of the pulse pressure, such as is found when a person has atherosclerosis, this was, until recently, considered to be of minor significance. However, the Department of Health (DOH) (2000) recommends that patients with a systolic blood pressure (SBP) of between 140 and 159 mmHg may require treatment, depending upon their overall risk of developing cardiovascular disease; those with a sustained SBP of 160 mmHg should be treated. Ramsay (1999) argues that an SBP treatment target of less than or equal to 140 mmHg should be the aim.

Connection

Chapter 5 (Coronary Heart Disease) describes the pathogenesis of atherosclerosis.

Elevation of the diastolic pressure is always associated with a rise in the systolic pressure, with an increase in diastolic measurement to 95 mmHg giving cause for concern and requiring investigation and vigorous management. The optimal treatment aim for people with raised diastolic readings is less than 85 mmHg and even lower (75–80 mmHg) for those with diabetes (British Hypertension Society, 2000).

A decrease in blood pressure is known as hypotension and, while some individuals, groups and cultures have a naturally lower systolic/diastolic blood pressure, which for them is normal, if the blood pressure falls quickly or dramatically it may be fatal if not reversed, for example, hypotension due to blood loss following extensive trauma. Hypotension, its causes and manifestations are outside the remit of this chapter.

Blood Pressure Classification

Measured in millimetres of mercury:

- Optimal blood pressure is classified as pressures below 120 systolic and below 80 diastolic.
- Normal blood pressure is classified as pressures below 130 systolic and below 85 diastolic.
- High–normal blood pressure is classified as pressures measuring in the range of 130 systolic and 85 diastolic to 139 systolic and 89 diastolic.

- Grade 1 (mild hypertension) is classified as pressures measuring in the range of 140 systolic and 90 diastolic to 159 systolic and 99 diastolic.
- Grade 2 (moderate hypertension) is classified as pressures measuring in the range of 160 systolic and 100 diastolic to 179 systolic and 109 diastolic.
- Grade 3 (severe hypertension) is classified as pressures measuring over 180 systolic and over 100 diastolic.
- Isolated systolic is classified as pressures measuring over 140 systolic and over 90 diastolic (Ide, 1997).

Hansson *et al.* (1998) draw attention to the fact that the phenomenon known as Isolated Systolic Hypertension is present in up to 30 per cent of individuals aged over 60 years and is due to a loss of elasticity in arterial walls and in particular those of the aortic arch. This type of hypertension may be initially slight and asymptomatic but with increasing age and severity of the blood pressure measurement, resultant organ damage, particularly to the retinas, may produce difficulty in performing the usual activities of living.

Epidemiology

In the UK, coronary heart disease (CHD) is a major cause of death and is related to high blood pressure in 14 per cent of male CHD deaths and in 12 per cent of CHD deaths in females (National Heart Forum, 2002). Most individuals are unaware that they have a problem, since hypertension is usually of gradual onset, until they experience a cardiovascular event such as myocardial infarction or stroke.

 **Connection**

Chapter 5 (Coronary Heart Disease) and Chapter 6 (Stroke) discuss hypertension as a predisposing factor in these disorders.

Almost one-third of females in the 45–54 years age group have hypertension with more than one-half in the age range 55 to 64 years. This rises to over three-quarters of women over 75 years having the disorder (Erens and Primatesta, 1999). Of those individuals known to have hypertension, 32 per cent and 23 per cent of males and females respectively were not receiving therapeutic medical control.

The incidence of hypertension varies throughout the world with only very few 'no hypertension' societies remaining (these being located around the Amazon basin). Most industrialized European and North American countries have very similar incidences of hypertension (15–30 per cent) with some sub-groups experiencing a greater risk, for example, black Americans (Cooper, 1999). A low level of hypertension (7–15 per cent) prevails amongst the South Chinese and rural African populations, with a high rate of 30–40 per cent being found in Russian and Finnish nationals and in the aforementioned US black people. Cooper (1999) asserts that the likelihood of the incidence of hypertension rising with distance from the equator (which has been documented in China) being linked to climate or temperature, is improbable given that the pattern is reversed in North America.

Calhoun and Oparil (1999) assert that gender differences in blood pressure can be identified at adolescence and persist throughout adulthood, with males in all ethnic groups having a higher SBP and Diastolic Blood Pressure (DBP) than women by 6–7 mmHg and 3–5 mmHg respectively. Through middle age, hypertension is more prevalent amongst men than women, but after the age of 59 years, the reverse becomes apparent. The influence of the menopause on BP is controversial; Lewis (1996) reported a four times greater incidence of hypertension in post-menopausal women than in pre-menopausal women (40 per cent as against 10 per cent) and even with adjustment for age and Body Mass Index (BMI), post-menopausal women were still twice as likely to develop hypertension as pre-menopausal females.

Aetiology

Since hypertension occurs internationally and is directly linked with premature death from cardiovascular, renal and other organ pathology, it attracts much research into risk factors amongst diverse populations. Poulter *et al.* (1997) assert that it is unlikely that hypertension is the result of a single pathological process. However, where researchers have determined contributory elements, it is essential that nurses use currently available information in order to help patients eliminate, as far as possible, those known factors, and to select a lifestyle that will stabilize blood pressure to measurements within the recognized normal limits.

Hypertension is subdivided into primary and secondary with 90 per cent of patients presenting with primary hypertension (also known as essential hypertension), which appears to have no known underlying medical cause (Van Muskirk, 1993). Of the remaining 10 per cent of adults who develop raised blood pressure, specific underlying medical disorders can be demonstrated as being causative. Secondary hypertension, where such an underlying pathological condition is found to be the cause, is mainly associated with:

- Renal disease, for example, renal artery stenosis
- Adrenal disease, for example, phaechromocytoma
- Hyperthyroidism
- Pregnancy.

Stadel (1981) reported that long-term (more than ten years) use of oral contraceptive drugs was implicated in secondary hypertension in females, but more recently, as a result of much study into these drugs, oral contraceptives currently prescribed have fewer such side effects.

The renal, adrenal and thyroid disorders that cause hypertension may be amenable to surgical or pharmacological treatment and that caused by pregnancy is self-limiting, but may still be life-threatening.

Associated Risk Factors

Although primary hypertension has no known single cause, a number of risk factors are seen as contributing to the disorder.

Primary hypertension – risk factors

- Obesity (Coombes, 2002)
- High sodium intake (Norman and Kaplan, 1999)
- Low potassium intake (Whelton, 1998)
- High alcohol intake (Cushman, 1999)
- Stress (O'Brien *et al.*, 1995)
- Physical inactivity (Simmons-Morton, 1999)
- Tobacco smoking (Medical Research Council [MRC], 1985)

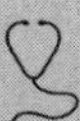

Nursing action points

- Assist individuals to utilize techniques that achieve weight control.
- Educate the public about the risks associated with high sodium and/or low potassium intake.
- Raise awareness of at-risk persons to the role of alcohol in the development of hypertension.
- Promote the benefits of relaxation techniques in the prevention and reduction of raised blood pressure.
- Discuss individualized exercise plans for persons with, or at risk of developing, hypertension.
- Alert patients to the effects of tobacco smoking on blood pressure.

Obesity

The National Audit Office (NAO) (2001) found from investigations into services for overweight and obese patients, that NHS provision was inconsistent.

Findings included the fact that almost 50 per cent of the adult population in England is overweight with a BMI of more than 25 kg/m^2, with 17 per cent of men and 21 per cent of women classified as obese, having a BMI of more than 30 kg/m^2. Obesity is defined as a BMI of 30 or greater. BMI is defined as weight (kilograms) divided by height in metres squared (kg/m^2). Additionally, about ten per cent of six year olds are now classified as clinically obese (Coombes, 2002). These figures explain why obesity is a major cause of death in the UK, accounting for over 30 000 deaths annually by its contribution to a wide range of diseases such as diabetes mellitus, coronary heart disease, stroke and renal disease.

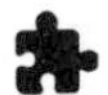

Connection

Chapter 13 (Diabetes Mellitus) discusses obesity and the distribution of body fat as predisposing factors in the development of diabetes.

The reasons for high rates of obesity in the UK and many other developed countries include the availability of cheap ready-made, high calorie foods, sedentary lifestyles and changes in attitude towards leisure activities such as sport and computer/television games (Coombes, 2002). Many view obesity as a self-inflicted problem with the solution lying solely with the obese person to lose weight. However, there needs to be a more positive attitude amongst health care workers, many of whom are well-placed to design weight-reduction programmes to meet the individual's needs. Coombes (2002) acknowledges that merely distributing diet sheets and advice and information is unproductive and that a two-way 'contract' needs to be established to monitor and support patients through an individually constructed programme of weight loss.

Nursing action points

- Educate the individual about limiting calorie intake across the nutritional perspective.
- Devise a diet that will reduce animal fat to a minimum but include vegetable fats of choice (in limited amounts) so that the diet remains attractive visually and psychologically and is not punitive.
- Establish regular mealtimes and encourage the patient not to snack between meals.
- Co-design an activity programme, for example, a brisk walk daily, which can be effective in helping the overweight patient make permanent and sustainable lifestyle changes that can achieve and maintain an acceptable BMI.

On average, for every kilogram of weight loss, a reduction of 3/2 mmHg in systolic and diastolic pressures occurs in hypertensive patients and a 1/1 mmHg reduction in normotensive patients (Wright, 1995). Regular monitoring and support in the early stages of any weight-reduction scheme (as seen in a number of commercial weight-loss regimes and products) can prove to be of benefit in lowering hypertension and related life-threatening disorders NAO, 2001).

High Sodium and Low Potassium

There is evidence that salt intake has a direct effect upon blood pressure; the findings of the Intersalt Cooperative Research Group (Intersalt) (1988) study indicated that the rise in blood pressure with advancing age resulted from the use of salt in the diet. Further large scale studies support this outcome by showing a reduction in blood pressure following salt restriction (MacGregor *et al.*, 1989; Neaton *et al.*, 1993).

The mechanism by which sodium increases blood pressure is unclear, but the improvement shown by restricting dietary sodium is unequivocal. The National Service Framework (DOH, 2000) draws attention to the need for a balanced diet for every member of the population, which includes a low salt intake. However, various mechanisms have been proposed to explain the purported influence of potassium on blood pressure: there appears to be suppression of the renin–angiotensin and sympathetic nervous systems, with direct arterial vasodilatation, resulting in a reduction of peripheral resistance.

Epidemiological studies are also consistent with the suggestion that low potassium may play a specific role in the strikingly high incidence and prevalence of hypertension in black and elderly people. Increasing potassium intake may play an important anti-hypertensive role in these particular sub-groups.

National Service Framework guidelines (DOH, 2000) include: educating the public about which foods contain high/low levels of sodium and potassium; setting clear goals based on theories of behavioural change, rather than providing information only; and the benefit of utilizing a small-group approach in helping patients maintain changes in nutritional habits.

Nursing action points

Since they can give personal contact over a sustained period of time with individuals and groups, community nurses, health visitors and school and practice nurses are in an excellent position to

- Provide information about risk factors.
- Promote healthy nutritional eating patterns.
- Offer feedback and support on any behavioural changes deemed necessary.

They are also in a position to:

- Collaborate with other Health Service users and providers to promote changes in the local environment that might influence sodium and potassium intake.
- Organize displays and blood pressure monitoring services in catering outlets and supermarkets.

High Alcohol Intake

Several epidemiological studies have indicated a close positive association between blood pressure and alcohol consumption (Klatsky *et al.*, 1977; MacMahon, 1987). The Intersalt (1988) study confirmed this relationship and found that the greater the alcohol consumption, the higher the blood pressure, although non-drinkers of alcohol appear to have a slightly raised blood pressure in comparison with moderate drinkers (Cushman *et al.*, 1998).

Excess intake of alcohol has also been associated with resistance to anti-hypertensive drug treatment. Jackson (2000) and Cushman *et al.* (1998) identify data that suggest a true interference with the hypotensive effects of appropriately-taken medication. They argue that a daily alcohol intake of more than three alcoholic drinks (one drink equal to 300 millilitres or being defined as 14 grams ethanol or equivalent to half a pint of beer) is associated with an almost doubling of the prevalence of hypertension and could account for up to 30 per cent of people with raised blood pressure, depending upon the dominance of heavy drinking within a population.

Cushman *et al.* (1998) propound that there are a number of potential mechanisms by which chronic overconsumption of alcohol results in hypertension, which include:

- Sympathetic nervous system stimulation with consequent effects on the renin–angiotensin–aldosterone mechanism. Insulin and cortisol secretions may also be affected.
- Inhibition of vascular relaxing substances with consequent development of a state of vasoconstriction.
- Calcium or magnesium depletion with consequent effects on muscle and nervous tissue.

Poulter *et al.* (1997) claim that nurses can encourage patients to adhere to their prescribed medication and reduce alcohol intake by offering realistic methods.

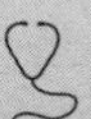

Nursing action points

- Tailor the quality of instructions given, to the individual.
- Ensure that the patient understands the reason for reducing alcohol intake and taking medicines as prescribed.
- Deal separately with problems associated with a complex regime.
- Put advice/instructions/information into writing.
- Be friendly, courteous, compassionate and nonjudgemental in approach.
- Encourage discussion and patient participation in decisionmaking regarding alcohol reduction.
- Suggest dilution of strong alcoholic drinks with carbonated water and changing to lower-alcohol-content beers for those who frequently socialize in public houses.
- Respond to complaints in a sensitive manner and avoid generating fear by constantly making reference to the effects of uncontrolled hypertension.

(Poulter *et al.*, 1997)

The overall aim of nursing interventions must be clearly communicated, that the patient is not being asked to cease all intake of alcohol, rather to moderate it to a safe level.

Stress

Stress may be defined as any external or internal pressure that causes personal conflict and demands a mental and/or physical reaction. It is largely accepted that essential hypertension is probably the culmination of several contributory factors of internal, for example, genetic, and external, for example, smoking, origins. While it has been widely suggested that psychological or environmental stress may play a part in the aetiology of hypertension, the links have not been positively identified, and although stressful events may cause an acute hypertensive response, there is doubt over any long-term significance.

However, Pickering *et al.* (1996), reported on some of the most persuasive evidence for the role of chronic stress in the development of hypertension in relation to occupational strain. They found that men in jobs that combined high personal demands with low control over decision-making, had a three times higher risk of hypertension and, having stayed in such a post for three years, had blood pressures of 11/7 mmHg higher than men employed in low strain jobs. They also found a significant correlation between exposure to job strain and left ventricular hypertrophy and increased risk of myocardial infarction. The effects that a given level of perceived stress will have on the heart and blood pressure will, to some degree, depend upon the susceptibility of the subject. Hampton (1999) suggests that individuals who display increased reactivity to stressful situations appear to be more likely to develop hypertension than those who respond in a calmer manner. This poses the concept of a 'hypertensive personality', in whom repressed hostility or anger results in increased sympathetic nervous system activity and a consequent rise in blood pressure. However, Pickering *et al.* (1996) identified studies that both supported and refuted this notion.

Physical Inactivity

Physical activity causes a sharp but transient rise in blood pressure as the cardiovascular system responds to sympathetic nervous stimulation. However, there is evidence that people who undertake regular exercise are fitter and healthier with lower blood pressures, than those who lead a sedentary lifestyle (O'Brien *et al.*, 1995).

Simmons-Morton (1999) asserts that 40 minutes of aerobic activity that raises heart and respiratory rates, engaged in at least three times per week has been shown to lower blood pressure. She gives examples of average effects of a net decrease of 2/3 mmHg in normotensive people to a net decrease of 10/8 mmHg in people with hypertension. The effect of exercise seen in hypertensive patients compares with that found in studies of hypertensive patients being treated with a single drug.

Exercise does not need to be intensive; indeed O'Brien *et al.* (1995) suggest that it may be harmful in people with pre-existing cardiovascular disease, where the incorporation of more gentle exercise, such as walking, into activities of living, would be more appropriate but still carry beneficial effects.

Nursing action points

- Advise patients to engage in moderate to vigorous aerobic-style exercise, two to three times per week to assist with anti-hypertensive therapy.
- Recognize that advice alone is rarely sufficient to induce behaviour change and discuss with the patient an individually tailored action plan that takes into consideration his or her personal preferences, such as a particularly enjoyable sport.
- Set realistic goals and attempt to overcome identifiable barriers.
- Seek ways in which the patient may be given positive reinforcement, for example, enjoying activity within a group setting, and enhancing social support where applicable.

The patient is more likely to follow an exercise plan if he or she can see or feel improvements for their personal efforts, so regular monitoring, for example, self-monitoring of heart rate during exercise, and follow-up by nurse-led blood pressure clinics are desirable, with the ultimate aim being that physical activity becomes part of permanent lifestyle behaviour.

Tobacco Smoking

While the smoking of tobacco is declining in many Western societies generally it has been identified that 37 per cent of men and women in the 16–24 year age group smoke tobacco and this figure is rising (Poulter *et al.*, 1997).

Sympathetic nervous system stimulation that occurs during smoking causes vasospasm and vasoconstriction with a rise in blood pressure. Continuous blood pressure measurement in heavy smokers shows that blood pressure is raised for most of the day, that is, during tobacco smoking, and Poulter *et al.* (1997) observed that more severe forms of hypertension are more likely to occur in the hypertensive smoker. The MRC (1985) hypertension trial confirmed that greater benefits can be obtained by the hypertensive patient who stops smoking than by taking anti-hypertensive drugs. Given that tobacco smoking also contributes to chronic bronchitis, stroke, myocardial infarction and a number of cancers, cessation can only prove to be beneficial.

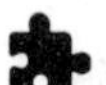 **Connections**

- Chapter 5 (Coronary Heart Disease) highlights the damaging effects of smoking on blood vessel walls.
- Chapter 9 (Chronic Obstructive Pulmonary Disease) discusses the association of tobacco smoking with the pathogenesis of chronic bronchitis and pulmonary emphysema.

Physiology of Blood Pressure Control and Maintenance

Blood pressure regulation depends upon a number of interrelated factors and their ability to respond in a flexible manner to internal and external stimuli.

Force of the Heart as a Pump

The left cardiac ventricle, on contraction, pumps blood through the arteries, arterioles and capillaries of the systemic circulation and the blood returns via the venous system, to the right side of the heart. The pressure at the arterial end is greater than at the venous end due to the force of contraction of the left ventricle and fluctuates between 120 and 80 mmHg with a mean value of about 100 mmHg (13.3 kPa) above atmospheric pressure. This is termed the arterial pressure or, simply, blood pressure. Venous blood pressure is that found in the great veins and right atrium and is approximately equal to atmospheric pressure, that is, 0 mmHg. The pressure difference between the two is the force that drives the blood through the systemic circulation.

Peripheral Resistance

The arteries and arterioles, having elastic fibres in their walls, can alter their internal diameter by constricting or relaxing these fibres; this is known as peripheral resistance (Swales *et al.*, 1991). The arteriolar involuntary muscle is usually partially contracted due to sympathetic nervous system action which maintains the tone of the walls of these vessels. A centre in the medulla oblongata in the brain stem, known as the vaso motor centre (VMC), is the origin of the constriction/dilatation mechanism. A reduced stimulus to the VMC will cause increased arteriolar vasoconstriction due to stimulation of the muscle fibres present in the arteriolar walls, resulting in their narrowing. Such narrowing causes a rise in blood pressure (Figure 4.1). An increase in VMC stimulation however, will cause relaxation of the muscle tone due to inhibition of the vasoconstriction mechanism. This will result in an increased diameter of the vessel walls and a consequent fall in blood pressure, provided other factors remain constant (Figure 4.2).

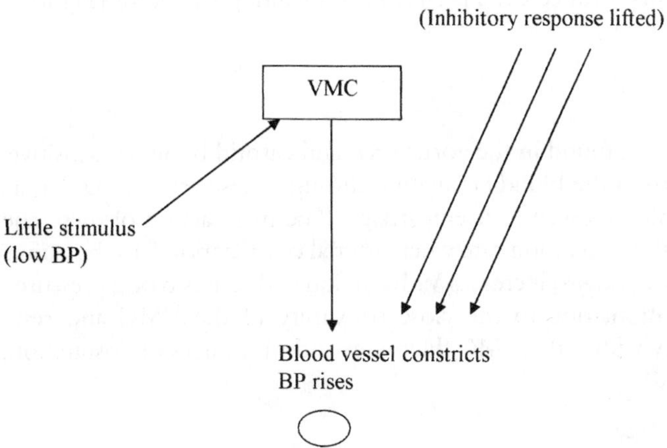

Figure 4.1 Arteriolar vasoconstriction due to reduced stimulus to the VMC

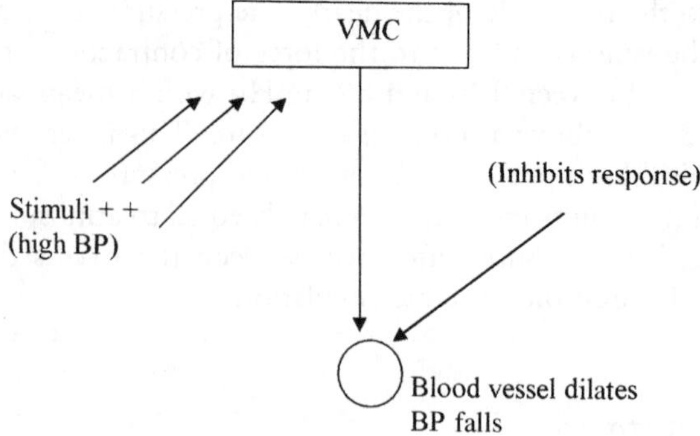

Figure 4.2 Blood pressure control

Baroreceptors

The aortic arch and carotid sinus have within their walls nerve receptors (baroreceptors), which are sensitive to the pressure of the blood passing over them. If that pressure rises then increased nerve impulses are transmitted to the VMC causing overriding of the inhibitory response with a dilatation of the peripheral arterioles and a resultant fall in blood pressure. If blood pressure over the baroreceptors is low, then the opposite occurs and vasoconstriction peripherally causes a consequent rise in blood pressure. This represents a feed-back system which helps to maintain the constancy of blood pressure by minimizing changes.

When a person changes position from lying to standing, cardiac output falls, but due to the baroreceptor/VMC system, blood pressure stays relatively constant. This system can be temporarily destabilized following a prolonged period of bed-rest (some weeks) and sudden movement from horizontal to vertical does not activate the compensatory mechanism, with the result that blood pressure is insufficient to maintain cerebral perfusion and fainting will occur (Figure 4.3).

Chemoreceptors

Further receptors, found in the aortic arch and carotid body, are sensitive to the levels of oxygen in the blood circulating through these arteries, also to a reduction in blood flow as seen in haemorrhage. The main action of these chemoreceptors is to raise respiration rate when arterial oxygenation falls, but stimulation by this hypoxic state also increases VMC action and causes blood pressure to rise. During respiration, due to the close proximity of the VMC and respiratory centres, activity within the VMC fluctuates and maximizes on inspiration.

Sensory Nerves

Some sensory activity (in particular, pain) can also affect VMC activity. Mild degrees of pain cause an increase in VMC activity and raised blood pressure,

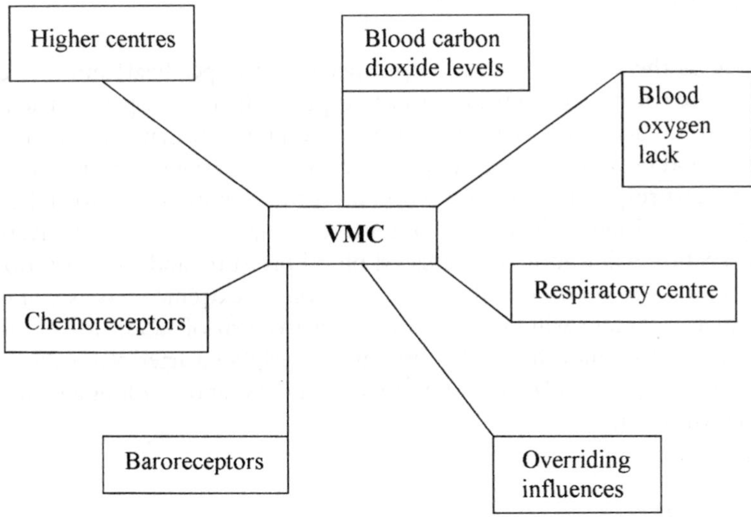

Figure 4.3 VMC influencing factors

whilst more severe pain stimulates the VMC inhibitory response and causes a severe drop in blood pressure, such that fainting may result. This mechanism is the basis of neurogenic shock, which is unrelated to hypovolaemia.

Any form of psychological stress or excitement can stimulate the higher centres of the cerebral cortex, which is usually associated with an increase in cardiac output. This combined effect also influences VMC inhibition (which is reduced) causing peripheral vasoconstriction and rising blood pressure.

Overriding Influences

Sometimes organ or tissue activity is increased and demands a greater blood supply locally. Surrounding mechanisms can override the VMC causing local vasodilatation and hyperaemia, but the VMC responds by vasoconstriction of other vessels in order to maintain overall peripheral resistance. Metabolites such as lactic acid, adenylic acid and potassium ions released from activated muscle cells during exercise can have similar overriding effects and cause increased blood flow to the demanding tissue.

Viscosity of Blood

This normally remains constant because of the solid components such as cells and plasma proteins, giving blood a viscosity of two and a half times that of water. Dilution or concentration of these solids will have an impact on peripheral resistance and hence on blood pressure.

Cardiac Output

Calculated as the stroke volume (output per ventricle per beat) multiplied by the heart rate (beats per minute), cardiac output is the output per ventricle per minute and the heart acts as a constant pressure-pump. It maintains a constant systemic blood flow against the peripheral arteriolar resistance. If the resistance rises, the heart responds by raising blood pressure, requiring it to work harder. As peripheral resistance changes do not affect cardiac output overall, arteriolar vasoconstriction will lead to an increased blood pressure, and vasodilatation to lowered blood pressure. Should vasoconstriction be extreme, vessels will close and circulatory failure will ensue due to a zero return of blood to the heart. Contraction of the smooth muscle fibres in the peripheral arteriolar walls is also influenced by intracellular calcium concentrations and prolonged smooth muscle constriction.

Blood Volume

Changes in the volume of circulating blood have a marked and rapid effect on blood pressure. The heart compensates for blood loss initially by beating more rapidly, sympathetic nervous system activity causes peripheral shutdown so that perfusion of the vital organs can be maintained and VMC activity causes widespread vasoconstriction in an attempt to maintain blood pressure. A characteristic clinical picture can be seen in a post-operative patient who is haemorrhaging, by a rapid, thready pulse, diminishing blood pressure as the system fails to compensate for the haemorrhage; cold, clammy skin as blood is diverted away from the periphery to vital organs, with eventual change in consciousness level as the brain becomes hypoxic and, if not reversed, death occurs. Increased blood volume that may occur as a result of badly managed intravenous infusion, will cause cardiac overload with increasing stress on the heart; pulmonary oedema; an initial rise in blood pressure with bradycardia until the compensatory mechanism fails to maintain circulation, which again will result in death.

Renin–Angiotensin System

An important enzyme/hormone mechanism that exerts a powerful control over blood pressure is the renin–angiotensin system. Renin is a protein-splitting enzyme, secreted from the juxtaglomerular apparatus of the kidney in response to reduced salt intake and poor renal blood flow. Sympathetic nervous system stimulation also causes renin release. It is responsible for a chain of reactions, converting the inactive renin substrate angiotensinogen to angiotensin I, which in turn is converted by angiotensin converting enzyme (ACE) to angiotensin II. The latter is a powerful vasoconstricting agent causing widespread vasoconstriction and rise in blood pressure. It also stimulates the adrenal zona glomerulosa to secrete aldosterone which creates a further blood pressure elevation response in relation to sodium retention. The thirst centre is also stimulated in an attempt to boost circulatory volume. While this system is not thought to be directly related to essential hypertension (some hypertensive groups have low levels of these chemicals, and drugs designed to block their function are not very effective in such people), there appear to be renin–angiotensin systems localized within the kidney and some arteries that do have some control over blood flow regulation.

Autonomic Nervous System

Stimulation of the sympathetic nervous system has both vasoconstrictive and vasodilation effects depending upon body organ demands at any particular time, for example, in response to stress, and has a considerable role in blood pressure regulation. While there is little evidence to suggest that the sympathetic nervous system and adrenaline/noradrenalin play a clear part in the development of hypertension, it is important to understand that there is an inter-relationship between the sympathetic nervous system and associated controlling mechanisms and drugs that block the action of one or the other can be effective in reducing blood pressure (Marieb, 2001; Foss and Farine, 2000; Cree and Rischmiller, 1991).

Other Factors

- Bradykinin is a vasodilating enzyme which is inactivated by ACE.
- Endothelin is a potent vasoconstrictor produced by the endothelium which has cardiovascular and non-cardiovascular functions.
- Natriuretic peptides may be described as inhibitory to the renin–angiotensin–aldosterone system, sympathetic nervous system and endothelin functions. They also play a part in increasing capillary permeability.
- Calcium and potassium are both associated with nervous system activity and muscle contraction. Their interaction with other factors is the subject of much research involving the predisposition to hypertension (Brown *et al.*, 1995).

Clinical Manifestations

People who are aware that they are at risk of developing hypertension may be more aware of potential symptoms. Many people, however, may be completely unaware of their hypertensive state, either having no symptoms at all or dismissing complaints such as headaches, vertigo, nosebleeds and fatigue (Thompson and Webster, 2000).

Investigative Tests

Hypertension has been justifiably described as 'the silent killer' (O'Brien *et al.*, 1995) since many people who have the disorder, even severely, are diagnosed incidentally, by routine medical examination for some other condition. Others may not be identified as hypertensive until a life-threatening heart attack or stroke has occurred and left the person with residual health problems. Both nurses and doctors can include specific questions when enquiring into a patient's health history.

Investigations into hypertension

- History
- Physical examination
- Urinalysis
- Blood tests
- X-rays
- Renal investigations
- Electrocardiograph and other cardiac investigations

History

This will include any past medical history that may have influenced blood pressure regulation, for example, pre-eclampsia during pregnancy; any medication that the patient has been, or is taking, and any family history that may reveal the presence of cardiovascular disease, diabetes, thyroid or renal disease which could influence the patient's risk. The patient's social history should also be obtained since dietary habits including salt, fat and alcohol intake, tobacco smoking and lifestyle, might indicate risk factors for hypertension.

Physical Examination

During assessment, the patient's physical presentation may reveal the likelihood of endocrine disorders such as Cushing's syndrome or thyroid disease for which more specific investigations will be ordered. Accurate measurement of the blood pressure is essential but, if raised, needs to be repeated, taken possibly by nursing staff to overcome the 'white-coat' (doctor-induced) hypertension measurement that occurs in 8–10 per cent of people being tested (Hurst, 2002).

The patient's weight and height should be measured and BMI recorded. Cardiovascular assessment may indicate heart arrhythmias and chest auscultation may reveal evidence of obstructive airways disease which may influence the category of any medication prescribed. General abdominal examination may reveal signs of chronic liver disease associated with high alcohol intake or, sometimes, polycystic kidneys or renal tumours may be detected. Central nervous system examination may indicate evidence of residual damage from a previous stroke and careful questioning may reveal short-term memory dysfunction associated with cerebral hypoxia.

Examination of the eyes via the ophthalmoscope will show any retinal changes associated with hypertension, including blood vessel tortuosity, 'silver wiring' effect, arteriovenous 'nipping', and later effects due to severe hypertension, for example, retinal haemorrhages, 'cotton-wool' spots and papilloedema (Jackson, 2000).

Urinalysis

Any abnormality found on routine testing should be investigated further. The findings may be simply an indication of a contaminated specimen, for example, from menstrual blood, but may be associated with more sinister pathology, for example, glucose in a previously undiagnosed diabetic person.

Blood Tests

- Serum cholesterol – to determine the risk of atheroma development.
- Serum sodium – raised levels may be found in chronic renal failure and in patients who have been prescribed large doses of diuretics.
- Serum potassium – low levels may be found in patients prescribed diuretics and also in hypo-aldosteronism. High levels of potassium may be found in people with renal failure and sometimes where ACE anti-hypertensive drugs are used.
- Serum urea and creatinine concentrations – renal disease can cause hypertension and vice versa. Creatinine levels may indicate the rapidity of renal function impairment and should be monitored regularly.
- Serum calcium and phosphate concentrations – these can be altered by chronic renal failure, primary hyper-parathyroidism or diuretics. The latter should be withheld before accurate levels of these salts can be ascertained.
- Plasma hormone concentrations – these may indicate an endocrine disorder.
- Serum uric acid – about 40 per cent of hypertensive patients have raised serum uric acid, but this can also be increased in conjunction with thiazide diuretics or elevated alcohol consumption.
- Full blood count – whilst this is a useful indicator of a number of health problems, it is not of great value in determining causes of hypertension, although it may show a raised red cell count resulting from chronic renal or airway disease (O'Brien *et al.*, 1995).

Changes in any of the above biochemical investigations suggest further tests that could be beneficial in determining any contributory pathology and may include renal tests.

Renal Tests

- Intravenous pyelography can indicate anatomical changes and the presence of filling defects.
- 24-hour urine collection for sodium, protein, catecholamines and/or urinary free cortisol.
- Magnetic resonance imaging and computed tomography may show phaechromocytoma.
- Renal ultrasonography may identify polycystic/hydronephrotic kidneys, or a small kidney reduced in size by renal artery disease.
- Renal angiography may provide evidence of renal artery stenosis.

In addition to the above, an important non-invasive test – ambulatory blood pressure measurement – which records a person's blood pressure intermittently over a 24-hour period – provides an accurate estimate of longer-term blood pressure and helps to avoid the difference of approximately 12/7 mmHg of recordings undertaken in a clinic (Hurst, 2002).

More sophisticated tests may be used, for example, echocardiography if earlier results indicate specific target organ damage.

Treatment

Depending upon the results of the examinations and investigations outlined above, the patient may be advised to follow lifestyle adaptations as discussed under risk factors and nursing action points/interventions, in combination with pharmacological prescription designed to suit the individual patient's needs. The usual approach to drug management of hypertension is a gradual introduction of either a thiazide diuretic or β blocker, as Hampton (1999) asserts that there is strong evidence for reduction of cardiovascular events with their use. However, Ramsay (1999) recognizes that preferential use of alternative anti-hypertensives should be adopted in certain circumstances such as the presence of complications from other diseases.

The use of one drug only controls hypertension in less than 50 per cent of those identified and more than 30 per cent of hypertensives will need three or more pharmacological preparations. Combinations of smaller doses of drugs with different modes of action have a cumulative effect and fewer side-effects than the maximum dose of a single drug. Common combinations for third-line prescriptions are:

- Diuretic with ACE inhibitor and calcium channel blocker, or
- Diuretic with β blocker and calcium channel blocker.

Pharmacological Preparations

- β blockers, for example, propranolol, lower blood pressure by inhibiting the action of catecholamines on β adrenoreceptors, by reducing cardiac output, suppressing the release of renin and/or affecting the VMC.
- Diuretics – these increase excretion of water and sodium, which decreases blood volume by reducing peripheral resistance. There are numerous types of diuretic but those most commonly used for hypertension are thiazides, for example, bendrofluazide and loop diuretics, for example, frusemide, the latter being less potent but very useful in patients with some cardiac or renal failure.
- ACE inhibitors, for example, lisinopril and captopril block the angiotensin converting enzyme system and bring about a reduction in blood pressure by reducing peripheral vascular resistance and by reducing renal reabsorption of sodium by aldosterone.
- Calcium channel blockers, for example, nifedipine, act by inhibiting the transfer of calcium ions across the cell membranes, eventually causing vasodilatation resulting in a lowering of blood pressure. Some, for example, verapamil, slow atrio-ventricular node conduction and reduce myocardial contractility. Diltiazam, the third sub-group of calcium channel blockers, has an effect on cardiac conduction and the smooth muscle of blood vessel walls. All of the calcium channel blocking drugs are well absorbed from the gastrointestinal tract and are metabolized in the liver.

Nursing Interventions

Encouraging Adherence to Treatment

Compliance is the extent to which a person's behaviour in relation to making lifestyle changes either adheres to, or defaults from, professional advice. Understanding of information and advice regarding empowerment of patients, while leading to informed consent, does not necessarily result in them acting in their own best interests. Poor compliance is a major therapeutic and economic problem in healthcare and is an important determinant of successful hypertensive therapy. Poulter *et al.* (1997) estimate that the numbers of patients prescribed a therapeutic drug regime who are lost to annual follow-up or who do not adhere appropriately to their prescriptions, must account for the greater proportion of the 50 per cent of hypertensive people who are treated but whose blood pressure is uncontrolled.

The task for nurses is to help patients to benefit fully from facilities offered for blood pressure control. Factors such as patient forgetfulness, poor comprehension of a complex therapeutic regime, poor or inadequate explanation by the prescription provider, cost of medication, unwelcome side effects and the belief that one course of medication will 'cure' the hypertension, all contribute to the patient not taking or continuing to take the prescribed treatment.

Stress Management

Whilst there may be only tenuous links between stress and hypertension, the increased feelings of calm and enhanced sense of well-being derived from relaxation techniques practised at regular intervals can only be of benefit to patients. Nurses should be able to direct patients towards a variety of known techniques such as aromatherapy, reflexology and yoga and, for some, strenuous sporting or exercising activities that result in an increased release of endorphins, which may produce a state of reduced anxiety and tension relief.

Assisting the Individual to Stop Smoking Cigarettes

Using techniques similar to those listed for aiding patients with reduction of alcohol intake, nurses can encourage smoking cessation. Additionally, nurses should appear as role models by not smoking themselves when near to patients, and avoid the hypocrisy of extolling the virtues of not smoking yet carrying packets of cigarettes visibly within uniform pockets (Kotcher and Kotcher, 1999). The MRC (1985) trial also identified smoke-filled areas and the odour of cigarette smoke on clothing worn by people nearby, as strong trigger factors to recommencing tobacco smoking, having previously ceased.

Patients need to be helped to identify situations that pose a high temptation to smoke and find enjoyable alternative venues/activities to replace these. As cigarette smoking is a major risk factor for a number of disease processes, in particular cardiovascular disease and chronic obstructive pulmonary disease, it has to be communicated to patients that smoking, either actively or passively, should be avoided whenever possible. Kotcher and Kotcher (1999) assert that benefits from cessation of smoking occur slowly over a period of about one year and those who continue to smoke reduce the beneficial cardiovascular effects of antihypertensive therapy.

Managing Elimination Problems

Diuretic drugs can result in the need to pass urine at socially inconvenient times. The nurse should advise the patient to take the drugs first thing in the morning. Discussing the person's daily routine and flexibility in the timing of treatment to adapt to the person's lifestyle can result in greater compliance with treatment.

Promoting Sleep and Relaxation

Relaxation and rest are important and daily routines should be examined to identify appropriate periods for resting. Night sedation may be required to ensure adequate sleep, although the nurse can encourage relaxation by suggesting such things as soaking in a warm bath. Referral to agencies teaching relaxation and stress management techniques may be of benefit to some people. Work may be a source of stress and patients should be encouraged to examine their work routines to assess the possibility of reducing work-related stress. Finding interest other than work may help the 'workaholic'. Sporting hobbies should be encouraged, as exercise will increase cardiac fitness as long as strenuous exercise is not undertaken without first seeking medical advice (Thompson and Webster, 2000).

Teaching Self-care

Because the therapeutic regimen is the responsibility of the patient in collaboration with the healthcare provider, education, goals and support can help the patient to achieve blood pressure control. Involving family members in education programmes enables them to support the patient's efforts to control hypertension. Written information about the expected effects and side effects of medication is very important. When side effects do occur patients need to understand the importance of reporting them and know where to contact the relevant person. Patients also need to be informed not to suddenly stop taking anti-hypertensive drugs, thus avoiding 'rebound hypertension'. Regular follow-up care is imperative so that the disease process can be assessed and treated (Smeltzer and Bare, 2000).

 **Connection**

Chapter 2 (Family-centred Care) discusses the positive aspects of involving family members in care for both the patients and their relatives.

Conclusion

Hypertension is a serious, indiscriminate disorder which lies undetected in many people until irreversible organ damage is evident. For this reason, it is often justifiably referred to as 'the silent killer'. Hypertension is relatively easily diagnosed, and nurses, if aware of its life-threatening trajectory, are well-placed to advise and encourage the general public to take advantage of blood-pressure testing.

Once diagnosed, if hypertensive people can conform to an individualized risk-reduction programme, then long-term problems associated with the disorder can be averted and blood pressure controlled.

A life-time measure of daily drug therapy and occasional medical investigations may appear unattractive, but the alternatives, for example, stroke and cardiac myopathies are appalling to most people. Nursing interventions in the form of education, advice and encouragement to engage in healthy lifestyle behaviours can make significant contributions to the management of hypertension and its short- and long-term effects.

References

British Hypertension Society 2000, *Management of Hypertension; Brief Summary.* www.Hyp.ac.uk/bhs/resources_manage_summary.htm

Brown, E. M., Vassiter, P. M. and Herbert, S. C. 1995, 'Calcium ions as extracellular messengers'. *Cell*, 83, 679–82.

Burt, V. L., Cutler, J. A., Higgins, M. and Horan, M. J. 1995, 'Trends in the prevalence, awareness, treatment and control of hypertension in the adult in the US population'. *Hypertension*, 26, 60–9.

Calhoun, D. A. and Oparil, S. 1999, 'Gender and blood pressure' in Izzo, J. and Black, H. R. 1999, *Hypertension Primer*. Dallas. American Heart Association.

Coombes, R. 2002, 'Trouble at large'. *Nursing Times*, 98 (46), 23-6.

Cooper, R. S. 1999, 'Geographical patterns of hypertension' in Izzo, J. and Black, H. R. *Hypertension Primer*. Dallas. American Heart Association.

Cree, L. and Rischmiller, S. 1991, *Science in Nursing*. Sydney. W. B. Saunders.

Cushman, W. C. 1999, 'Alcohol use in blood pressure' in Izzo, J. and Black, H. R. *Hypertension Primer*. Dallas. American Heart Association.

Cushman, W. C., Cutler, J. A. and Hanna, E. 1998, 'The prevention and treatment of high blood pressure study: effects of an alcohol treatment programme on blood pressure'. *Archives of International Medicine*, 152, 1197–200.

Department of Health (DOH) 2000, *National Service Framework for Coronary Heart Disease*. London. Department of Health.

Erens, B. and Primatesta, P. (eds) 1999, *Health Survey for England; Cardiovascular Disease*. London. The Stationery Office.

Foss, M. and Farine, T. 2000, *Science in Nursing and Health Care*. Harlow. Prentice Hall.

Hampton, J. R. 1999, 'Evidence in cardiovascular medicine'. *The Practitioner*, 243 (1603), 718–27.

Hansson, L., Hedner, T. and Himmelmann, A. 1998, 'The growing importance of systolic blood pressure'. *Blood Pressure*, 7, 131.

Hurst, R. 2002, 'Managing hypertension, measurement and prevention'. *Nursing Times*, 98 (38), 38–40.

Ide, B. 1997, 'Cardiovascular system' in Thompson, J. M., McFarland, G. K., Hirsch, J. E. and Tucker, S. M. (eds). *Mosby's Clinical Nursing*. 5th edn. London. Mosby.

Intersalt Cooperative Research Group 1988, 'Intersalt, an international study of electrolyte excretion and blood pressure. Results for 24 hour urinary sodium and potassium excretion'. *British Medical Journal*, 297, 319–28.

Izzo, J. L. and Black, H. R. 1999, *Hypertension Primer*. Dallas. American Heart Association.

Jackson, R. 2000, 'Guidelines on preventing cardiovascular disease in clinical practice'. *British Medical Journal*, 3201 (7236), 659–61.

Klatsky, A. L., Friedman, G. D. and Siegelaub 1977, 'Alcohol consumption and blood pressure'. *New England Journal of Medicine*, 296, 1194–2000.

Kotcher, T. and Kotcher, J. M. 1999, 'Smoking and hypertension' in Izzo, J. and Black, H. R. 1999, *Hypertension Primer*. Dallas. American Heart Association.

MacGregor, G. A., Markandu, N. D., Sagnella, G. A., Singer, D. R. and Cappuccio, F. P. 1989, 'Double-blind study of three sodium intakes and long term effects of sodium restriction in essential hypertension'. *Lancet*, ii, 1244.

MacMahon, S. 1987, 'Alcohol consumption and hypertension'. *Hypertension*, 9, 111–21.

Marieb, N. E. 2001, *Human Anatomy and Physiology*. 5th edn. London. Addison-Wesley.

Medical Research Council (MRC) 1985, 'MRC trial of treatment of hypertension in older adults; principal results'. *British Medical Journal*, 304, 405–12.

National Audit Office (NAO) 2001, *Tackling Obesity in England*. London. National Audit Office.

National Heart Forum 2002, *Coronary Heart Disease: Estimating the Impact of Changes in Risk Factors*. London. The Stationery Office.

Neaton, L., Grim, R. H. and Prineas, R. J. 1993, 'Treatment of mild hypertension study: final results'. *Journal of the American Medical Association*, 270, 713.

Norman, M. and Kaplan, M. D. 1999, 'Salt and blood pressure' in Izzo, J. and Black, H. R. 1999, *Hypertension Primer*. Dallas. American Heart Association.

O'Brien, E. T., Beevers, D. G. and Marshall, H. J. 1995, *ABC of Hypertension*. London. BMJ Publishing.

Pickering, T.G., Devereaux, R. B. and James, G. D. 1996, 'Environmental influences on blood pressure and the role of job strain'. *Journal of Hypertension (Supplement)*, 14, S179–86.

Poulter, N., Sever, P. and Thom, S. 1997, *Managing Hypertension in Subgroups*. Surrey. Whitfield.

Ramsay, L. 1999, 'British Hypertension Society guidelines for hypertension management 1999: summary'. *British Medical Journal*, 319 (7210), 630–5.

Simmons-Morton, D. 1999, 'Physical activity, fitness and blood pressure' in Izzo, J. and Black, H. R. 1999, *Hypertension Primer*. Dallas. American Heart Association.

Smeltzer, S. and Bare, B. 2000, *Textbook of Medical–Surgical Nursing*. Philadelphia. Lippincott.

Stadel, B. V. 1981, 'Oral contraceptives and cardiovascular disease'. *New England Journal of Medicine*, 305, 672.

Swales, J. D., Sever, P. S. and Peart, W. S. 1991, *Clinical Atlas of Hypertension*. London. Gower Medical.

Thompson, D. R. and Webster, R. A. 2000, 'The cardiovascular system' in Alexander, M. F., Fawcett, J. N. and Runciman, P. J. *Nursing Practice – Hospital and Home*. 2nd edn. London. Harcourt Publishers Ltd.

Van Muskirk, M. C. 1993, 'Monitoring blood pressure'. *American Journal of Nursing*, 93 (6), 44–7.

Whelton, P. K. 1998, 'Potassium and blood pressure' in Izzo, J. and Black, H. R. 1999, *Hypertension Primer*. Dallas. American Heart Association.

Wright, J. T. 1995, 'The antihypertensive and lipid lowering heart attack prevention trial'. *American Journal of Hypertension*, 8, 27A.

5

Coronary Heart Disease

PHILIPPE MARIE AND NORMA WHITTAKER

Coronary heart disease (CHD) is the most important cause of death and the single biggest cause of premature death in modern industrialized countries (Lorimer, 1997). It accounts for up to 28 per cent of all deaths in the United Kingdom (UK) (Office of Health Economics, 1992). A government action plan for tackling poor health and improving health specifically highlights the need to reduce the death rate from CHD (Department of Health [DOH], 1999). Several modifiable risk factors for CHD are well-recognized and healthcare professionals have an important role to play in its prevention, as well as, the diagnosis and management of the disorder (Lindsay and Gaw, 1997). The National Service Framework for CHD (DOH, 2000) reaffirms the government's eagerness to tackle the problem. The purpose of the framework is to transform the prevention, diagnosis and treatment of CHD. It is viewed as a means of helping professionals to give better, fairer and faster care everywhere. It is quite important that prevention is seen as a significant measure to be adopted (standards three and four) if heart disease is to be reduced in the population as a whole (standards one and two).

Contents

Learning Objectives

By the end of the chapter you should be able to demonstrate knowledge of:

- The epidemiology of CHD.
- Risk factors associated with CHD.
- The pathophysiology of CHD and the different clinical manifestations of angina and myocardial infarction.
- The range of diagnostic tests and treatment options.
- The significant roles that nurses have in primary health promotion and the overall management of patients with CHD.

Definition

The term coronary heart disease is synonymous with coronary artery disease and ischaemic heart disease and may be used interchangeably. Ischaemia refers to a lack of blood supply and coronary artery disease refers to the arteriosclerotic and atherosclerotic changes taking place in the coronary arteries that supply the myocardium (Timby *et al.*, 1999). CHD refers to the effects of the accumulation of atherosclerotic plaques in coronary arteries that leads to a reduction in the blood flow to the myocardium (Tortora and Grabowski, 2000). The disease may not be diagnosed until individuals are in late middle age but the vascular changes most likely begin at a much younger age (Timby *et al.*, 1999).

The pathophysiological events that occur with CHD range from reversible injury of the muscle cells to the irreversible destruction of all cellular components in an area of tissue. Ischaemia results from an imbalance between the flow of blood to the myocardium and the metabolic needs of the myocardium. Myocardial ischaemia is by definition reversible. In acute myocardial infarction the ischaemia is severe and prolonged and irreversible injury or infarction of tissue results (Jenson, 1995).

Epidemiology

In addition to geographical variations, CHD is also influenced by ethnic origin and social class.

 **Connection**

Chapter 1 (Social and Environmental Influences on Health and Well-being) and Chapter 3 (Health Issues Related to Ethnic Minority Groups) highlight differences in the prevalence of some diseases among certain groups in the general population.

Rates of CHD in the most deprived groups are much greater than in the affluent groups, which is a reversal of the previous situation. When CHD first emerged as an important cause of death it was found predominantly in social class one. Lifestyle modifications by people in this group diminished their risk of CHD but as the disease emerges in the Third World, it is once again those in social class one who are susceptible. The mortality rates from CHD in 1994 for men and women in 32 countries showed a wide variation. The highest rates were found in Eastern Europe, Northern Ireland and Scotland and the lowest rates in Spain, France and Japan. Mortality rates are generally much higher for men than women. This distinction is present at all ages but is less marked after the menopause. Coronary morbidity and mortality in women generally lag behind those for men by about ten years but, beyond the seventh decade in life, become similar in men and women (Lorimer, 1997).

Deaths from CHD fell during the 1970s and 1980s in most Western countries and England was no exception; numbers dropped by 38 per cent between the early 1970s and the late 1990s. Across the European Union (EU), however, England has one of the worst rates of CHD for people aged less than 65 years (DOH, 1999). Coronary artery disease is responsible for over 450 deaths per day (one every three minutes) in the UK. Each year in the UK alone, 320 000 people consult for angina and 300 000 experience myocardial infarction (Jackson, 2000).

Aetiology/Risk Factors

Atherosclerosis is the most common aetiological factor leading to CHD and, although several theories have been postulated to explain the pathogenesis of atherosclerosis, the aetiology of this condition remains unclear (Abraham and Wyper, 1995).

Contributory Factors

There are quite a number of factors that have been identified as increasing an individual's risk of developing CHD. These factors can be divided into two groups, those that are controllable and those that are not.

Controllable predisposing factors associated with CHD

- Obesity
- Cigarette smoking
- Physical inactivity
- Excessive alcohol consumption

- Salt intake
- Hyperlipidaemia
- Diabetes mellitus
- Hypertension
- Stress
- Oral contraceptives

Non-controllable predisposing factors associated with CHD

- Genetic predisposition
- Age and gender
- Race/ethnicity

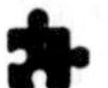 **Connection**

Chapter 4 (Hypertension) discusses the shared risk factors of obesity, smoking, physical inactivity, excessive alcohol consumption and salt intake.

Controllable Risk Factors

Hyperlipidaemia

Hyperlipidaemia refers to the elevation of cholesterol and triglyceride levels within the blood. Cholesterol is essentially a form of fat or lipid and can be derived from animal dietary sources or manufactured by the liver and intestine. Triglycerides are derived from fatty acids found in adipose tissue or the diet (Abraham and Wyper, 1995). Cholesterol and triglycerides both have important functions in the body. Cholesterol is an essential component of cell membranes, functioning to provide stability while permitting membrane transport; it is a precursor to adrenal steroids, sex hormones and to bile and bile acids. Triglycerides are the major source of energy for the body. Cholesterol and triglycerides are insoluble molecules and must be transported in the circulation as lipoproteins (Fair and Burke, 1995). Most lipids, such as cholesterol and triglycerides, are hydrophobic and to be transported in watery blood must be made water soluble by combining them with proteins produced by the liver and intestine. The combinations that are formed are lipoproteins.

Different types of lipoprotein are produced, which vary in density and functions. Roughly these lipoproteins can be classified into low-density lipoproteins

(LDLs) and high-density lipoproteins (HDLs). When present in excessive numbers LDLs also deposit cholesterol in and around smooth muscle fibres in arteries, forming fatty atherotic plaques that increase the risk of CHD. Some LDLs contain a docking protein that binds to LDL receptors; people who have too few LDL receptors cannot remove LDL from the blood effectively, consequently their plasma LDL level is abnormally high and they are more likely to develop atheromatous plaques (Tortora and Grabowski, 2000). People who consume a high-fat diet may saturate all available cholesterol receptors, which also results in hyperlipidaemia (Timby *et al.*, 1999). Furthermore, eating a high-fat diet increases the production of very low-density lipoproteins, which in turn elevates the LDL level and increases plaque formation (Tortora and Grabowski, 2000).

High-density lipoproteins remove excess cholesterol from body cells and transport it to the liver for elimination. HDLs are thought to be protective, as they prevent or delay atherogenesis. A 10 per cent reduction in serum cholesterol has been associated at a five year follow-up with a 54 per cent reduction in the incidence of CHD at 40 years, 27 per cent at 60 years and 19 per cent reduction at 80 years (Law *et al.*, 1994). Although the benefit seems to be greater in the age group younger than 40, these figures clearly illustrate the importance of reducing cholesterol levels in the blood for all at-risk age groups.

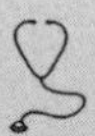

Nursing action points

- Encourage patients/clients to check the labels on food for the fat content. Nowadays food manufacturers are compelled by law to label their products in terms of their fat and cholesterol contents.
- Explain the difference between saturated and unsaturated fats to patients. Saturated fat is found mainly in animal products such as fatty cuts of beef, lamb, pork and dairy products such as cheese and butter; it is also found in margarine and lard.
- Explain to patients that polyunsaturated fat is less harmful than saturated fat and is found mainly in vegetable products such as sunflower oil, soya and corn.

Diabetes Mellitus

Both insulin-dependent and non-insulin-dependent diabetes are associated with a markedly increased risk of CHD. Diabetes is a particularly strong cardiovascular risk for women and has been shown to diminish the relative protection against cardiovascular disease that the female hormones confer. CHD is the leading cause of death in diabetic patients. Diabetes mellitus, especially type II, non-insulin-dependent diabetes is associated with more profound abnormalities in cardiovascular risk factors and therefore should not be regarded as a less threatening condition with less serious consequences in terms of CHD risk (Lindsay, 1997). Coronary atherosclerosis has been found to be two to three times more prevalent in people with diabetes, regardless of blood lipid levels. The mechanism whereby impaired glucose tolerance increases the risk of CHD is unclear. A predisposition to vascular degeneration has been noted in people with diabetes and abnormal lipid metabolism may also play a role in the development of atheromas (Abraham and Wyper, 1995). Intensive glycaemic control in non-insulin diabetes has been shown to be associated with reduced cardiovascular disease mortality (United Kingdom Prospective Diabetes Study [UKPDS], 1998).

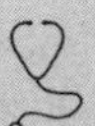

Nursing action point

- Recommend a weight reducing and lipid lowering diet, which also maintains carbohydrate balance, to people with diabetes. Weight control has been shown to improve glucose control.

(Lindsay, 1997)

Hypertension

The relationship between hypertension and CHD has been attributed to acceleration of the process that results in coronary atherosclerosis (Abraham and Wyper, 1995). Hypertension is believed to damage blood vessel walls, precipitating atheroma formation. This in turn causes narrowing of the blood vessel wall, thereby increasing peripheral resistance, which in turn increases the workload of the heart. Hypertension on its own is a serious predisposing factor to coronary artery disease. Concomitantly with diabetes it is even a bigger threat to the cardiovascular system (Fuller *et al.*, 1998; UKPDS, 1998). Since both conditions have controllable risk factors, the health education aspect of the management must be given a high priority.

Stress

An activity regarded as stressful by one person may be seen as a positive challenge by another and therein lies the difficulty in assessing stress as a risk factor. The possible mechanisms by which stress exerts its negative effects on CHD are by increasing the blood pressure and heart rate, increasing plasma cholesterol levels and having adverse effects on coagulation and fibrinolysis (Lindsay, 1997).

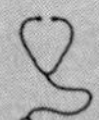

Nursing action points

- Assess the level of stress perceived by the individual.
- Introduce individual strategies for stress reduction. These can improve individual well-being greatly.

Oral Contraceptives

The use of oral contraceptives has been associated with an increased risk of CHD (Abraham and Wyper, 1995). In women aged 30–39 years the risk of fatal and non-fatal myocardial infarction was three times that of non-users. For women aged 40–44 years, the risk of fatal myocardial infarction was 5.7 times that of non-users, while the risk of non-fatal myocardial infarction was 4.7 times greater. Concurrent smoking acts synergically with the risk from oral contraceptives, with the greatest risk occurring in women smokers over 35 years.

Oral contraceptives:

- Increase the risk of arterial and venous thromboembolism.
- Promote atherogenesis through unfavourable effects on blood pressure, serum lipids and glucose tolerance.

(Newton and Froelicher, 1995)

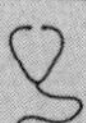

Nursing action points

- Adopt a multifaceted approach to reducing the risks associated with CHD.
- Address all the major risk factors.

Non-controllable Risk Factors

Genetic Predisposition

A family history of CHD puts men and women at greater risk. The clustering of risk factors such as hypertension, diabetes and obesity is also common. Most of these groupings are as a result of interactions between genetic and environmental influences, so it is difficult to determine the relative effect of genetic factors, except in those with familial hypercholesterolaemia (Lindsay, 1997).

A history of myocardial infarction in a first degree relative doubles the risk and in two or more first degree relatives triples the risk of a myocardial infarction. The risk is strongest when the myocardial infarction occurred before age 55. The risk associated with a family history is independent of other risk factors (Newton and Froelicher, 1995). The genetic component of CHD is thought to be the influence of many genes, rather than a single gene (Lindsay, 1997).

Age and Gender

CHD increases with age in both men and women. It is rare in the first two decades in life, becoming much more prevalent after 30 and much more marked in males than in females below 60 years. Beyond 60 years CHD in women increases at an accelerated rate (Lindsay, 1997). After the age of 70 both sexes are equally affected (Tunstall-Pedoe, 1985). It is unclear whether atherosclerosis is a result of the ageing process *per se*, or the cumulative effect of the known risk factors exerting their influence over time (Lindsay, 1997).

Race/Ethnicity

British Asians and Afro-Caribbeans are more prone to ischaemic heart disease than the average population (Webster, 1997). It could be that this is because both communities have a greater incidence of diabetes and hypertension, which are both high risk factors for ischaemic heart disease.

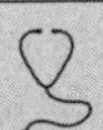

Nursing action point

- Identify high risk groups and make them a priority for risk assessment and management.

Anatomy and Physiology

The Heart

The heart is a muscular pump consisting of two upper chambers, the atria and two lower chambers, the ventricles (Figure 5.1). It is hollow, cone shaped, about the size of a fist and weighs between 300 and 350 grams. As it rests on the superior surface of the diaphragm, the heart lies anterior to the vertebral column and posterior to the sternum. The lungs flank the heart laterally and partially obscure it (Marieb, 2001).

The heart is enclosed in a double walled sac, the pericardium. This consists of a tough fibrous connective tissue outer layer, and a thin transparent inner layer of simple squamous epithelium called the serous pericardium. The fibrous pericardium prevents over-distension of the heart and anchors the heart within the mediastinum (Seeley *et al.*, 1992). The serous pericardium has two layers. The parietal layer lines the internal surface of the fibrous pericardium, while the second layer, the visceral layer or epicardium, is an integral part of the heart wall. The bulk of the heart is made up of the myocardium which is composed mainly of cardiac muscle. The endocardium is a glistening white sheet of endothelium that lines the heart (Marieb, 2001). The right and left sides of the

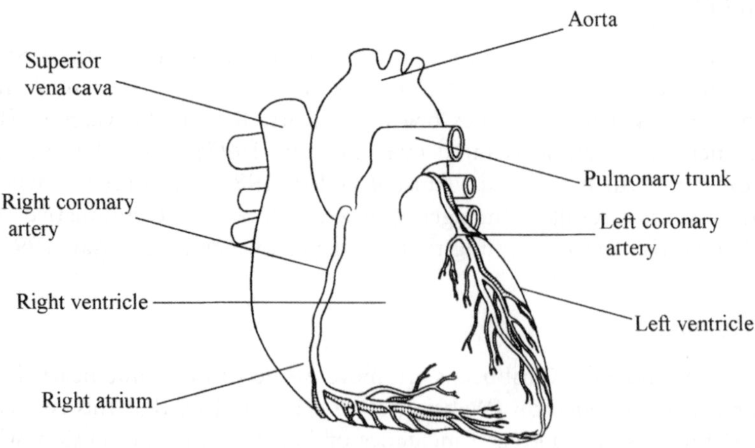

Figure 5.1 The heart

heart are divided by the septum. Inside the heart, there are four valves designed to allow unidirectional flow of blood through the heart (Seeley *et al.*, 1992).

Coronary Arteries

The walls of arteries have three layers as follows:

- Tunica adventia or outer layer of fibrous tissue
- Tunica media or middle layer of smooth elastic tissue
- Tunica intima or inner lining of squamous epithelium.

(Wilson and Waugh, 1998)

The arterial supply of the coronary circulation is provided by the right and left coronary arteries, both of which arise from the base of the aorta and encircle the heart in the atrioventricular groove. The left coronary artery runs towards the left side of the heart and then divides into its main branches, the anterior interventricular artery and the circumflex artery. The right coronary artery courses to the right of the heart, where it also divides into two branches, the marginal artery and the posterior interventricular artery (Marieb, 2001). There are few connections between the main coronary arteries, therefore blockage of one of its branches will cause a diminished blood supply (ischaemia) to the portion of cardiac muscle supplied by that vessel and may result in angina pectoris or a myocardial infarction. Such blockage may be caused by a coronary artery spasm, a thrombus or more commonly atherosclerosis (Abraham and Wyper, 1995).

Pathophysiology

Arteriosclerosis

As cells within the arterial tissue layers degenerate due to ageing, calcium is deposited within the cytoplasm, which causes the arteries to become less elastic. As the left ventricle contracts, sending oxygenated blood from the heart, the rigid arterial walls fail to stretch, potentially reducing the volume of oxygenated blood reaching the organs (Timby *et al.*, 1999).

Atherosclerosis

Atherosclerosis is a form of arteriosclerosis in which the thickening and hardening of the vessel walls are caused by soft deposits of intra-arterial fat and fibrin that harden over time (Haak *et al.*, 1994). Hyperlipidaemia triggers atherosclerotic changes. Microscopic injury in blood vessel walls may occur because of carbon monoxide from cigarette smoke, catecholamine release from stress, hyperglycaemia from diabetes mellitus, or increased pressure from hypertension. The body responds to the injury by activating the inflammatory response. Monocytes migrate to the site of the injury and deposit themselves under the endothelial cells of the tunica intima. The monocytes then attract and accumulate lipid material. The enlarging lesion elevates the endothelium and narrows the lumen (Timby *et al.*, 1999).

The first lesion to form within the coronary arterial wall is called a fatty streak and begins to appear as early as 15 years of age. Lipid filled cells or foam cells invade the intimal wall and produce a fatty streak. As the disease progresses, raised thick fibrous plaques form and with increasing size limit the luminal capacity of the vessel. Calcified fibrous plaque or complicated plaque is an advanced stage of atherosclerosis. This calcified deposit can rupture and hence greatly increase the risk of spasm, thrombus formation and embolization. It is this final type of atherosclerotic lesion that gives rise to the symptoms of CHD. The arterial lumen becomes so narrowed that a great imbalance exists between the myocardial oxygen supply and myocardial demand. Manifestations of myocardial ischaemia do not usually occur until the artery is about 75 per cent occluded (Abraham and Wyper, 1995).

Manifestations of myocardial ischaemia

- Angina pectoris
- Myocardial infarction
- Sudden death

Angina Pectoris

Angina is a clinical diagnosis based on the doctor's interpretation of the person's history.

> **Types of angina**
>
> - Stable angina
> - Variant angina
> - Unstable angina

Stable Angina

Stable angina is ischaemic cardiac pain, which may be perceived in many ways, that is brought on by effort and relieved by rest. It is precipitated by predictable factors and relieved promptly by rest and/or sublingual nitrates (Jackson, 2000).

Variant Angina

Variant angina is thought to develop from intermittent coronary artery spasm with or without atherosclerotic heart disease. Pain can develop during normal activities and is not necessarily precipitated by exercise or stress and often occurs at the same time of day or night (Abraham and Wyper, 1995).

Unstable Angina

Unstable angina describes a clinical presentation between stable angina and myocardial infarction (Jackson, 2000). This type of angina is characterized by an increase in the severity, frequency and duration of symptoms without infarction (Abraham and Wyper, 1995). Unstable angina is a manifestation of myocardial ischaemia that may signify impending infarction (Haak *et al.*, 1994).

Myocardial Infarction

Unlike the temporary ischaemia that causes angina and reversible cell injury, the prolonged ischaemia that causes infarction leads to irreversible hypoxia and cell death. Thrombus formation resulting from abnormal platelet aggregation seems to be the most probable cause of eventual arterial occlusion. Evidence indicates that the fissuring and rupturing of atherosclerotic plaques stimulate platelet aggregation, platelet thrombus formation and abnormal vasomotor tone on the plaque location (Abraham and Wyper, 1995).

The degree of damage to the heart caused by slowly developing atherosclerotic constriction of the coronary vessels or by sudden occlusion is determined to a great extent by the degree of collateral circulation that is already developed or that can develop in a short period of time after the occlusion (Guyton, 1992). The deprivation of oxygen to the myocardial cells can lead to a number of changes. First there may be lactic acid formation because of anaerobic metabolism, which can further compromise the myocardium, leading to heart failure. The damaged tissue also releases catecholamines such as adrenaline and noradrenaline. These can lead to an imbalance in the sympathetic and parasympathetic activity which can cause a variety of arrhythmias, the most dangerous being ventricular fibrillation. The excess secretion of catecholamines can also raise the level of glucose in the blood. This may last for several weeks. The damaged cells will also release a series of enzymes, namely creatine kinase (CK), lactate dehydrogenase (LDH), and serum glutamic oxalcetic transaminase (SGOT), also known as aspartate aminotransferase (AST). These can be assessed in order to confirm the diagnosis of myocardial infarction (Haak *et al.*, 1994; Jenson, 1995).

Clinical Manifestations of Myocardial Ischaemia

Pain

The coronary blood supply may be sufficient at rest, but an increase in demand due to effort may not be met, leading to ischaemia (Stevens and Lowe, 1995). As the heart is deprived of blood, it is deprived of oxygen and pain ensues.

The characteristics of typical angina pectoris

- Chest pain or discomfort that appears during periods of activity or stress.
- Sudden pain or pressure, which may be most severe over the heart (pericardial) or under the sternum (substernal).
- Pain that may radiate to the shoulders and arms, especially on the left side, or to the jaw, neck or teeth.
- Discomfort other than pain, including, indigestion, burning, squeezing or crushing tightness in the upper chest or throat (Timby *et al.*, 1999).
- The duration of the pain is usually brief.
- Apprehension, nausea and diaphoresis may be noted but are not common.
- Angina is not usually described as a sharp pain.

(Abraham and Wyper, 1995)

Symptoms of acute myocardial infarction

- Sudden severe chest pain which is similar to angina pectoris but is more severe and persistent and is not relieved by nitrates.
- The pain may be described as heavy and crushing and radiation to the neck, jaw, back, shoulder or left arm is common.
- A sensation of unrelenting indigestion is often stimulated by an infarction.
- Nausea and vomiting may occur because of reflex stimulation of vomiting centres by pain fibres.
- Vasovagal reflexes from the region of the infarcted myocardium may also affect the gastrointestinal tract.
- Catecholamine release results in sympathetic stimulation, producing diaphoresis and peripheral vasoconstriction that cause the skin to become cool and clammy.
- Fever may develop in the first 24 hours and persist for a few days because of inflammatory reaction in the myocardium.
- Blood pressure may initially decrease followed by a temporary increase in blood pressure and heart rate.
- Some individuals, especially the elderly or those who have diabetes mellitus may experience no pain, thereby having a 'silent' infarction.

(Haak et al., 1994)

Many patients die suddenly and unexpectedly of CHD. Death can occur within the first minutes or hours following a myocardial infarction. Ventricular fibrillation occurs in a substantial percentage of individuals following myocardial infarction and is the commonest cause of death. It usually occurs very soon after the onset, especially in the first hour. It does not require a large area of muscle to be affected to cause ventricular fibrillation. Most patients appear to be making good progress when cardiac arrest due to ventricular fibrillation occurs. If it is corrected promptly, the outcome is usually good. Patients with a history of prior myocardial infarction and ventricular tachycardia occurring beyond the first 24 hours after an infarction are a high risk group for sudden death (Oldroyd, 1997).

Complications following acute myocardial infarction include:

- Arrhythmias
- Cardiogenic shock
- Ventricular rupture
- Ventricular aneurysm
- Arterial embolism
- Venous thrombosis
- Pulmonary embolism

- Pericarditis
- Mitral insufficiency

(Timby *et al.*, 1999)

Investigative Tests

History

History taking is vital so that a clear picture is obtained regarding factors such as the nature of the pain, the time the pain commenced, its duration, whether it happened at rest, whether it was associated with exertion or emotional upset and whether it was accompanied by nausea and vomiting. The patient may disclose relevant information about lifestyle such as smoking and stress, or may also reveal a history of hypertension or diabetes.

Investigative tests

- Electrocardiogram
- Thallium
- Positron emission tomography
- Cardiac enzymes
- Cardiac catheterization
- Coronary arteriography
- Serum electrolytes
- Blood gases
- Blood sugar

Electrocardiogram (ECG)

A full 12 lead ECG is a recording of the electrical activity of the heart muscle. Since in many cases of angina, ischaemia is only brought about by effort or exercise, the resting ECG is less useful in patients with angina than in those with myocardial infarction. It is important however that an ECG is performed when a patient complains of chest pain. Electrographically, there is a clear distinction between stable angina and variant angina (Haak *et al.*, 1994). The latter shows ST segment elevation whereas the former shows ST segment depression.

In patients with normal ECG an exercise treadmill can be used as a screening tool. In this case the patient is fitted with electrodes before the exercise so that continuous ECG recordings of the heart are obtained as the patient undergoes increasing levels of effort. The occurrence of chest pain during the exercise can then be correlated with changes on the ECG, which demonstrate the lack of oxygen to the heart muscle. Following myocardial infarction, 12 lead ECGs help to locate the affected area. Ischaemic and injured myocardial tissue causes ST and T waves changes. As the myocardium heals the ST segment and T waves gradually return to normal, but abnormal Q waves usually persist (Haak *et al.*, 1994).

Ambulatory ECGs for 24–48 hours can be useful when physical limitation prohibits exercise testing, when pain occurs at night or when chest pain is linked to arrhythmias. Dobutamine stress echocardiography has also been shown to be a valuable alternative for such individuals. Intravenous dobutamine is gradually increased in dosage, increasing heart rate in a similar way to exercise testing. Continuous ECG and echocardiograph monitoring is performed. Ischaemic myocardium shows reduced thickening and transient movement abnormalities whereas normal myocardium increases in movement and shows thickening. Hibernating myocardium can also be assessed (Jackson, 2000).

Thallium

Nuclear scanning has a limited role in addition to exercise ECG. Radio isotope imaging with thallium may be used to diagnose coronary artery disease. Thallium-201 is taken up by the perfused myocardium. Infarction is a 'cold' area that fails to fill in. Exercise may cause a cold area that fills in later, which is a sign of reversible ischaemia. Partial filling suggests ischaemia adjacent to infarction (Jackson, 2000).

Positron Emission Tomography (PET)

This is an expensive technique that uses positron emitters with very short half-life as tracers. It provides the opportunity of measuring regional blood flow accurately. It can identify areas of 'hibernating' myocardium that are still viable but unable to function because of severely limited blood supply. Prognosis in affected patients would be improved by intervention (Jackson, 2000).

Cardiac Enzymes

Intracellular enzymes are released when ischaemia disrupts cell membranes. Changes in cardiac enzymes after a myocardial infarction follow a characteristic pattern over time and are of considerable value in making a diagnosis. The enzymes are usually measured in the first three days following a suspected myocardial infarction. CK levels rise rapidly after muscle damage and peak at approximately 24 hours, allowing a rapid diagnosis of suspected myocardial infarction. AST and alanine transaminase (ALT) are measured, as increased AST with a normal ALT indicates cardiac muscle damage. Sometimes patients may be seen two to three days after a possible infarction. LDH will still be increased when the others have returned to normal. The diagnosis of suspected infarction can still be made. Creatine kinase MB isoenzyme (CKMB) is a specific isoenzyme found in cardiac muscle and a raised level implies cardiac damage, whereas a raised CK may follow muscle damage anywhere in the body (Lorimer, 1997).

Cardiac Catheterization

The most frequent use of cardiac catheterization is to confirm or define the extent of CHD. Cardiac catheterization provides a means of measuring fluid pressures within the chambers of the heart and collecting blood samples for analysis of oxygen and carbon dioxide content. Under fluoroscopy, a long flexible catheter is inserted from a peripheral blood vessel in the groin, arm or neck into one of the great vessels and then into the heart. Cardiac catheterization may be carried out on the left side of the heart by way of an artery or the right side by way of a vein. Vital information about the heart structure and functions can be obtained as it allows visualization of heart chambers. Pressures in each chamber and across the valves can be precisely measured, as can the timing of events in the cardiac cycle and a comparison made of the oxygen content in various chambers. As this is a highly invasive and technical operation demanding quite a lot of expertise, it is carried out in a specially equipped laboratory. It is normally carried out under local anaesthetic (Jowett, 1997). Cardiac catheterization can cause life-threatening arrhythmias leading to ventricular fibrillation and cardiac arrest. This is one of the reasons why it must be carried out in a specially equipped laboratory where resuscitation procedure can be undertaken (Abraham and Wyper, 1995; Timby *et al.*, 1999). Day case procedures are increasingly employed (Jackson, 2000).

Coronary Arteriography

The most common use of a left-sided cardiac catheterization is to determine the degree of blockage of the coronary arteries by performing arteriography while the catheter is in place. Radio-opaque dye is injected into the coronary arteries through a fine catheter inserted into the femoral or brachial artery and passed up to the aortic ring. The right side of the heart is not studied. Occlusive heart disease is indicated if one or more coronary arteries appear narrow or do not fill (Lorimer, 1997).

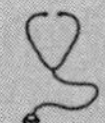

Nursing action points

- Ensure that the patient has clear instructions about restricted food and fluid intake. For example, no food for four hours prior to the procedure and no fluids for two hours.
- Prepare the skin over the catheter insertion site by washing and removal of hair if deemed appropriate.

- Ask the patient about any known allergies if a contrast medium is to be used during the catheterization.
- Check and document the presence and quality of peripheral pulses and skin colour and temperature prior to the procedure.
- Reassure the patient prior to and during the procedure as anxiety is often experienced.
- Monitor the patient throughout the procedure.
- Inspect the site of the catheter insertion for bleeding, tenderness, haematoma formation or inflammation.
- Check temperature following catheterization and warn the patient that the temperature may be elevated for a few hours after the test.
- Keep the patient on bed rest for at least two hours following the procedure.
- Advise the patient to avoid flexion or bending of the arm or leg used for catheter insertion.
- Monitor peripheral pulses, colour and the warmth of limbs. Absence of peripheral pulse, cool toes, pale or cyanotic arms and legs indicate arterial occlusion, usually from a blood clot.
- Immediately report the above signs. In conjunction with a rapid or irregular pulse rate a medical emergency is indicated.

(Timby *et al.*, 1999)

Serum Electrolytes

The electrolyte balance in the body can change rapidly. The cardiac patient is particularly subject to changes in potassium and sodium. Small increases or decreases in potassium affect heart function. Decreased cardiac output results in decreased renal blood flow which in turn results in an increase in blood urea nitrogen (Goe, 1997).

Blood Gases

Tissue oxygenation, carbon dioxide removal and the acid-base status are analysed. Monitoring the arterial oxygen saturation and the mixed venous saturation reflect the relationship between oxygen supply and demand and the extent of overall tissue utilization. Blood pH may be affected during a myocardial infarction resulting in metabolic acidosis (Guyton and Hall, 2000).

Blood Sugar

Mild hyperglycaemia would be expected during stress states. Hyperglycaemia is often precipitated by myocardial infarction (Goe, 1997).

Treatment

- Prevention
- Suppression of pain
- Medication
- Coronary angioplasty
- Coronary artery bypass graft

Primary Prevention

Primary prevention should focus upon reducing the identified risk factors associated with CHD.

Prevention of an Angina Attack

Patients can learn to control their level of activity to avoid excessive demand on the heart. Heavy labouring and stressful jobs are likely to induce pain and this can lead to early retirement or working reduced hours. In some cases help may be required in the home.

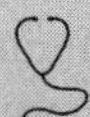

Nursing action points

- Fully inform patients about the risk factors in order for an informed choice to be made with regard to behaviour modification.
- Advise the patient to take medication prior to sexual intercourse.
- Advise the patient that the bedroom and sheets should be warm and sex should be avoided within one hour of a large meal or hot bath.
- Advise the patient to stop driving if angina occurs when driving.

(Jackson, 2000)

Medication

- Aspirin
- Nitrates
- Beta-blockers
- Calcium channel blockers
- Vasodilators
- Thrombolytics
- Diuretics

Aspirin

A review of the trials of aspirin in patients with stable angina showed a reduction in the risk of vascular death, stroke and myocardial infarction of 25 per cent. An initial dose of 300 mg maximizes the inhibition of platelet aggregation and 75 mg daily then maintains it. Clopidogrel, 75 mg daily is an alternative where aspirin is contraindicated (Jackson, 2000).

Nitrates

Nitrates are vascular smooth muscle relaxants. Nitrates act by dilating peripheral veins thereby reducing venous return to the heart (preload). This then reduces the workload of the heart, thus reducing oxygen demand. Nitrates can also help by reducing spasm in the coronary arteries thereby improving the blood flow to the heart muscle. These drugs cannot achieve vasodilatation in blood vessels already affected by the atherosclerosis and arteriosclerosis (McKenry and Salerno, 1995). Nitrates are also inhibitors of platelet aggregation that may be important in unstable angina.

Sublingual Nitrates

Glycerine trinitrate (GTN) acts within two minutes and its effect lasts for 30 minutes. It can be used to relieve pain or as a prophylaxis. During an attack, it can be taken repeatedly every five minutes until the pain is relieved (Henney *et al.*, 1995). GTN can be administered via a spray or as a tablet. A sustained release formulation of GTN is available. This is placed between the upper lip and the gum and it lasts up to four hours. It can be useful in unstable angina. Long acting nitrates, for example, isosorbide mononitrate give more constant blood levels. Topical nitrates may help nocturnal pain, when put on at night and removed in the morning (Jackson, 2000).

Nursing action points

- Inform patients of the common side effects of GTN, which include a throbbing headache and hypotension. These are due to the vasodilatory effect but can be minimized or avoided if the tablet is removed or swallowed once relief is obtained.
- Instruct patients about the safekeeping of tablets. This includes keeping the container in a cool and dark place as heat and light deactivate the tablets.
- Instruct patients not to place cotton-wool in the container, as it will absorb the chemicals, deactivating the tablets.

- Instruct patients to discard the tablets eight weeks after opening the container, as potency may be lost.

  (Henney et al., 1995)

- Advise patients that an active GTN tablet has a burning effect on the tongue and instruct the patient to get a new supply, if this is not experienced.

  (Jackson, 2000)

Beta-blockers

Common Beta (β)-blockers used are: atenolol (tenormin), metorprolol (lopressor), and propranolol (inderal). These drugs are called β-blockers because they block the beta receptors in the heart thereby intercepting the action of catecholamines on these receptors. This leads to reduction in heart rate, myocardial contractility, and blood pressure. Oxygen demand is thereby reduced. The reduced heart rate means that there is more time for the heart to fill up, leading to increased oxygen delivery to the heart (Prosser *et al.*, 2000). Beta-blockers should not be suddenly withdrawn because rebound effects can occur, leading to unstable angina or myocardial infarction. Side effects include tiredness and depression, impotence, bradycardia, exacerbation of asthma, hypotension, dyspnoea and cold peripheries (Jackson, 2000).

Calcium Channel Blockers

Calcium itself is very important for the electrical excitation of cardiac cells and the contractility of myocardial muscle cells. Calcium channel blockers interfere with the flow of calcium into smooth muscle, myocardial cells and conducting tissue. This results in relaxation of the smooth muscle of the coronary arteries, reduction in myocardial contractility and oxygen consumption (Kuhn, 1994). Three calcium blockers which are frequently used in angina management are verapamil, ditiazem and nifedipine. The side effects of calcium antagonists include flushing, headaches and constipation (Jackson, 2000).

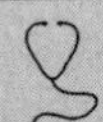

Nursing action points

- Be aware of the side effects of any prescribed drug being administered and inform the patient.
- Advise patients not to stop taking their medication without medical advice.

Vasodilators

Vasodilators relieve chest pain by dilating coronary arteries and re-establishing blood flow around thrombi.

Thrombolytics

These may be used to treat myocardial infarction as they re-establish blood flow to ischaemic areas by dissolving thrombi. The best result is achieved when administered within the first hour of the attack. Thrombolytic agents administered after six hours are deemed ineffective as most of the muscle damage may have already occurred. Using thrombolitic agents such as urokinase or streptokinase has been known to open up to 80 per cent of occluded coronary arteries. This method of treatment carries a significant risk of bleeding and is not recommended for certain patients such as those with a history of gastric or duodenal bleeding ulcer, recent surgery or recent stroke.

Diuretics

Diuretics decrease the work of the heart by promoting the excretion of sodium and water, thus reducing the circulating blood volume (Timby *et al.*, 1999).

Coronary Angioplasty

This is a procedure which is used both in the management of persistent angina and myocardial infarction. It can be performed even on patients over the age of 65 years with very good results. The complication rate in both young and old patients is the same but the death rate is higher in the older patients. Some of the remarkable benefits of angioplasty are that it is much less traumatic than coronary artery bypass graft and patients have a much shorter stay in hospital. The selection of patients for the procedure is based upon careful assessment of the nature of the lesion through coronary angiography. Ideally the patient has a single non-calcific coronary artery lesion, which is less than 10 ml long (Grines *et al.*, 1993).

Percutaneous transluminal coronary angioplasty (PTCA) is a procedure by which coronary arteries narrowed by atheromatous plaques can be dilated. A small balloon tipped catheter, about 1 ml in diameter, is passed under radiographic guidance into the coronary system and pushed through the occluded artery until the balloon portion of the catheter straddles the partially occluded point. The balloon is then inflated with high pressure, which stretches the diseased artery almost to the point of bursting. Blood flow through the vessel may be increased three- to four-fold. More than 75 per cent of patients are relieved of coronary ischaemic symptoms for several years by this procedure (Guyton and Hall, 2000). This method of intervention has been known to open up to 95 per cent of blocked coronary arteries within 60 minutes (Grines *et al.*, 1993).

Another procedure employs a laser beam from the tip of a coronary artery catheter, which when aimed at the atherosclerotic lesion, literally dissolves the lesion without significantly damaging the basic arterial wall (Guyton and Hall, 2000). This is used when plaques are no longer soft and pliable (Timby *et al.*,

1999). Stents are metal cages that are expanded by a balloon to compress the stenosis. They are used to prevent acute vessel closure following PTCA when a dissection has occurred and to reduce the risk of re-stenosis (Jackson, 2000).

Coronary Artery Bypass Graft (CABG)

A coronary artery bypass graft procedure increases the supply of blood to the myocardium by bypassing the occluded portion of the vessel with a donor vessel. The donor vessel is taken from the saphenous vein in the leg or from the internal mammary artery. When using a saphenous vein, one end is grafted to the aorta and the other is sutured below the blockage in the coronary artery. The left internal mammary artery is diverted from the muscle of the chest wall and attached to the affected coronary artery beyond the area of stenosis. One or more bypasses are done at the same time. Circulation in the leg used for retrieval is compromised for several weeks. Elastic stockings are prescribed (Keith, 1997).

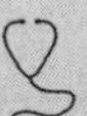

Nursing action points

- Reinforce information making sure the patient understands procedures.
- Give consistent information and answer queries which will help to allay the patient's fears and anxiety.
- Support and keep relatives equally informed so that they can be of assistance to the patient.

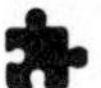

Connection

Chapter 2 (Family-centred Care) discusses how keeping relatives informed can do much to reduce their anxiety.

Nursing Interventions

Health Education

Nurses are well placed to educate individuals with regard to the identified risk factors (refer to the section on risk factors).

Fruit and Vegetables as Part of the Diet

Evidence for a protective effect of specific antioxidants, particularly vitamins E and C and beta-carotene is incomplete. Further research is necessary before recommendations for specific antioxidants can be made. There is good evidence, however, that a diet rich in a range of vegetables and fruit is beneficial and lowers the risk of CHD. National and international recommendations suggest increasing fruit and vegetable intakes to at least five portions a day (National Heart Forum, 1997). Health promotion strategies should focus upon highlighting the benefits of increasing fruit and vegetable intake.

Health education should address cultural differences particularly when targeting high risk groups.

First aid treatment of a myocardial infarction

1. It is important to create a sense of calm and not to panic.
2. Call for an ambulance. The earlier the patient gets to hospital the better because early medication and intervention are vitally important and can be the difference between life and death.
3. If the patient is well enough, an aspirin can be given to suck. The patient can also be given a tranquillizer if one has been previously prescribed.

The priorities in hospital are to:

1. Control the pain
2. Limit the damage
3. Prevent complications.

The Control of Pain

Pain is very often associated with anxiety and it is not a pain that can be relieved by GTN. Morphine may be prescribed for the relief of pain and apprehension and its vasodilatory effects (Abraham and Wyper, 1995). The role of the nurse is paramount in assessing the patient's perception of pain and the extended role also involves the administration of intravenous morphine or diamorphine (Jowett and Thompson, 1995).

Cardiac Monitoring

By far the most common complication that can happen following a heart attack is cardiac arrhythmia, which can seriously compromise the already ischaemic heart. Following myocardial infarction it is preferable for patients to be cared for in a coronary care unit. Coronary care nurses are highly trained and play a vital part in the effective monitoring of patients. In their extended roles nurses closely monitor heart rate and rhythms to identify complications such as ventricular tachycardia. These arrhythmias are treated promptly by defibrillation and anti-arrhythmic medication (Jowett and Thompson, 1995; Teo *et al.*, 1993).

Mobilizing the Patient following a Myocardial Infarction

Bed rest followed by a gradual return to the activities of living, reduces the demands placed upon the compromised heart. Transfer to a general ward may be welcomed by some, but may leave some patients feeling vulnerable, away from the high ratio of nurses to patients found in coronary care units. The former group may need to be encouraged to slow down and mobilize gradually, while the latter may lie rigid in bed, unwilling to mobilize at all. The role of the cardiac rehabilitation nurse is to expand and bring together the information given to patients by the many people responsible for their care prior to discharge. The specialist nurse must take care not to de-skill the ward nurses but encourage them to develop their rehabilitation role. The return to normal mobilization and self-care is gradual and determined to a great extent by the presence or absence of pain. The patient may be discharged having been given clear guidelines concerning increased activity and instructions concerning medication (Keith, 1997).

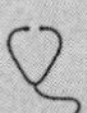

Nursing action points

- Note the presence of any risk factors.
- Assess the level of anxiety.
- Determine the patient's perception of the pain by asking the patient to describe it.
- Note whether the pain is relieved with medication.
- Report any changes in vital signs or cardiac arrhythmias.
- Observe the patient for associated signs, such as diaphoresis, vomiting, pallor, cold clammy skin, laboured respirations.

(Abraham and Wyper, 1995)

Anxiety and Depression

An important aspect of care is to monitor the patient's psychological and emotional state. Thirteen per cent of males and 24 per cent of females reported moderate to severe levels of anxiety during their hospital stay following myocardial infarction. In its severe form, it has been associated with depression and terrifying panic attacks. As many as 30 per cent of patients with normal coronary arteries on angiography also experienced panic attacks. Acute anxiety can often be resolved with reassurance and psychotherapy: referrals to professionals who specialize in the treatment of such problems should be considered

(Taylor and Arnow, 1988). One of the most important considerations in trying to help such patients is timing. The best time to decide whether further treatment is necessary is after the patient has been home for two weeks. During that time the patient would have been able to settle down in the home environment and to be relaxed.

Depression can hinder patients' participation in lifestyle change programmes and depressed patients may not have the energy, enthusiasm, concentration and determination to understand and pursue recommended changes. Intervention such as lifestyle changes, in particular exercise, has consistently been proved to be a good ancillary treatment for depression and anxiety (Benight and Taylor, 1994). Reducing anxiety by promoting a relaxed environment is an important aspect of nursing care. Assessing the patient's level of knowledge and keeping the patient fully informed will not only help to reduce anxiety but also enable the patient to provide informed consent and self care afterwards. It is also important to communicate with relatives accompanying the patient as they are likely to be anxious.

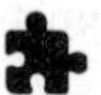

Connection

Chapter 2 (Family-centred Care) discusses how illness in a family member can be detrimental to the health and well-being of the relatives.

Many patients with CHD suffer from depression while trying to come to terms with the condition. It is claimed that depression occurs in 10 to 20 per cent of post-myocardial infarction patients (Shuster *et al.*, 1992) and according to Eaker (1989), depression can affect morbidity and mortality. The depression may also be caused by some of the drugs used to manage their condition. For instance, between 10 and 35 per cent of patients on beta-blockers experience depression or other symptoms of psychological distress (Petruzello *et al.*, 1991).

The symptoms are quite varied and may include emotional problems such as anxiety, loss of interest, withdrawal from others and preoccupation with death, together with cognitive problems, such as feeling worthless or guilty, hopelessness, despair, poor concentration and suicidal feelings. Other common symptoms of depression include trouble sleeping, loss of appetite, lack of energy and lack of interest in sex.

Return to Sexual Activity

Both the patient and his or her partner may be concerned that intercourse will impose too great a strain on the heart. The physical effort used in intercourse is much the same as walking up two flights of stairs, but the strain on the heart is much greater if intercourse is very vigorous or intensely emotional. Patients can be advised that a return to gentle sexual activity is usually quite safe within a short period following the myocardial infarction, provided that recovery has been good. Doctors and nurses often fail to mention this subject spontaneously and yet one of the greatest worries that many patients have after a myocardial infarction is about the return to sexual activity (Julian and Marley, 1991).

Rehabilitation Programmes

There are two essential components to such programmes, counselling and physical retraining. Both should start before discharge from hospital. This involves a structured programme of exercises tailored to the individual. At the sessions, the patient's personal problems are discussed, attempts are made to deal with stress and relaxation exercises are taught (Julian and Marley, 1991).

Conclusion

Coronary heart disease is a serious medical condition caused by the effects of the accumulation of atherosclerotic plaques in coronary arteries that lead to a reduction in blood flow to the myocardium. The indirect costs of CHD are significant, with 12 per cent of the working days that are lost in the UK through sickness being due to CHD (Jackson, 2000). In both sexes the prevalence increases with age. Though the overall death rate is declining, the number of women dying from cardiovascular disease is increasing and nurses should strive to increase the general population's awareness of this factor. Some people experience no signs or symptoms; others experience angina pectoris, myocardial infarction or sudden death. People who possess combinations of certain risk factors are more likely to develop CHD. As a number of these risk factors are modifiable, the risk of developing CHD can be reduced by changing certain behaviour. Nurses are well placed to assist individuals make decisions about their own health through providing information about the risks and the benefits of adopting healthier lifestyles. The association of CHD with other significant disorders such as diabetes, stroke and hypertension means that it cannot be considered in isolation. As the proportion of elderly in the population increases, CHD will become more common and the need for effective evidence-based strategies for investigation, diagnosis and treatment will become even more important.

References

Abraham, T. and Wyper, M. A. 1995, 'The Patient with Cardiovascular Problems' in Long, B. C., Phipps, V. and Cassmeyer, V. L. (eds) *Adult Nursing. A Nursing Process Approach.* London. Mosby-Times Mirror International Publications Ltd.

Benight, C. C. and Taylor, C. B. 1994, 'The effects of exercise on improving anxiety, depression, emotional well-being and elements of type A behaviour' in Department of

Health (DOH) 1999, 'Saving Lives: Our Healthier Nation'. http://www.archive.official-documents.co.uk/document/cm43/4386/4386.htm

Department of Health (DOH) 2000, *The National Service Framework for Coronary Heart Disease*. London. The Stationery Office.

Eaker, E. D. 1989, 'Psychological factors in the epidemiology of coronary heart disease in women'. *Psychiatric Clinics of North America*, 12, 167–73.

Fair, J. M. and Burke, L. E. 1995, 'Cholesterol Education' in Woods, S. L., Sivarajan Froelicher, E. S., Halpenny, C. J. and Underhill Motzer, S. *Cardiac Nursing*. 3rd edn. Philadelphia. Lippincott Company.

Fuller, J., Stevens, L. K., Chaturvedi, N. and Holloway, J. F. 1998, 'Anti-hypertensive therapy in diabetes mellitus'. *Cochrane Database of Systematic Reviews. The Cochrane Library*, Issue 4. Oxford. Update Software.

Goe, M. R. 1997, 'Laboratory Tests Using Blood' in Woods, S. L., Sivarajan Froelicher, E. S., Halpenny, C. J. and Underhill Motzer, S. *Cardiac Nursing*. 3rd edn. Philadelphia. Lippincott Company.

Grines, C. L., Browne, K. F. and Marco, J. 1993, 'A comparison of immediate Angioplasty with thrombolytic therapy for acute Myocardial Infarction'. *The Primary Angioplasty in Myocardial Infarction Study Group. New England Journal of Medicine*. March, 328 (10), 673–9.

Guyton, A. C. 1992, *Human Pathophysiology and Mechanisms of Disease*. London. W. B. Saunders Company.

Guyton, A. C. and Hall, J. E. 2000, *The Textbook of Medical Physiology*. 10th edn. London. W. B. Saunders Company.

Haak, S. W., Richardson, S. J., Davey, S. S. and Parker-Cohen, P. D. 1994, 'Alterations of Cardiovascular Function' in McCance, K. L. and Heuther, S. E. (eds) *Pathophysiology. The biological basis for Disease in Adults and Children*. 2nd edn. London. Mosby-Yearbook Inc.

Henney, C. R., Dow, R. J. and MacConnachie, A. M. 1995, *Drugs in Nursing Practice*. Edinburgh. Churchill Livingstone.

Jackson, G. 2000, *Angina*. London. Martin Dunitz Ltd.

Jenson, S. K. 1995, 'Pathophysiology of Myocardial Ischaemia and Infarction' in Woods, S. L., Sivarajan Froelicher, E. S., Halpenny, C. J. and Underhill Motzer, S. *Cardiac Nursing*. 3rd edn. Philadelphia. Lippincott Company.

Jowett, N. I. 1997, *Cardiovascular Monitoring*. London. Whurr Publishers Limited.

Jowett, N. I. and Thompson D. R. 1995, *Comprehensive Coronary Care* 2nd edn. London. Scutari Press.

Julian, D. and Marley, C. 1991, *Coronary Heart Disease. The Facts*. Oxford. Oxford University Press.

Keith, E. M. 1997, 'Cardiac rehabilitation' in Lindsay, G. M. and Gaw, A. (eds) *Coronary Heart Disease Prevention*. London. Churchill Livingstone.

Kuhn, M. A. 1994, *Pharmacotherapeutics: A Nursing Process Approach*. 3rd edn. Philadelphia. F. A. Davies.

Law, M. R., Wald, N. J. and Thompson, S. G. 1994, 'By how much and how quickly does reduction in serum cholesterol concentration lower risk of ischaemic heart disease?' *British Medical Journal*, 308, 367–72.

Lindsay, G. 1997, 'Risk Factor Assessment' in Lindsay, G. M. and Gaw, A. (eds) *Coronary Heart Disease Prevention*. London. Churchill Livingstone.

Lindsay, G. M. and Gaw, A. (eds) 1997, *Coronary Heart Disease Prevention*. London. Churchill Livingstone.

Lorimer, A. R. 1997, 'Coronary Heart Disease: Pathology and Epidemiology and Diagnosis' in Lindsay, G. M. and Gaw, A. (eds) *Coronary Heart Disease Prevention.* London. Churchill Livingstone.

Marieb, E. N. 2001, *Human Anatomy and Physiology.* 5th edn. London. Pearson Education Inc. publishing as Benjamin Cummings.

McKenry, L. and Salerno, E. 1995, *Pharmacology in Nursing.* London. Mosby.

National Heart Forum 1997, *Preventing Coronary Heart Disease. The Role of Antioxidants, Vegetables and Fruit.* National Heart Forum. London. The Stationery Office.

Newton, K. M. and Froelicher, E. S. 1995, 'Coronary Heart Disease Risk Factors' in Woods, S. L., Sivarajan Froelicher, E. S., Halpenny, C. J. and Underhill Motzer, S. *Cardiac Nursing.* 3rd edn. Philadelphia. Lippincott Company.

Office of Health Economics 1992, *Compendium of Health Statistics.* 8th edn. London. OHE.

Oldroyd, K. G. 1997, 'Medical Management of Coronary Heart Disease' in Lindsay, G. M. and Gaw, A. (eds) *Coronary Heart Disease Prevention.* London. Churchill Livingstone.

Petruzello, S. J., Landers, D. M., Hatfield, B. D., Kubitz, K. A. and Salazar. 1991, 'A meta analysis of the anxiety-reducing effects of acute and chronic exercise; Outcomes and mechanisms'. *Sports Medicine*, 11, 143–8.

Prosser, S., Worster B., MacGregor, J., Dewar, K., Runyard, P. and Fegan, J. 2000, *Applied Pharmacology.* Edinburgh. Mosby.

Seeley, R. R., Stephens, T. D. and Tate, P. 1992, *Anatomy and Physiology.* 2nd edn. London. Mosby Year Book.

Shuster, J. L., Stern, T. A. and Tesar, G. E. 1992, 'Psychological Problems and their Management' in Wenger, N. K. and Herrenstein, H. K. (eds), *Rehabilitation of the Coronary Patient.* 3rd edn. 483–510. New York. Churchill Livingstone.

Stevens, A. and Lowe, J. 1995, *Pathology.* Mosby, London.

Taylor, C. B. and Arnow, B. 1988, *The Nature and Treatment of Anxiety Disorders.* New York. Free Press.

Teo, K. K., Yusuf, S. and Furberg, C. D. 1993, 'An overview of results from randomised controlled trials. Effects of prophylactic anti-arrhythmic drug therapy in acute myocardial infarction'. *An overview of results from randomised controlled trials. JAMA. Journal of the American Medical Association.* 6 October. 1589–95.

Timby, B. K., Scherer, J. C. and Smith, N. E. 1999, *Introductory Medical–Surgical Nursing.* 7th edn. Philadelphia. Lippincott Williams and Wilkins.

Tortora, G. J. and Grabowski, S. R. 2000, *Principles of Anatomy and Physiology.* 9th edn. Chichester. John Wiley and Sons Ltd.

Tunstall-Pedoe, H. 1985, 'Monitoring trends in cardiovascular diseases and risk factors'. The WHO MONICA Project. *WHO Chronicle*, 39, 3–5.

United Kingdom Prospective Diabetes Study (UKPDS) Group 1998, 'Tight blood pressure control and risk of macrovascular and microvascular in type 2 diabetes'. UKPDS 39.1. *British Medical Journal*, 317, 703–13.

United Kingdom Prospective Diabetes Study (UKPDS) Group 1998, 'Intensive blood-glucose control with sulfonylureas or insulin compared with conventional treatment and risk of complications in patients with type 2 diabetes'. UKPDS 33. *Lancet*, 352, 837–53.

Webster, R. A. 1997, 'The experience and health care needs of Asian coronary patients and their partners: methodological issues and preliminary findings'. *Nursing in Critical Care*, 2, 215–23.

Wilson, K. J. W. and Waugh, A. 1998, *Ross and Wilson Anatomy and Physiology in Health and Illness.* 8th edn. London. Churchill Livingstone.

6 Stroke

Philippe Marie and Norma Whittaker

Stroke is the third leading cause of death in developed countries and the single most common nervous system disorder (Schenk, 1995; Marieb, 2001). The lack of blood supply to the brain can be caused by an interruption in blood supply or by bleeding into or around the brain. The severity of the attack and the long term neurological deficits are very much dependent on the degree of deficiency of blood, the part or parts of the brain affected, the effectiveness of early medical interventions and treatment and rehabilitation. Nurses have a role to play in primary prevention, as a number of factors have been identified that increase the risk of stroke. The approach to care is essentially a multidisciplinary one in which nurses play a significant role.

Given the impact of stroke on mortality and morbidity, it is a major area of concern, emphasized in government initiatives such as, *Saving Lives: Our Healthier Nation* (Department of Health [DOH], 1999) and in the *National Service Framework for Older People* (Standard Five) (DOH, 2001). As many of the people who suffer from stroke are elderly, this is a particularly relevant government initiative. The framework is a key document for moving forward with the development of services for older people. It recognizes the importance of working across all sectors of health and social care. The aim is to reduce the incidence of stroke in the population and ensure prompt access to integrated services for those people who have a stroke (DOH, 2001).

Contents

Learning Objectives

By the end of this chapter you should be able to demonstrate knowledge of:

- Factors associated with the epidemiology and aetiology of stroke.
- The differences between ischaemic and haemorrhagic strokes, identifying the mechanisms involved.
- The pathophysiology of stroke and the associated clinical manifestations.
- The range of common investigations.
- Various modes of treatment.
- The overall contributions of the nurse in the acute and rehabilitation phases of stroke recovery.

Definition

Stroke is the result of an acute lack of blood to some part of the brain. The term stroke is synonymous with cerebral vascular accident (CVA) and the terms may be used interchangeably. Clinically, stroke refers to the sudden dramatic development of focal neurological deficits (Allan, 2000).

Epidemiology

There has been a fall in death rate from stroke over recent years, but mortality is still alarmingly high. Every five minutes someone in England and Wales has a stroke. It is estimated to be responsible for 13 per cent of all deaths in this country, which represents about 60 000 deaths a year. Every year about 110 000 people in England and Wales have their first stroke and 30 000 people go on to have further strokes (DOH, 2001). About 10 000 of these are under the age of 55 (Clacton and District Stroke Association, 2000), and 1000 people under the age of 30 years have a stroke (DOH, 2001).

There is a variation in the mortality rate between ethnic groups in this country depending on the country of origin. Data from the Health Survey for England show that amongst African-Caribbean and South Asian men the prevalence of stroke was between about 40 per cent and 70 per cent higher than that of the general population after adjusting for age (DOH, 2001). In south London the incidence of stroke is higher in people of black ethnic origin, but the case fatality is higher in whites. The majority of survivors have considerable long-term morbidity (Wolfe, 2002).

Stroke has an extensive impact on both the individual and on the community at large. At any given time there are 25–30 patients with stroke as their primary diagnosis in the average hospital (DOH, 2001). Stroke patients occupy around 20 per cent of all hospital beds and 25 per cent of long-term beds. The cost to the NHS is about 2.3 billion pounds a year, which is twice that spent on coronary heart disease (Marshall, 1999).

Aetiology

The three main causes of stroke are:

- Cerebral thrombosis
- Cerebral embolus
- Cerebral haemorrhage

Strokes are caused by either a blockage, leading to ischaemic strokes, in up to 80 per cent of cases or by rupture of an artery in up to 20 per cent of cases, causing haemorrhagic strokes (Bougousslavsky *et al.*, 1988).

Ischaemic stroke can be caused by the following:

- A thrombus
- An embolus

Common causes of vascular occlusions leading to ischaemia are cerebral thrombi and cerebral emboli. Arteries can also be blocked by local pressure in the brain. Swollen brain cells, or fluid in the extracellular space can press on an artery blocking blood flow with the same end result (Guyton and Hall, 2000).

Cerebral Thrombosis

A thrombus is a blood clot usually made up of a solid mass of platelets, fibrin and other components of the blood. Thrombi often occur in larger vessels, for example the internal carotid arteries, and are associated with localized damage to the artery wall at the point of the occlusion. Atherosclerosis and hypotension are important underlying predisposing factors, but other types of vascular injury, for example arteritis, can initiate thrombosis (Campbell, 2002).

Atheroma tends to occur at points of arterial branching and tortuosity, which are areas of haemodynamic stress on the arterial wall, turbulent blood flow, and blood stasis. Thrombosis occurs on atheromatous plaques that have ulcerated as a result of plaque fracture, necrosis, or intraplaque haemorrhage and also in areas of turbulent or sluggish blood flow in relation to atheromatous stenotic areas that are severe enough to have a haemodynamic effect. Thrombi may occlude arteries, embolize to distal sites, be lysed, become incorporated into the plaques themselves or enlarge proximately and/or distally (Warlow, 2000).

Cerebral vascular accident secondary to thrombosis is most commonly seen in the 60–90-year-old group and the onset of symptoms tends to occur during sleep or soon after arising. This is thought to be related to the fact that elderly people have decreased sympathetic activity, and because recumbency causes a lowering of blood pressure, which can lead to brain ischaemia. These individuals often have postural hypotension and poor reflex response to changes in position (Schenk, 1995).

Cerebral Embolism

Embolism is the second most common cause of CVA. Patients who have a CVA secondary to embolism are usually younger. Most commonly, emboli originate from a thrombus in the heart, which is usually caused by rheumatic heart disease with mitral stenosis and atrial fibrillation (Schenk, 1995). Poor blood flow from a weakened pump following myocardial infarction can also encourage thrombus formation. Air or fat, for example from a fractured femur, can also act as an embolus (Allan, 2000). Emboli usually affect small vessels and are commonly found at points of bifurcation where the vessels narrow. They most commonly occur in the middle cerebral artery and can occur at any time (Schenk, 1995). Bits of fatty atheromatous plaques can break off from the lumen of an artery and are transported by the blood flow to a narrowed artery in the brain.

Transient Ischaemic Attacks

Transient ischaemic attacks probably represent thrombotic particles causing intermittent blockage of circulation or spasm. In a true transient ischaemic attack, all the neurological deficits must be completely clear within 12 hours, leaving no residual dysfunction. A transient ischaemic attack indicates the presence of cardiovascular pathology (Mittleman *et al.*, 2001). Approximately 35 per cent of completed thrombotic strokes are preceded by transient ischaemic attacks (Boss, 1994).

The attacks most commonly due to atherothrombembolism are associated with diseased arteries, disorders of the heart or small vessel disease within the brain. A transient fall in blood pressure, for example due to postural hypotension, cardiac arrhythmias, a hot bath or a heavy meal, can also cause transient ischaemic attacks, but only if one or more of the arteries to the brain are extremely stenotic or occluded (Warlow, 2000).

Transient ischaemic attack (TIA)

- TIA is a precursor of ischaemic stroke.
- Ischaemic stroke can happen without prior warnings of TIAs.
- The signs and symptoms of ischaemic stroke are usually the same, as the patient would have encountered in previous TIAs.
- These could be different if a different artery is involved.

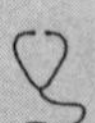

Nursing action points

- Be aware of patients who have an increased risk of experiencing a stroke. These include:
  - ☐ Patients suffering from cardiac disorders.
  - ☐ Patients undergoing prolonged surgery.
  - ☐ Patients with circulatory problems.

Cerebral Haemorrhage

Haemorrhagic strokes are the result of bleeding into the brain tissue or into a space such as the subarachnoid space (Smeltzer and Bare, 2000). Intracranial haemorrhage is the third most frequent cause of cerebral vascular accident. The most common predisposing factors for cerebral haemorrhage are hypertension, ruptured aneurysms or arteriovenous malformation, and haemorrhage associated with bleeding disorders (Boss, 1994).

Intracerebral haemorrhage, bleeding into the brain substance, is most common in patients with hypertension and cerebral atherosclerosis because degenerative changes from these diseases cause rupture of the vessel. In people younger than 40, intracerebral haemorrhages are usually caused by arteriovenous malformations, haemangioblastomas and trauma. Other causes include certain types of arterial pathology, brain tumour and the use of medications, for example, anticoagulants and amphetamines. The bleeding is usually arterial and occasionally ruptures the wall of the lateral ventricle, which is invariably fatal. Cerebral haemorrhage has a death rate of 50 to 75 per cent; many people die on the day of the bleed and most die within a month (NHS Direct, 2002).

Extradural haemorrhage (epidural haemorrhage) is usually due to a skull fracture and is a neurosurgical emergency. Subdural haemorrhage is basically the same as an epidural haemorrhage, except that in subdural haematoma a bridging vein is torn and a longer period is required for the haematoma to form and put pressure on the brain. Subarachnoid haemorrhage may occur as the result of trauma or hypertension but the most common cause is a leaking aneurysm in the area of the circle of Willis (Smeltzer and Bare, 2000). It can also be the result of the rupture of a congenital arteriovenous malformation.

Both cases are consequences of developmental abnormality giving rise to a weak vascular wall (Schenk, 1995). In both cases there can be early warning signs that affect the sufferer prior to a full haemorrhagic stroke. Both the aneurysm and the arteriovenous malformation can either bulge or bleed slightly to compress surrounding nerves and blood vessels so as to cause headaches or other neurological problems, without necessarily causing a full stroke.

Lacunar infarcts

Lacunar strokes are small deep infarcts, usually less than 1.5 centimetres in diameter and involve the small perforating arteries predominantly in the basal ganglia, thalamus, internal capsules, cerebral peduncle and pons. Higher cortical function is normal and the patient is conscious (Warlow, 2000). Lacunar strokes are associated with hypertension. Because of the subcortical location and small area of infarction, theses strokes may have pure motor and sensory defictis (Boss *et al.*, 1994).

Risk Factors

Certain predisposing factors increase the likelihood of cerebrovascular disease. The probability of reducing the prevalence of stroke by control of the risk factors has been calculated to be as high as 80 per cent, particularly among patients with atrial fibrillation, based on randomized therapeutic trials (Lechner *et al.*, 2001). These risk factors can be classified as those which can be modified and those which cannot be modified (Gorelick *et al.*, 1999).

Modifiable risk factors		*Non-modifiable risk factors*
Lifestyle	*Medical conditions*	
Cigarette smoking	Hypertension	TIA
Excessive alcohol consumption	Diabetes mellitus	Family history
Obesity	Heart problems and atrial fibrillation	Age
Lack of exercise		Gender
Socio-economic factors		Race/ethnicity

Cigarette Smoking

Other factors remaining constant, cigarette smoking increases the risk of stroke by about one and a half times (Shinton and Beevers, 1989). Stroke risk begins to decrease almost immediately after ceasing to smoke. After five years, ex-smokers have the same risk as non-smokers. Studies show that stroke risk decreases by half between two and five years after cessation, regardless of the age at which smoking started or the number of cigarettes smoked per day (Wannamethee *et al.*, 1995). Women over 30 who smoke and take high-oestrogen birth-control pills are 22 times more likely to develop a stroke than someone who does not smoke (Shinton and Beevers, 1989).

Alcohol Consumption

Alcohol consumed in small amounts (one to two drinks a day) can have a protective effect against ischaemic stroke. Heavy drinking (five drinks a day) by contrast, significantly increases the risk of stroke. While the exact relationship between alcohol consumption and stroke is unknown, it can produce irregular cardiac rhythms, contribute to high levels of triglycerides, can cause heart failure and induce hypertension (Gorelick *et al.*, 1999).

Socio-economic Factors

There is some evidence that people of lower income and educational levels have a higher risk of stroke (Irish Heart Foundation, 2002a). People in socio-economic group V have a 60 per cent higher chance of having a stroke and 50 per cent higher mortality rate from stroke in comparison with those in socio-economic group I (DOH, 2001).

Nutrition

Bananas may lower stroke risk. People whose diets are low in potassium could be at an increased risk of stroke according to American scientists. In a study of 5600 men and women over the age of 65, it was discovered that those with the lowest intake of potassium were, in the worst cases, two and a half times more likely to suffer a stroke (BUPA, 2002). A large study carried out in New Orleans found that people who eat fruit and vegetables that are high in folic acid, for example, broccoli and beans, were 20 per cent less likely to have a stroke. They were also 13 per cent less likely to have a myocardial infarction, and have lower systolic blood pressure and lower cholesterol levels than those on low folate diets. Further research is needed to determine the optimal dose of folic acid (NHS Information Authority, 2002).

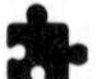 **Connection**

Chapter 4 (Hypertension) discusses the shared risk factors of obesity and physical inactivity.

Heart Problems and Atrial Fibrillation

People with heart problems, for instance, damaged heart valves – especially cardiac valve disease – have twice the risk of stroke as those with a normal heart. The mitral and aortic valves have been known to increase the formation of clots, which can then travel to block an artery in the brain, resulting in a stroke. A stroke patient with such defective valves has to be given anticoagulants or antiplatelet drugs to prevent formation of such clots. Atrial fibrillation is an irregular and ineffective heartbeat, which causes pooling of the blood in the left atrium and increases clot formation. It is very often seen in patients with rheumatic heart disease and in patients with congestive cardiac failure. It has been known to increase the risk of a stroke by about six times (Wolf *et al.*, 1991).

Treatment to restore normal rhythm is by administration of antiarrhythmic drugs, such as digitalis and cardioversion. Administration of the latter when the patient is receiving digitalis is risky and has to be carried out by cardiologists in a well-controlled environment with proper resuscitation equipment readily available. Administration of anticoagulants such as warfarin and antiplatelets such as aspirin are also recommended (Atrial Fibrillation Investigators, 1994).

Non-modifiable Risk Factors

Previous Stroke and TIA

These are very significant risk factors in that they are evidence that underlying pathology already exists. Somebody who has had a TIA is ten times more likely to have a full blown stroke than someone who has not had a TIA (Chelsea Community Hospital Health Advantage, 2002).

Family History

People who have a family history of stroke have a greater tendency to develop a stroke than the average population (Irish Heart Foundation, 2002a).

Age and Gender

The risk of stroke almost doubles for each decade of life after the age of 55 years. While stroke is common among the elderly, substantial numbers of people under the age of 65 also have strokes. Overall, men have about a 19 per cent greater risk of stroke than women and among people under the age of 65, the risk for men is even greater when compared with that of women (Irish Heart Foundation, 2002a). Although men are more prone to stroke than women, the number of women suffering from a stroke is larger than the number of men because women outlive men into old age (Wolf *et al.*, 1991).

Race/Ethnicity

British Asians and Afro-Caribbeans are more prone to stroke than the average population and it is more likely to be fatal. It could be that this is because both communities have a greater incidence of diabetes and hypertension, which are both high risk factors for stroke (Stroke Association, 2002a).

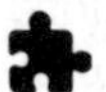 **Connection**

Chapter 1 (Social and Environmental Influences on Health and Well-being) and Chapter 3 (Health Issues Related to Ethnic Minority Groups) highlight differences in the prevalence of certain diseases among some groups within the general population.

Anatomy and Physiology of the Brain

The brain is a pinkish grey organ that weighs approximately 1.4 kilograms. It receives 15–20 per cent of the total cardiac output (Sunderland, 1994). The brain consists of four principle parts:

- Brain stem
- Cerebellum
- Diencephalons
- Cerebrum

The Brain Stem

The brain stem is continuous with the spinal cord and consists of the medulla oblongata, pons and the midbrain. Posterior to the brain stem is the cerebellum. Superior to the brain stem is the diencephalons, consisting primarily of the thalamus and hypothalamus and including the epithalamus and subthalamus. The cerebrum spreads over the diencephalons like a mushroom cap and occupies most of the cranium (Tortora and Grabowski, 2000).

The brain stem has a variety of very important functions. Some of its main functions are found in the control it provides for the rate and force of the heart and the rate and depth of respiration. It also controls the muscular walls of the small blood vessels causing vasoconstriction or dilatation and there are reflex centres in the medulla oblongata that initiate coughing, sneezing and vomiting.

The Cerebellum

The cerebellum, which means little brain, communicates with other regions of the central nervous system through three nerve tracts called the cerebral peduncles. One of the main functions of the cerebellum is to provide smooth and co-ordinated movements (Seeley *et al.*, 1992).

The Thalamus

The thalamus has about a dozen nuclei and has many important functions. For instance it contains geniculate bodies which are important visual and auditory relay centres. The thalamus also plays a key role in mediating sensation, motor activities, cortical arousal, learning and memory (Marieb, 2001).

The Hypothalamus

The hypothalamus is linked to the posterior lobe of the pituitary gland by nerve fibres and to the anterior lobe by a complex system of blood vessels. Through these connections the hypothalamus controls the output of hormones from both lobes of the gland (Wilson and Waugh, 1998). It is vitally important to the overall maintenance of body homeostasis, including control of the autonomic nervous system, hunger and thirst, body temperature, emotional reactions, sexual behaviour and circadian rhythms (Guyton and Hall, 2000).

The Cerebrum

The cerebrum forms the bulk of the brain. It consists of a thin layer of grey matter, the cerebral cortex and an inner layer of white matter called the cerebral medulla. There are three main varieties of activity associated with the cerebral cortex:

- Mental activities involved in memory, intelligence, sense of responsibility, thinking, reasoning, moral sense and learning are attributed to the higher centres.
- Sensory perception, including the perception of pain, temperature, touch, sight, hearing, taste and smell.
- Initiation and control of voluntary muscle contraction.

(Wilson and Waugh, 1998)

Arterial Blood Supply to the Brain

The greater part of the brain is supplied with arterial blood by an arrangement of arteries called the circulus arteriosus or the circle of Willis (see Figure 6.1). Four large arteries contribute to its formation:

- Two internal carotid arteries
- Two vertebral arteries

Anteriorly, two anterior cerebral arteries arise from the internal carotid arteries and are joined by the anterior communicating artery. Posteriorly, two vertebral arteries join to form the basilar artery. After travelling a short distance the

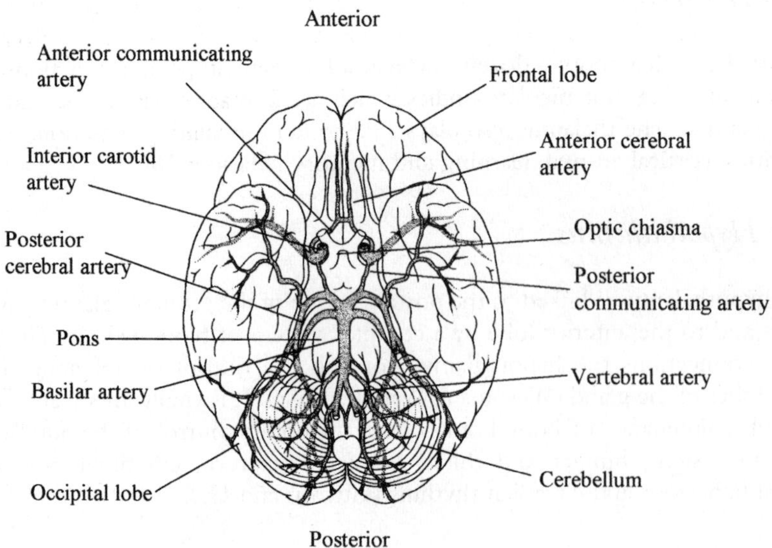

Figure 6.1 The brain and its blood supply

basilar artery divides to form two posterior cerebral arteries, each of which is joined to the corresponding internal carotid artery by a posterior communicating artery, completing the circle. The arrangement in the circle of Willis is such that the brain as a whole receives an adequate blood supply when a contributing artery is damaged and during extreme movements of the head and neck (Wilson and Waugh, 1998). In many individuals, parts of this arterial ring are hypoplastic and fewer than half are of the standard pattern. Nonetheless, unless affected by disease, it can form an excellent collateral channel for blood to the brain if one or more of the four main extracranial arteries is occluded (Warlow, 2000).

This ensures that the brain is well supplied with nutrients and oxygen. The brain requires 20 per cent of the body's oxygen supply, despite constituting only 2 per cent of the body's total body weight (Chipps *et al.*, 1992). Because cerebral tissues have no oxygen and glucose reserves, inadequate blood supply to the brain tissue results in irreversible damage. If blood flow to the brain is interrupted even briefly, unconsciousness may result (Tortora and Grabowski, 2000).

Pathophysiology

A stroke is usually the result of

- Ischaemia due to the blockage of a cerebral blood vessel.
- Haemorrhage due to a ruptured cerebral blood vessel.

The brain is very dependent on oxygen and has no reserve oxygen supply. When anoxia occurs as in a cerebral vascular accident, cerebral metabolism is promptly altered and cell death and permanent damage can occur within 3–10 minutes. Any condition that alters cerebral perfusion will cause hypoxia or anoxia. Hypoxia first leads to cerebral ischaemia. Short term ischaemia (less than 10–15 minutes) causes temporary deficits but no permanent deficits. Long-term ischaemia causes permanent cell death and results in cerebral infarction, with accompanying cerebral oedema. The area of the brain affected depends on which cerebral vessels are involved and this in turn determines the type of permanent focal deficits. The vessels most commonly affected are the middle cerebral artery and the internal carotid artery. Permanent focal deficits may be unclear initially because of generalized cerebral ischaemia that may later resolve (Schenk, 1995).

Ischaemic infarctions are not usually demonstrable on gross examination for 6–12 hours. The initial change of the affected area is a slight discolouration and softening, with the grey matter taking on a muddy colour and the white matter losing its normal fine-grained appearance. After 48–72 hours, necrosis, circumlesional swelling and disintegration of the affected area are evident. Eventually there is liquefaction and formation of a cyst surrounded by a firm glial tissue (Campbell, 2002).

The rupture of blood vessels causes disruption of the flow of blood to a selected area, focal ischaemic changes and infarction of brain tissue. The sudden release of blood leads to unconsciousness and causes a rapid rise in cerebrospinal fluid pressure with displacement of the brain. Bleeding into the brain tissue itself can cause damage by dissecting the brain along the fibre tracts. In addition, haemorrhage may produce a filling of the ventricular system or produce a haematoma that distorts brain tissue. Blood is a noxious agent and as it is haemolysed it irritates blood vessels, the meninges and brain. The presence of blood and the release of vasoactive substances promote arterial spasm, which can further decrease cerebral perfusion. Vasospasm usually occurs four to ten days after the haemorrhage and is a serious complication, potentially causing focal neurological decline, ischaemia of the brain and infarction (Schenk, 1995).

Clinical Manifestations

Neurones surrounding the ischaemic or infarcted area undergo changes that lead to oedema, causing further compression of capillaries. Cerebral oedema peaks at about 72 hours and takes about two weeks to subside. Most people survive an initial hemispheric ischaemic stroke unless massive cerebral oedema occurs. Massive brainstem infarcts, caused by basilar thrombosis or embolism, are almost always fatal (Boss *et al.*, 1994). Clinical manifestations of ischaemic stroke vary depending on the artery obstructed, the size of the area of inadequate perfusion and the amount of collateral (secondary or accessory) blood flow (Smeltzer and Bare, 2000). With haemorrhagic strokes, clinical manifestations vary, depending upon the location and size of the bleed. If a deep unresponsive state occurs the prognosis is grave; however, if the person survives, recovery of function is frequently possible (Boss *et al.*, 1994). The onset of symptoms in cerebral infarction is normally quite sudden or occurs during sleep, but there may be a worsening over a few hours; occasionally the clinical picture develops over a few days but rarely longer. Clinically it is difficult to distinguish between primary intracerebral haemorrhage and ischaemic stroke. Severe headache and coma within a few hours of onset, however, is unusual in ischemic stroke (Warlow, 2000). Subarachnoid haemorrhage typically causes a sudden severe headache, often accompanied by vomiting (Allan, 2000).

Neurological deficits of stroke

- Motor loss
- Communication loss
- Perceptual disturbances
- Sensory loss
- Cognitive impairment and psychological effects

Motor Loss

A disturbance of voluntary motor control on one side of the body may reflect damage to the upper neurones on the opposite side of the brain. Hemiplegia (paralysis of one side of the body) is the most common motor dysfunction. Hemiparesis (or weakness of one side of the body) is another sign. Flaccid paralysis and loss of, or decrease in, the deep tendon reflexes are seen initially. When the deep tendon reflexes reappear, usually within 48 hours, there is increased tone and spasticity (Smeltzer and Bare, 2000).

Dysphagia (Difficulty in Swallowing)

Up to 50 per cent of stroke patients have dysphagia immediately after the stroke. Dysphagia can occur when one side of the mouth is weak, leading to difficulty in chewing and swallowing, and drooling. One or both sides of the mouth can be affected by paralysis, increasing the risk of aspiration when trying to swallow liquids or food (Irish Heart Foundation, 2002b).

Bladder and Bowel Deficits

These include:

- Urinary and/or bowel incontinence
- Urinary frequency
- Urinary urgency

(Allan, 2000)

Communication Loss

Dysfunction of language may include:

- Dysarthria – poor, unintelligible speech caused by paralysis of the muscle responsible for speech.
- Dysphasia or aphasia – defective speech or loss of speech, which is mainly expressive or receptive.
- Apraxia – inability to perform a previously learned action, though the patient understands its purpose and has no motor or sensory loss.

Perceptual Disturbances

Perception is the ability to interpret sensation. Stroke can result in visual perceptual dysfunctions, disturbances in visual–spatial awareness and sensory loss. Homonymous hemianopia (loss of half the visual field) may occur, and may be temporary or permanent.

Sensory Loss

This may take the form of slight impairment of touch or may be more severe, with loss of proprioception (the ability to perceive position and motion of body parts) as well as difficulty in interpreting visual, tactile and auditory stimuli.

Cognitive Impairment and Psychological Effects

Damage to the frontal lobe may result in impairment of learning capacity, memory or other higher cortical intellectual functions. Such dysfunction may be reflected in limited attention span, difficulties in comprehension, forgetfulness and lack of motivation, which may cause patients to experience frustration in their rehabilitation programmes. Depression, emotional lability, hostility, resentment, frustration and lack of cooperation are also common (Smeltzer and Bare, 2000).

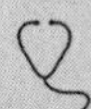

Nursing action points

- Place objects within the patient's visual field.
- Place objects within reach on the unaffected side.
- Approach the patient from the side of intact field of vision.
- Encourage the patient to exercise the affected side.

- Encourage the patient to strengthen the unaffected side by exercising.
- Provide the patient with alternative methods of communication.
- Allow the patient time to respond.
- Test the patient's pharyngeal reflexes before offering food.
- Assist the patient with meals, offer food to the unaffected side of the mouth.
- Reorient to time, place and situation frequently.
- Provide familiar objects.
- Repeat and reinforce instructions frequently.
- Support the patient during uncontrollable outbursts.

(Smeltzer and Bare, 2000)

Investigative Tests

A whole battery of investigations can be undertaken during stroke management. Investigations are necessary to confirm diagnosis and assess effectiveness of treatment as well as monitoring the patient's progress.

History

Any patient with neurological deficits requires a careful history and a complete physical and neurological examination. Initial assessment will focus on the individual's ability to maintain a patent airway, due to loss of gag or cough reflexes and altered respiratory pattern (Smeltzer and Bare, 2000).

Diagnostic tests

- Computerized axial tomography
- Magnetic resonance imaging
- Cerebral angiography
- Transcranial Doppler ultrasonography
- Single photon emission tomography
- Electroencephalogram
- Lumbar puncture
- Electrocardiogram and chest x-ray
- Blood testing

Computerized Axial Tomography (CT Scan)

The most reliable way in which primary intracerebral haemorrhage can be differentiated from ischaemic stroke is by unenhanced CT scan within hours of stroke onset (Warlow, 2000). Contrast enhancing agents may normalize density of small hypodense infarct (Campbell, 2002). CT scan can also provide information as to the location and size of the haemorrhage. Structural abnormalities such as aneurysms can also be detected (Smith *et al.*, 2001). Early differentiation between haemorrhage and ischaemia is crucially important because of the potential use of anticoagulant and antiplatelet drugs.

Magnetic Resonance Imaging (MRI)

This uses radio frequency waves in conjunction with strong magnetic field to give detailed structures of an organ, rather similar to a CT scan. It is able to detect ischaemic stroke much earlier than CT scan and with greater accuracy (Szabo *et al.*, 2001). It produces very accurate pictures of the brain. It can detect the presence, location and size of aneurysms and arteriovenous malformations, which as pointed out before are potential sources of haemorrhages.

Cerebral Angiography

Angiography is a radiological technique that demonstrates cerebrovascular blood flow. A small catheter is inserted into the femoral artery and passed to the level of the cerebral circulation and a contrast dye is then injected. Serial x-ray films are then taken, which demonstrate the flow of the dye through the cerebral vasculature and provide information on the patency, location and size of the vessels (Sunderland, 1994). Cerebral angiogram demonstrates displacement or blockage of cerebral vessels (Timby *et al.*, 1999). Cerebral angiogram is not usually indicated during the acute phase of ischaemic stroke since the result is unlikely to influence the immediate management and the procedure itself can make the patient worse (Warlow, 2000).

Transcranial Doppler Ultrasonography

This test determines the size of intracranial vessels and the direction of blood flow and locates obstructed cerebral vessels. This is an imaging procedure in which high frequency or ultrasound waves are used to detect blockages in the carotid artery. Ultrasound waves generated by a probe strategically placed on the neck near the carotid artery travel through the neck to bounce off travelling blood cells. Reflected sound waves at a different frequency generated by the moving blood cells are then picked up by the probe, enabling blood flow to be interpreted. As it is a non-invasive technique, it carries no risk to the patient (Kee, 1995). This test can help a vascular surgeon to advise people with either a TIA or mild stroke as to whether surgery to the carotid artery in the neck would protect against further TIA or stroke (Irish Heart Foundation, 2002c).

Single Photon Emission Tomography

This also determines cerebral blood flow.

Electroencephalogram

Electroencephalogram reveals reduced electrical activity in the involved area but is not a specific diagnostic test (Timby *et al.*, 1999).

Lumbar Puncture

If subarachnoid haemorrhage is diagnosed and the patient is alert, obeying commands and has no focal deficits, lumbar puncture is indicated. If a subarachnoid haemorrhage has occurred, the cerebrospinal fluid will be blood stained.

Electrocardiogram and Chest X-ray

Since both ischaemic heart disease and stroke have similar pathogenesis, it is possible that the patient has an underlying heart problem.

Blood Testing

A rapid way of detecting whether someone has had a stroke may soon be available through a blood test. Researchers have found a pattern of proteins in blood that only occurs in someone who has had a stroke. This discovery means that it may be possible to make an earlier diagnosis, thus enabling treatment to begin sooner (syn.X Pharma Inc., 2001).

Treatment and Management

Primary Preventative Measures

 **Connection**

Chapter 4 (Hypertension) highlights the risk factors associated with stroke.

Secondary Prevention

Aims of treatment:

- To prevent further brain damage
- Treatment of pre-existing contributory disorders
- Provide supportive care
- Regain functional independence

(Allan, 2000)

Conservative Management – Medication

Anticoagulants

Anticoagulation therapy has been used in an attempt to improve the patient's recovery, however, there is some doubt as to its usefulness, as a risk of further haemorrhage into the infarcted brain has been identified (Allan, 2000).

Thrombolytics

The use of thrombolytic agents, especially recombinant tissue plasminogen activator (rTPA) has been shown to produce a sustained, significant neurological improvement if administered within a few hours of infarction. As it is contraindicated in cerebral haemorrhage and in anticoagulant therapy, patients must meet eligibility criteria (Campbell, 2002).

Antifibrinolytics

Antifibrinolytic agents have been used in patients following subarachnoid haemorrhage. Their use is thought to prevent re-bleeding by delaying dissolution of the clot around the aneurysm, but their effect in the overall outcome is questionable.

Antiplatelets

Antiplatelets include aspirin, dipyridamole, ticlopidine and clopidogrel; patients suffering from TIAs may benefit from the use of these drugs. The International Stroke Trial Collaborative group has found that the combination of aspirin and dipyridamole can reduce the risk of a second stroke after 24 months by 38 per cent (Sudlow and Wardlow, 1997). According to Taylor (1996), the best time to start treatment is during the first three hours after a stroke. A CT scan must be done to rule out cerebral haemorrhage, in which case antiplatelets are contraindicated. With regard to the secondary prevention of stroke, clinical trials have shown the benefits of ticlopidine and clopidogrel to be superior to those of aspirin (Hass *et al.*, 1989; CAPRIE Steering Committee, 1996).

Treatment of Pre-existing Contributory Disorders

These may be treated with drug therapy, for example antihypertensive drugs and diuretics (Allan, 2000). Other potential medications include calcium channel blockers, anticonvulsants, corticosteroids, narcotic analgesia and analgesic/ antipyretics (Campbell, 2002). Following stroke, administration of low-molecular-weight heparin (LMWH) and early mobilization for the appropriate patients should be instigated to prevent complications such as deep vein thrombosis (Kay *et al.*, 1995).

Haematological investigations may include coagulation studies; because of the use of anticoagulants and antiplatelet drugs it would be necessary to monitor clotting time to avoid complications such as haemorrhage. Other tests may include full blood count and blood gases (Kee, 1995).

Surgical Interventions

Carotid Endarterectomy

Endarterectomy is the resection and removal of the lining of an artery (Timby *et al.*, 1999). Carotid endarterectomy involves the removal of stenosing or ulcerating atheromatous lesions at the bifurcation of the common carotid arteries (Allan, 2000). It can be beneficial for patients who have already had a stroke or experienced warning signs of a stroke and who have stenosis of 70–99 per cent. The degree of stenosis is normally expressed as a percentage of the normal diameter of the opening. In these patients it can reduce the risk of a second stroke by as much as 80 per cent (European Carotid Surgery Trialists' Collaborative Group, 1998).

Superficial Temporal to Middle-artery Anastomosis (ST-MCA bypass)

This provides an artificial collateral blood supply to the affected part of the brain.

Treating Subarachnoid Haemorrhage

An effective way to stop re-bleeding is to place a metal clip across the neck of the aneurysm. This is a major neurological procedure and is not suitable for all patients, owing to their general condition or the location of the aneurysm (Allan, 2000).

Nursing Interventions

Stroke Units

Research has proved that stroke units reduce both death and disability. But according to the latest audit of stroke services from the Royal College of Physicians, around 6000 people are dying each year and a similar number are left disabled, because they do not receive treatment in a stroke unit. The audit found that only 27 per cent of stroke patients are spending most of their stay in a stroke unit. While the number of stroke units has increased it is evident that many units do not have the capacity to meet demand (Stroke Association, 2002b).

Organization of Stroke Care

- Health education
- Acute care
- Rehabilitation
- Continuing care

Health Education

In many cases stroke can be prevented and, in the event of a stroke occurring, its impact upon the individual can be minimized. This can be achieved by a number of interventions including lifestyle changes and medical and technological interventions. A recent survey suggests that people in Northern Ireland are largely ignorant of the causes and effects of stroke, even though it is the single biggest reason for disability in the community and costs the Health Service millions of pounds every year (Northern Ireland Chest Heart and Stroke Association, 2002). The role of the nurse in educating patients, however, does not stop at the primary prevention level. Education goes on after the individual has sustained a stroke. This helps to prevent or minimize further complications.

Acute Care

The number of symptoms and the severity vary considerably and nursing management is based on the problems identified during initial and ongoing assessments. Certain procedures, such as airway maintenance, continuous monitoring of heart rate and administration of oxygen should be undertaken as soon as the patient arrives in the accident and emergency department. In the majority of cases, hypertension returns to normal within 90 minutes of the stroke without any pharmacological intervention. Fever and hyperglycaemia should be treated, as both worsen stroke outcome.

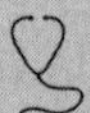

Nursing action points

- Maintain a clear airway.
- Monitor the level of consciousness.
- Monitor vital signs.
- Assess for total incontinence and implement the appropriate care to maintain hygiene.
- Assess for degree of impaired mobility and implement care to prevent complications of joint stiffening and muscle contracture.
- Assess the risk for impaired skin integrity.
- Assess self-care deficit.

- Assess impaired verbal communication and adopt/alternative ways of communication.
- Refer to a speech therapist.
- Assess the psychological impact of the stroke upon the patient.
- Allow time to talk to the patient and be prepared to discuss worries relevant to sexual dysfunction.

Airway. About 50 per cent of patients with strokes have difficulty in swallowing during the first 48 hours (Marshall, 1999). This must be assessed and monitored regularly to prevent aspiration. An appropriate feeding regimen can be administered should the problem persist. Suction should be available and fluid balance maintained.

Levels of Consciousness. This is assessed partly by using the Glasgow coma scale and a full neurological examination. Essentially, recording levels of consciousness is about determining the patient's ability to be aware of his or her environment and to react to a variety of stimuli such as verbal stimulation or pain (Guyton and Hall, 2000).

Monitoring of Vital Signs. Pulse is observed for regularity, strength and rhythm. Respiration should be observed for rate, rhythm, depth and sound. Ineffective breathing can also be recognized by cyanosis. Increased intracranial pressure will result in blood pressure and pulse changes.

Total Incontinence. An indwelling catheter may be inserted. Bowel incontinence is related to unconsciousness and immobility. Suppositories or enemas may be prescribed.

Impaired Mobility. Prevention of the potential problems of immobility should have a high profile. Active and passive exercises should be demonstrated to the patient and he or she encouraged to exercise the affected and unaffected parts. The patient should be positioned to avoid contractures and the affected limb supported and correctly positioned. Correct posture and movement of limbs and joints should start on day one to try and prevent spasticity with limb and trunk contractures that will interfere with future rehabilitation. Referral to a physiotherapist should be made. Mobilization should be an early goal of care; use of mobilization devices may assist in this aim.

Risk for Impaired Skin Integrity. The skin should be kept clean and dry, with pressure area risk assessment being carried out according to local policy.

Self-care Deficit. This may be related to unilateral use of the hands, visual deficits or impaired physical mobility. It is important to set realistic goals and to encourage the patient. Modify clothing and utensils to accommodate the patient's neurological deficits.

Impaired Communication. Referral to a speech therapist needs to be made, and alternatives to verbal communication should be offered. Speak slowly and clearly to the patient and allow him or her time to respond, while not inviting lengthy responses (Timby *et al.*, 1999).

Depression. Depression is common and antidepressants may help if the depression dominates the person's life. Positive reinforcement as progress is made will help.

Sexual Dysfunction. Sexual functioning can be profoundly affected by stroke. Often stroke is such a catastrophic illness that the patient experiences loss of self-esteem and value as a sexual being. Although research in this area is limited, it appears that while sexual function is considered to be important, most have sexual dysfunction. The patient and his or her partner may benefit from a referral to a counsellor who might discuss alternative approaches to sexual expression (Smeltzer and Bare, 2000).

Rehabilitation

Rehabilitation begins the moment the patient comes into care; it is the process of minimizing the effects of stroke and reducing the impact of the stroke on the individual and/their family. Proper positioning in a wheelchair and treating depression are regarded as part of rehabilitation. Part of rehabilitation is aimed at helping the person adapt to the neurological deficits. There is some evidence that parts of the brain that are not damaged by the stroke take over some of the functions that have been damaged (neuroplasty). Some of the physiotherapy, speech therapy and occupational therapy is based upon this possibility. There is evidence that more intensive rehabilitation can lead to a more rapid recovery of function within the first six months compared with those who do not receive intensive rehabilitation. However, recovery evens out after six months. Part of a therapist's role is to tailor therapy to the individual in hospital or at home. Most gains in function in the first 30 days after stroke are due to spontaneous recovery. Successful rehabilitation depends on:

- The extent to which the brain is affected
- The person's attitude
- The rehabilitation team's skill
- The support of family and friends

(Irish Heart Foundation, 2002d)

The goal of rehabilitation is to reduce dependence and improve physical ability; nurses have a crucial role to play in preventing complications such as stiff joints, pressure sores and chest infections. Patient and family education is a fundamental component of rehabilitation, and nurses should make ample time for teaching about stroke, its causes, prevention and the rehabilitation process (Smeltzer and Bare, 2000).

Continuing Care

The recovery and rehabilitation process may be prolonged, requiring patience and perseverance on the part of the patient and family. Depending upon the specific neurological deficits the patient at home may require the services of a number of healthcare professionals. The nurse frequently plays a coordinating role. The family will require assistance in planning and providing aspects of care. Long-term care requirements should be within the care management arrangements described in the National Service Framework for Older People (Standard Two). Patients and their carers should have access to a stroke care coordinator who can provide advice, arrange reassessment when needs or circumstances change, coordinate long-term support or arrange specialist care (DOH, 2001). Caregivers often require reminders to attend to their health and well-being as the burden placed upon them can be great.

Hospital outreach teams deliver care in the patient's home. A speech therapist who visits the home allows the family to be involved and gives practical instructions to help the patient. Community-based stroke clubs allow the patient and family to share their experiences. All nurses coming into contact with the patient should encourage the patient to keep active, adhere to the exercise programme and remain as self-sufficient as possible (Smeltzer and Bare, 2000).

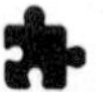 **Connection**

Chapter 2 (Family-centred Care) discusses how the health of carers can be compromised by the burden of caring for a relative.

Conclusion

There is an increased interest in stroke disorders, with the development of rapid access clinics, acute stroke units, stroke rehabilitation units, stroke physicians, stroke nurse specialists and nurse consultants working in this area of practice. Underpinning these service developments is an increased understanding of the pathophysiology of stroke, together with some evidence on how best to manage stroke. The development of national clinical guidelines by the Intercollegiate Working Party for Stroke (1999) representing healthcare professionals, service users and the voluntary sector has been well received by those caring for stroke victims and their families. The inclusion of stroke in the *National Service Framework for Older People* has also emphasized the benefits of an integrated stroke service (DOH, 2001). Meanwhile the role of nurses at the preventative level should be intensified in an attempt to reduce the incidence of this disorder, which results in so many deaths and disabilities. People should be made aware of the risk factors, in particular the controllable ones. They should also be made aware of recent technological advances and expertise, which can be helpful in secondary prevention. Stroke should not be considered in isolation: related disorders such as ischaemic heart disease, diabetes and hypertension, should also be given close attention (Gorelick *et al.*, 1999).

There have been numerous reports that have identified the need to improve acute stroke management and all have reported major deficiencies in stroke management (Ebrahim and Redfern, 1999). There is also the need to develop further stroke units so that some of the most advanced treatment can be effectively administered. These include easy access to a CT scan for all stroke patients and the administration of anticoagulants and thrombolytic therapy. Significant gains in patient outcomes can be achieved in the weeks and months following the stroke with a therapeutic regimen executed by healthcare professionals and the patient's family and friends. Rehabilitation begins from the time of the onset of the stroke and is actively carried out once the patient is medically stable. Rehabilitation is complex and requires a multidisciplinary approach. It is a planned, goal-directed activity that requires assessment and reassessment using standard measures to monitor progress and must include the patients and their families and friends. Patient outcomes can be improved and many patients are able to return to independent lives.

References

Allan, D. 2000, 'The Nervous System' in Alexander, M. F., Fawcett, J. N. and Runciman, P. J. *Nursing Practice – Hospital and Home*. 2nd edn. London. Harcourt Publishers Ltd.

Atrial Fibrillation Investigators 1994, 'Risk factors for stroke and efficacy of anti-thrombotic therapy in atrial fibrillation'. *Archives of Internal Medicine*, 154, 1449–57.

Boss, B. J. 1994, 'Concepts of Neurologic Dysfunction' in McCance, K. L. and Heuther, S. E. (eds), *Pathophysiology. The Biological Basis for Disease in Adults and Children*. 2nd edn. London. Mosby-Year Book Inc.

Boss, B. J., Sunderland, P. M. and Heath, J. 1994, 'Alterations of Neurologic Function' in McCance, K. L. and Heuther, S. E. (eds), *Pathophysiology. The Biological Basis for Disease in Adults and Children*. 2nd edn. London. Mosby-Year Book Inc.

Bougousslavsky, J., Van Melle, G. and Regli, F. 1988, 'The Lausanne stroke registry: analysis of 1000 consecutive patients with first stroke'. *Stroke*, 19, 1083–92.

BUPA 2002, 'Bananas may lower stroke risk'. http://www.bupa.co.uk/health_information/htrd/health_news/130802stroke.html

Campbell, V. G. 2002, 'Neurological System' in Thompson, J. M., McFarland, G. K., Hirsch, J. E. and Tucker, S. M. (eds), *Mosby's Clinical Nursing*. 5th edn. London. Mosby Inc.

CAPRIE Steering Committee, 1996, 'A randomised, blind, trial of clopidogrel versus aspirin in patients at risks of ischaemic events (CAPRIE)'. *Lancet*, 348, 1329–30.

Chelsea Community Hospital Health Advantage 2002, 'Mini-strokes are not mini-problems'. http://www.cch.org/hlthmat/pg2a_0800.htm

Chipps, E. M., Clanin, J. N. and Campbell, V. G. 1992, *Neurologic Disorders*. London. Mosby-Year Book.

Clacton and District Stroke Association 2000, http://www..stosyth.gov.uk/defaultasp?calltype=strokemar01

Department of Health (DOH) 1999, 'Saving lives; our healthier nation.' http://www.archive.official-documents.co.uk/document/cm43/4386/4386.htm

Department of Health (DOH) 2001, *National Service Framework for Older People*. London. Department of Health.

Ebrahim, S. and Redfern, J. 1999, *Stroke Care. A Matter of Chance: A National Survey of Stroke Services*. London. Stroke Association.

European Carotid Surgery Trialists' Collaborative Group 1998, 'Randomised Trial of Endarterectomy for recently symptomatic carotid stenosis: final results of MRCP European Carotid Surgery Trial (ECST)'. *Lancet*, 351, 1379–87.

Gorelick, P. B., Scacco, R. L., Smith, D. B. *et al.* 1999, 'Consensus statement: Prevention of a first stroke'. *Journal of the American Medical Association*, 281, 24–31.

Guyton, A. C. and Hall, J. E. 2000, *Textbook of Medical Physiology*. 10th edn. London. W. B. Saunders Company.

Hass, W. K., Easton, J. D., Adams, H. P. Jr. *et al.* 1989, 'A randomised trial comparing ticlopidine hydrochloride with aspirin for the prevention of stroke in high-risk patients'. Ticlopidine Aspirin Stroke Study Group. *New England Journal of Medicine*, 321, 501–7.

Intercollegiate Working Party for 'Stroke' 1999, 'National clinical guidelines for stroke'. http://www.nelh.nhs.uk/guidelinesdb/html/AFstroke.htm

Irish Heart Foundation 2002a, 'Stroke risk factors'. http://www.irishheart.ie/patientqueries/stroke4.htm

Irish Heart Foundation 2002b, 'Stroke'. http://www.irishheart.ie/patientqueries/stroke2.htm

Irish Heart Foundation 2002c, 'Stroke symptoms/warning signs'. http://www.irishheart.ie/patientqueries/stroke5.htm

Irish Heart Foundation 2002d, 'Stroke rehabilitation'. http://www.irishheart.ie/patientqueries/stroke3.htm

Kay, R., Wong, K. S., Yu, Y. L. *et al.* 1995, 'Low-molecular-weight heparin for the treatment of acute ischaemic stroke'. *New England Journal of Medicine*, 333, 1588–93.

Kee, J. L. 1995, *Laboratory and Diagnostic Tests with Nursing Implications*. 4th edn. Connecticut. Appleton & Lange.

Lechner, H., Linhofer, H. and Gerhard, S. 2001, 'Basis for primary prevention of stroke under a social health act'. *The Journal of Stroke and Cerebrovascular Diseases*, 10, 4. http://www2.strokejournal.org/scripts/om.dl1/serve?action=searchDB&searchD B for=art2art

Marieb, N.E. 2001, *Anatomy and Physiology*. 5th edn. London. Addison Wesley Longman.

Marshall, J. 1999, 'PCGs should take lead role in stroke units'. http://www.healthinfocus.co.uk

Mittleman, M. A., Voetsch, B. and Caplan, L. R. 2001, "Triggers of ischaemic stroke. Results from the stroke onset pilot study". *Stroke*, 32, 66–7.

NHS Direct 2002, '*Online health encyclopaedia – stroke*'. http://www.nhsdirect.nhs.uk/nhsdoheso/display.asp?sSection=Introduction&Topiic=Stroke&

NHS Information Authority 2002, 'Can broccoli and beans cut the risk of stroke?' http://www.nelh.nhs.uk/hth/broccoli_beans.asp

Northern Ireland Chest, Heart and Stroke Association, 2002, 'People unaware of stroke dangers – survey'. http://www.nichsa.com/html/pressroom/news-153.html

Schenk, E. 1995, 'The Patient with Neurological Problems' in Long, B. C., Phipps, W. J. and Cassmeyer, V. L. (eds), *Adult Nursing. A Nursing Process Approach.* London. Times Mirror International Publishers Ltd.

Seeley, R. R., Stephens, D. T. and Tate, P. 1992, *Anatomy and Physiology.* 2nd edn. London. Mosby-Year Book Inc.

Shinton, R. and Beevers, G. 1989, 'Meta-analysis of relation between cigarette smoking and stroke'. *British Medical Journal,* 298, 789–94.

Smeltzer, S. C. and Bare, B. G. 2000, *Bruner & Suddarth's Textbook of Medical–Surgical Nursing.* 9th edn. Philadelphia. Lippincott, Williams and Wilkins.

Smith, W. S., Johnston, S. C., Tsao, J. W. *et al.* 2001, 'Safety and speed of CT imaging protocol for the entire cerebrovascular axis during acute stroke'. *Stroke,* 32, 345.

Stroke Association 2002a, 'Stroke awareness campaign'. http://www.stroke.org.uk/noticeboard/asianstroke.htm

Stroke Association 2002b, 'Stroke – it's just not good enough'. http://www.stroke.org.uk/Campaign/campindex.html *Stroke,* 19, 1083–92.

Sudlow, C. L. M. and Wardlow, C. P. 1997, 'International incidence collaboration. Comparable studies on the incidence of stroke and its pathological types; results from an international collaboration'. *Stroke,* 28, 491–9.

Sunderland, P. M. 1994, 'Structure and Function of the Nervous System' in McCance, K. L. and Heuther, S. E. (eds), *Pathophysiology. The Biological Basis for Disease in Adults and Children.* 2nd edn. London. Mosby–Year Book Inc.

Syn.X Pharma Inc. 2001, 'What's new at Syn.X'. http://www.synxpharma.com/news_2001_1.html

Szabo, K., Behrens, S. and Hirsh, J. 2001, 'Subgroup analysis of patients with severe acute neurological ischaemic syndromes without diffusion weighted magnetic resonance imaging abnormalities'. *Stroke,* 32, 318.

Taylor, T. N., Davis, P. H. *et al.* 1996, 'Life time cost of stroke in the United States'. *Stroke,* 27, 1459–66.

Timby, B. K., Scherer, J. C. and Smith, N. E. 1999, *Introductory Medical–Surgical Nursing.* 7th edn. Philadelphia. Lippincott, Williams and Wilkins.

Tortora, G. J. and Grabowski, S. R. 2000, *Principles of Anatomy and Physiology.* 9th edn. New York. John Wiley and Sons.

Wannamethee, S. G., Shaper A. G., Whincup, P. H. and Walker, M. 1995, 'Smoking cessation and the risk of stroke in middle-aged men'. *Journal of the American Medical Association,* 55–160.

Warlow, C. P. 2000, 'Cerebrovascular Disease' in Ledington, J. G. G. and Warrell, D. A. (eds), *Concise Textbook of Medicine.* Oxford. Oxford University Press.

Wilson, K. J. W. and Waugh, A. 1998, *Ross and Wilson Anatomy and Physiology in Health and Illness.* London. Churchill Livingstone.

Wolf, P. A., Abbott, R. D. and Kannel, W. B. 1991, 'Atrial fibrillation as an independent risk factor for stroke: the Framingham Study'. *Stroke,* 22, 983–8.

Wolfe, C. 2002, 'The incidence, natural history, resource use and outcome of stroke'. UK Department of Health Research. http://www.doh.gov.uk/research/rd3/nhs.randd/timeltdprogs/cvd/is10a.htm

7

Multiple Sclerosis

Norma Whittaker

Multiple sclerosis (MS) is a chronic disease of the central nervous system and the most common cause of disability in young people. It is a degenerative disease for which there is no cure, although recent evidence suggests that it may be possible to influence the course of the disease (Pinn, 1997). MS represents a significant healthcare problem; the annual cost of care for MS in the United Kingdom (UK) is estimated at £1.2 billion (Watkiss and Ward, 2001).

Contents

- Definition
- Epidemiology
- Aetiology
- Anatomy and physiology relative to the cerebral neurones
- Pathophysiology
- Clinical manifestations
- Psychological aspects
- Diagnostic investigations
- Treatment
- Nursing interventions

Learning Objectives

By the end of the chapter you should be able to demonstrate knowledge of:

- Factors associated with the epidemiology and aetiology of MS.
- The potential effects upon the individual of demyelination of neurones.
- The relapsing remitting nature of MS.

- How MS is diagnosed and treated.
- The roles of other agencies.
- Nursing interventions that reflect the need to empower patients while acknowledging the chronic nature of the disorder.
- The role of the specialist nurse.

Definition

Multiple sclerosis is a chronic, complex neurological disease of unknown origin characterized pathologically by the widespread occurrence in the nervous system of patches of demyelination followed by gliosis. In most cases there is improvement after the initial manifestation of the disease and periods of exacerbation and remission are a feature of the disease (Walton, 1977).

Epidemiology

Multiple sclerosis affects an estimated 86 000 people in the UK; around 100 people out of every 100 000 in the UK will develop MS at some time (Barnes and Jones, 1996). The annual incidence is around five per 100 000 (Allen and Lueck, 1999). Approximately 2400 new cases are diagnosed each year; a typical general practitioner (GP) with a list of 2000 patients being likely to have two to four patients with MS (Pinn, 1997). The lifetime risk of developing MS for someone growing up in the UK is 1 in 800 according to Hopkins (1993).

The usual age of onset is after puberty until the fourth decade, the onset of symptoms occurring between 20 and 40 years of age in most patients. The disease is rare in childhood and uncommon in old age (Chipp *et al.*, 1992). The peak age for diagnosis is 30; it remains high in the fourth decade of life and then starts to decline (Watkiss and Ward, 2001). Current diagnostic criteria exclude the diagnosis of MS after the age of 59 years (Poser *et al.*, 1983). A review of 800 patients in Ontario, however, highlighted the fact that 40 had developed the first symptoms of MS after the age of 50 years. The majority had not been initially diagnosed as suffering from MS (Mattison, 1996). More women than men are affected: a female to male ratio of 1.5 : 1 is most common in temperate climes (Allen and Lueck, 1999; Campion, 1997a).

Types of Multiple Sclerosis

- Benign
- Relapsing/remitting
- Secondary progressive
- Primary progressive

The clinical course of MS ranges from mild, infrequent attacks that have little impact upon the individual, to severe disability in a short period of time. The disease progresses in four ways and may be classified accordingly.

Benign

A very mild form of the disease, which affects approximately 20 per cent of people diagnosed with MS. This form is characterized by minor relapses, often with long periods of remission and no disability. The person may have an attack and then experience nothing more for several years. Diagnosis in this case can only be made retrospectively (Sutton, 1998).

Relapsing/Remitting

This is most common in young people. The majority of people with MS have this type initially. Relapses are unpredictable. During a relapse, earlier symptoms may occur or new symptoms develop over a few days. These may last for a few days, weeks or months followed by a period of remission. Recovery from a relapse is dependent on the level of damage, the area affected and other variables. The person may have three or more attacks in a year and may require short hospital admissions. Remission periods vary, lasting weeks or years. During a remission the individual may have few or no symptoms (Campion, 1997a).

Secondary Progressive

This is the most common type affecting approximately 40 per cent of those diagnosed with MS (see Figure 7.1). Over half of all people with relapsing/remitting MS eventually move into a secondary progressive stage after a period of 15–20 years following the initial onset of the disease (Revesz *et al.*, 1991). Attacks may continue over time with individuals noticing a gradual progression of symptoms. There is less recovery from a relapse and 25 per cent of people will develop disability severe enough for them to require a wheelchair. A gradual decline may, however, take 20–30 years.

Primary Progressive

Approximately 15 per cent of people with MS follow this course. The average age when diagnosed is 40 years and the disease follows a progressive course from the onset. There are no periods of relapse and remission and there is a steady deterioration. The way in which the disease progresses is variable and symptoms can plateau at any time (Campion, 1997a).

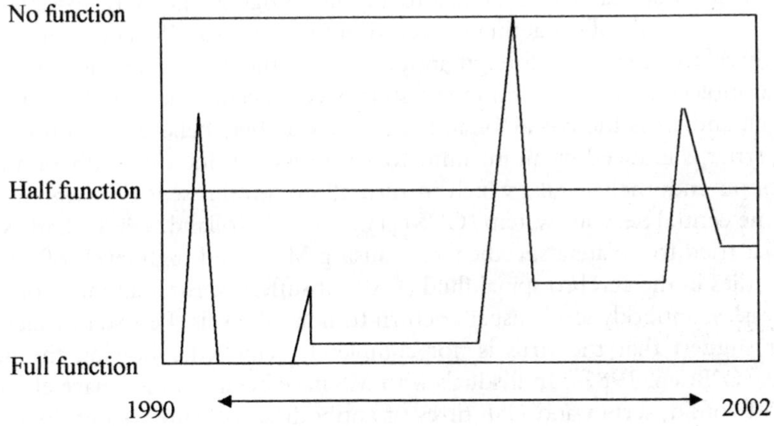

Figure 7.1 A pattern of relapse and remission of symptoms

Aetiology

While a number of theories have been proposed as to the cause of MS, all remain unproven. There is evidence that susceptibility to the disease is linked to the individual's genetic make-up and environmental factors (Sadovnick *et al.*, 1988; Lindsay and Bone, 1991). Researchers suggest that in genetically susceptible people the disease results from an abnormal autoimmune response to some agent, possibly a virus or environmental trigger (Halper and Holland, 1998). A popular theory is that a viral infection occurs very early in life and MS only develops if there is a deficit in the person's immune system.

Theories as to the Causes of MS

- Viral
- Immunological
- Myelin loss
- Genetic
- Social and physical
- Epidemiological

Viral

Evidence suggests that MS is some form of disease affecting the immune system that finds its origin in a viral infection. There may be some genetic defect in the immune system, which permits the persistence of viruses. It may be that a virus lies dormant within the body and in later life attacks the myelin sheath directly or stimulates an autoimmune response to the myelin. Certain viral proteins appear to be similar to myelin antigens and it is possible that viruses are capable of triggering the reaction that leads to MS. The immune system therefore reacts to a foreign antigen and to the myelin because they have similar molecular features. Immune system T-cells become activated by a myelin antigen and cross the blood–brain barrier. Researchers believe that a breach of the barrier is induced by an inflammatory process that increases adhesion molecules on endothelial cells, which in turn allows myelin sensitive lymphocytes into the central nervous system (CNS) (Halper and Holland, 1998). Early studies that tried to isolate a specific virus causing MS found high levels of measles antibodies in the cerebro spinal fluid (CSF) of sufferers. After an infection such as measles, antibody levels usually return to normal levels. Persistently elevated levels suggest that the virus is not completely removed following the initial attack (O'Brien, 1987). Individuals with MS have been found to have elevated, up to twofold, serum and CSF titres of antibodies, to many viruses, including measles, mumps, herpes simplex type 1, rubella and parainfluenza (Thompson *et al.*, 1993) (Schenk, 1993).

Immunological

Some support the view that MS is an autoimmune disease, influenced, for example, by hormonal changes at puberty (Pinn, 1997). Most individuals with MS have been found to have abnormalities of the CSF indicative of autoimmune disease (Schenk, 1993). Approximately 90 per cent of people with the disease have been found to have particularly increased immunoglobulin (IgG) and oligoclonal bands. Suppressor lymphocyte function is altered and acute deteriorations are accompanied or possibly preceded by defective immunoregulation, allowing unimpeded damage to the myelin membrane and oligodendrocytes. A rebound elevation in suppressor function accompanies remission (Thompson *et al.*, 1993).

Myelin Loss

The normal role of T-lymphocytes is to recognize foreign particles. There are T-cells, which are known as auto-reactive T-cells, circulating in healthy individuals, that recognize 'self'. In a healthy individual T-cells are strictly regulated by the immune system. In MS this control fails, and the auto-reactive T-lymphocytes become stimulated and breach the normally impenetrable blood–brain barrier, coordinating an attack on myelin, by recruiting macrophages and secreting inflammatory cytokines. This inflammatory response damages myelin in scattered areas throughout the CNS, and the characteristic lesions of MS occur (Watkiss and Ward, 2001).

Genetic

It has been found that relatives of persons with MS have a much higher incidence of the disease than the general population. Several studies have demonstrated an increased risk among siblings and even distant relatives (Schenk, 1993). First-degree relatives of a family member with MS have a 15 times greater incidence of the disease than the general population. A person with an identical twin with MS has a 20 per cent chance of developing it – 300 times greater than in the general population (Thompson *et al.*, 1993).

Some individuals, as well as being exposed to a virus, may have an inborn or acquired vulnerability to the disease. Immunologists have found that particular human leucocyte antigens (HLAs) were found more frequently in MS sufferers (O'Brien, 1987). The function of HLA is participation in immune responsiveness. HLA typing undertaken on Northern Europeans with MS has shown an excess of HLAs in comparison with the incidence of these antigens in the general population. This cannot be taken as a reliable diagnostic test, however, as these antigens can be found in healthy individuals and 30 per cent of MS sufferers may not be positive for these antigens. Some indigenous populations (Zulus, for example) are commonly positive in certain HLAs but MS is rare (Hopkins, 1993).

Social and Physical

Mayer (1981) correlated both social and physical factors with the areas of high prevalence of the disease. Climatic and geographical factors such as latitude, hours of sunshine and mean annual temperature were highly correlated with the prevalence rate, as were a series of factors associated with the social and economic development of the areas. The geographical relationship of the disease with nutrition and diet has been explored. It has been suggested that susceptibility to demyelination may be due to an increase in the proportion of saturated fatty acids in cerebral lipids relative to unsaturated fatty acids (Dick, 1976). A high correlation between the geographical distribution of MS and the consumption of animal fat was highlighted by Swank (1950). Epidemiological data, however, is not on a large enough scale or sufficiently detailed to be convincing, according to Acheson (1985). It has also been suggested that there may be a fault with the way in which MS sufferers metabolize essential fatty acids. Many patients have been found to have low levels of linoleic acid, leading to treatment with dietary supplements, such as oil of evening primrose, which has a high content of linoleic acid. The possible link with certain animal diseases that have similar characteristics to MS has also been investigated (O'Brien, 1987). The general hypothesis that MS is an acquired exogenous (environmental) disease, the acquisition of which takes place years before the clinical onset, is reinforced by data that suggest that risk factors may be altered by migration at an appropriate age. There is evidence of 'epidemics' of the disease. A significant number of cases occurred in the Faroe Islands during the period 1943–70 following war-time British army occupation. There was no evidence of MS before this period in the islands and it was thus hypothesized that MS may be transmitted, which suggests a viral agent (Robinson, 1988).

Epidemiological

There is a large variation in the worldwide distribution of MS and epidemiologists have sought to identify relating environmental, genetic and other predisposing factors to the international differences in the prevalence of MS. The frequency of MS increases with distance from the equator in both the Northern and Southern hemispheres. Researchers have identified significant correlations between the prevalence of MS and the degree of geographical latitude; the prevalence of MS approaching zero in the tropics and increasing to the north and south. A north–south pattern of MS prevalence is observed in Europe. In the case of the UK, Scotland (particularly north-east Scotland) has a relatively high rate of MS mortality and prevalence. Specifically, there has been clustering of MS in the Orkneys over and above that which would have been predicted in relation to the latitude hypothesis (O'Brien, 1987).

The prevalence of MS then is very low in warm climates and increases in temperate and colder climates. Given the geographical distribution of MS one way to find out more about the disease has been to observe migrants from low-risk areas to high-risk areas and vice versa. Such studies help researchers to investigate whether the disease is genetically determined, in which case migration would have little impact on individual risk, or environmentally determined. The epidemiological evidence points to an environmental influence, the prevalence of which increases with distance from the equator (or a protective influence with a reciprocal distribution) and which is operative during childhood and adolescence (Acheson, 1985). Studies have shown that persons who move from areas of higher prevalence to areas of lower prevalence after 15 years of age retain the risk of MS at the level of their previous environment. Individuals below 15 years of age acquire the risk prevalence of the new environment (Chipp *et al.*, 1992). For example, those who migrate in early childhood to low-risk zones, such as South Africa, acquire the lower risk of their new home. However, other studies have shown that in high-risk areas, the illness can still be acquired in adult life (Hopkins, 1993).

Anatomy and Physiology Relative to the Cerebral Neurones

The nervous system is the system of communication between the various parts of the body. It is the mechanism whereby sensations of all kinds are received from the environment and from the tissues and organs of the body itself. It is also responsible for the interpretation of these sensations and for initiating action by sending impulses to other parts of the nervous system and other organs of the body.

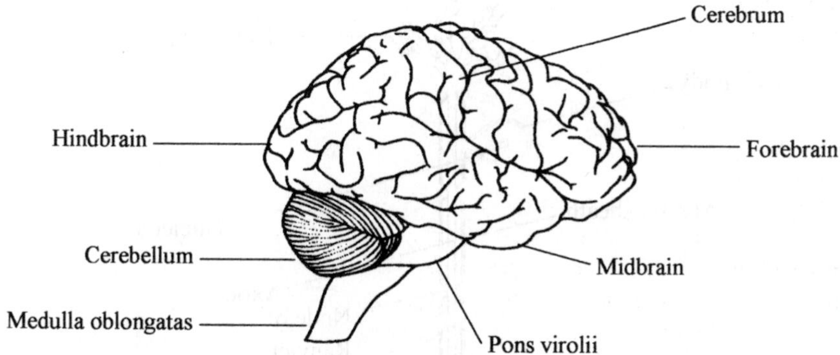

Figure 7.2 The brain

The nervous system can be divided into

- The central nervous system, consisting of the brain (Figure 7.2) and spinal cord.
- The peripheral nervous system, including the autonomic nervous system.

(Jackson and Bennett, 1988)

There are two distinct classes of cell in the nervous system:

- Neurones
- Glial cells.

Neurones

The neurone is the basic unit of the nervous system. A typical neurone has four morphologically defined regions:

- Cell body
- Dendrites
- Axon
- Pre-synaptic terminals (see Figures 7.3 and 7.4).

Each region has a distinct function in the generation of signals (Kandel, 1995).

The Cell Body

This is the metabolic centre of the cell, containing the nucleus, which stores the genes of the cell, and the rough and smooth endoplasmic reticulum, which synthesizes the proteins of the cell (Kandel, 1995). Nerve cell bodies form the grey matter of the brain and spinal cord. The cell body is comparatively large, though its size and shape vary according to the position of the cell and its function. The cell body usually gives rise to two types of outgrowth, the dendrites and the axon. Neurones can be divided according to the arrangement of the

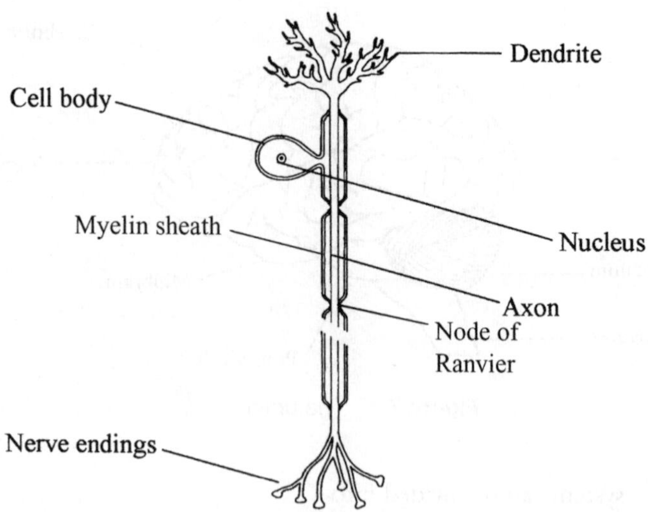

Figure 7.3 Sensory neurone

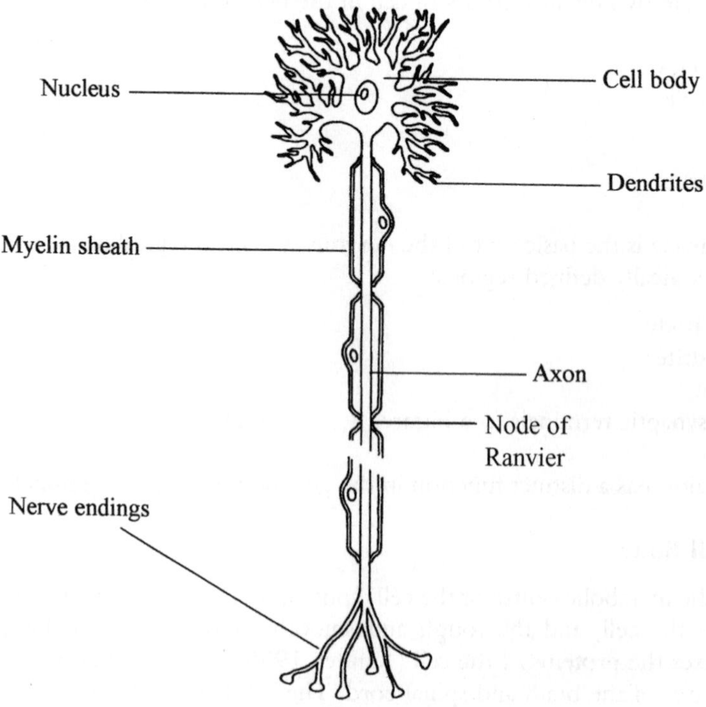

Figure 7.4 Motor neurone

axon and the dendrites as follows:

- A multipolar neurone has one axon and many dendrites arising from the cell body (Jackson and Bennett, 1988). These are the most numerous types: the dendritic processes vary in number and their degree of branching. Most of the neurones in the CNS are multipolar (Seeley *et al.*, 1989).
- A bipolar dendrite has one axon and just one dendrite, that is, one process at each end of the cell. The dendrite is often specialized to receive the stimulus and the axon conducts action potentials to the CNS. Bipolar neurones are components of some sensory organs, such as olfactory receptors of the nasal cavity and rods and cones of the eye (Seeley *et al.*, 1989).
- A unipolar neurone has one process arising from the cell body, which then divides into two branches, the axon and the dendrite (Jackson and Bennett, 1988). Most sensory neurones are unipolar (Seeley *et al.*, 1989).

Dendrites

Most neurones have several dendrites and these branch out in tree-like fashion, serving as the main apparatus for receiving signals from other nerve cells.

The Axon

There is usually only one axon, and it is tubular in shape. It grows out from a specialized region in the cell body. The diameter of axons varies. The axon is the main conducting unit of the neurone, capable of conveying electrical signals along distances that range from as short as 0.1 millimetre to as long as 2 metres. Many axons split into several branches, conveying information to different targets.

The electrical signals propagated along the axon are called action potentials. To ensure high-speed conduction of action potentials, large axons are surrounded by a fatty insulating sheath called myelin (Kandel, 1995). This myelin sheath is produced by Schwann cells, which surround the nerve fibres and the sheath, providing a covering. This layer of cells is called the neurilemma (Jackson and Bennett, 1988). This sheath is interrupted at regular intervals by the nodes of Ranvier, and it is at these uninsulated sites along the axon that the action potential becomes regenerated (Kandel, 1995). At these gaps the nerve fibre is in contact with the surrounding tissues and can take in nutrients and excrete waste materials. Myelinated nerves form the white matter of the brain and spinal cord. Myelinated nerves pass nerve impulses much more quickly than non-myelinated nerves (Jackson and Bennett, 1988).

Pre-synaptic terminals

Near its end the axon divides into fine branches that make contact with other neurones. The point of contact is the synapse. The cell transmitting a signal is called the pre-synaptic cell and the cell receiving the signal is the post-synaptic cell. Specialized swellings on the axon's branches serve as the transmitting site in the pre-synaptic cell. These pre-synaptic terminals do not communicate anatomically with the post-synaptic cell. Instead the two cells are separated at the synapse by a space (Kandel, 1995).

Glial Cells

Nerve cell bodies and axons are surrounded by glial cells. There are between 10 and 50 times more glial cells than neurones in the CNS of vertebrates. There are three predominant types of glial cells:

Oligodendrocytes

Oligodendrocytes are small cells with many processes. In white matter these participate in myelination; in grey matter they surround the cell bodies of neurones, providing support. A single oligodendrocyte forms myelin sheaths around many axons by wrapping its plasma membrane around the axons (Kandel, 1995).

Schwann Cells

These cells surround and form myelin sheaths around the larger nerve fibres in the peripheral nervous system. They are functionally similar to oligodendrocytes. Schwann cells are vital to the process of peripheral nerve fibre regeneration (Marieb, 2001). Each of several Schwann cells, positioned along the length of a single axon, forms a segment of myelin. The sheath assumes its form as the inner tongue of the Schwann cell turns around the axon several times, wrapping it in concentric layers of membrane. The intervals between the segments of myelin are the nodes of Ranvier (Kandel, 1995).

Astrocytes

Astrocytes are characterized by their star-like shape and by the broad end feet of their processes. They are the most abundant and most versatile glial cells. Their numerous radiating processes cling to neurones and cover nearby capillaries, supporting and bracing the neurones and anchoring them to the blood capillaries, their nutrient supply lines. Astrocytes have roles to play in making exchanges between capillaries and neurones, guiding the migration of young neurones and helping to determine capillary permeability. They also control the chemical environment around neurones, most importantly 'mopping up' leaked potassium ions and recapturing and recycling released neurotransmitters. Glucose provides the fuel source for producing the ATP (adenosine triphosphate) needed to carry out their activity. The electrical charge and ion types outside nerve fibres must be just right for nerve impulses to be conducted (Marieb, 2001).

The roles of glial cells

- They serve as supporting elements, providing structure and firmness to the brain.
- They separate and occasionally insulate groups of neurones from each other.
- Two types of glial cells produce myelin.
- Some glial cells are scavengers, removing debris after injury or neuronal death.
- They buffer and maintain concentrations of potassium ions in the extracellular space; some also take up and remove chemical transmitters released by neurones during synaptic transmission.
- During development of the brain, certain classes of glial cells guide the migration of neurones and direct the outgrowth of axons.
- Some glial cells help with the formation of a special, impermeable lining in the capillaries and venules of the brain, creating a blood–brain barrier, which prevents toxic substances in the blood entering the brain.
- There is some evidence, albeit inconclusive, to suggest that some glial cells play a role in nourishing nerve cells.

(Kandel, 1995)

Pathophysiology

Axons (nerve fibres) are protected by a segmented myelin sheath that is maintained by 'supportive' cells such as oligodendrocytes.

The functions of myelin are

- To act as an insulator
- To protect from pressure or injury
- To supply nutrients to the fibre
- To speed up the flow of the nerve impulses through the axon.

Any damage to the myelin will delay or interrupt the transmission impulses as they travel from the brain, down through the spinal cord and out to various parts of the body. In the early stages of MS there is the capacity for myelin to regenerate, although it rarely grows back as before. This probably plays a part in the disease remission. Axonal loss can also occur and, as this is irreversible, accounts for permanent disability (Watkiss and Ward, 2001).

Multiple foci of demyelination are distributed randomly within the white matter of the brainstem, cerebellum, spinal cord, optic nerve and cerebrum.

They occur randomly, but typically in the periventricular area of the brain in close proximity to blood vessels. There may be more than one active plaque at any one time, but the numbers of lesions do not necessarily equate with the extent of disability or severity of symptoms (Watkiss and Ward, 2001).

The external surface of the brain appears normal, but brain weight may be diminished and the ventricles may be enlarged. Proliferation of astrocytic processes, which transform the lesion into a glial scar, is the most characteristic feature. During the demyelination process (primary demyelination), myelin is removed, with the release of free fat. This triggers local inflammation, marked by an accumulation of lymphocytes, which cluster around the plaque and cause swelling to occur (Thompson *et al.*, 1993). Lymphocyte proliferation at the lesion releases cytokines and antibodies, further destroying myelin (Halper and Holland, 1998). As the lesions age, the lipid products of myelin breakdown are removed by phagocytosis. Myelin is replaced with a distinct fibrous plaque. The fact that the myelin does not grow back suggests that oligodendrocytes are destroyed early in the process. The demyelination leads to four significant central disturbances: a decrease in nerve conduction velocity, nerve conduction block (frequency related), differential rate of transmission impulses and complete failure of impulse transmission. These disturbances and the wide distribution of degeneration account for the variety of clinical signs and symptoms experienced (Thompson *et al.*, 1993). The primary process of demyelination and the formation of plaques or lesions leave the axons exposed but initially appear not to damage them. Remission of symptoms occurs when demyelinated areas are healed by sclerotic tissue, however, symptoms become permanent when the nerve fibre degenerates. The plaques are multiple in space, being scattered throughout the CNS and in time, as the disease progresses. The plaques are confined to the CNS rather than the peripheral nervous system; in the latter the myelin sheaths are of a different chemical makeup (O'Brien, 1987).

Concurrent processes of demyelination

- Breakdown of myelin structure
- Lysis of oligodendrocytes
- Activation of astroglial processes

Clinical Manifestations

The range of symptoms is vast because plaques of demyelination can occur anywhere in the CNS, and in cranial nerves containing oligodendroglial cells. Three main groups of symptoms predominate however, due to demyelination in the optic nerve, the brain stem or the spinal cord (Sutton, 1998) (see Table 7.1).

Table 7.1 Classification of symptoms

Cerebral	*Brainstem*	*Cerebellum*	*Spinal*
■ Optic neuritis ■ Seizures ■ Hemiparesis ■ Hemisensory loss ■ Dysphasia ■ Emotional and intellectual changes	■ Dysarthria ■ Nystagmus ■ Vertigo ■ Diplopia ■ Weakness of abducion of one eye ■ Facial weakness ■ Internuclear ophthalmoplegia	■ Motor ataxia ■ Hypotonia ■ Asthenia ■ Charcot's triad may be observed	■ Spastic paresis ■ Lhermitte's sign ■ Heaviness and dragging of one or both legs ■ Paresthesia ■ Bladder dysfunction

Chipp *et al.*, 1992; Hopkins, 1993.

Demyelination in the Optic Nerve

This is called optic neuritis and is a common presenting symptom. Blurring or loss of vision, loss of intensity of colours or loss of visual acuity may feature and there may also be localized pain.

Demyelination may occur in the olfactory and auditory nerves, the only other cranial nerves where oligodendroglial cells are present. Unilateral deafness is sometimes a problem and special tests of olfaction may show evidence of plaques.

Brainstem

As the brainstem is the pathway for many nerves, demyelination may result in a variety of symptoms. Problems with balance coordination of limbs, intention tremor, and speech and swallowing problems are common occurrences.

Spinal Cord

Lower damage may result in difficulty in walking and tingling, pain and burning sensations in the legs. This may also link to spasticity due to increased muscle tone. Similar symptoms will occur in the arms or torso when higher damage has occurred. Bladder problems are common; approximately 59 per cent of people with MS experience some difficulty (Kraft, 1986).

Paroxysmal Symptoms

These come on suddenly, might occur frequently and generally disappear quickly (for example, trigeminal neuralgia).

Unthoff's Phenomenon

An increase in body temperature following exercise or a warm bath will cause a temporary worsening of symptoms.

Charcot's Triad

Dysarthria, intention tremor and nystagmus.

Lhermitte's Sign

On bending the head forwards a shower of tingling spreads down the arms to the hands and sometimes to the trunk and legs.

Fatigue

This is an overwhelming type of exhaustion that can occur after minor exertion. This is a common symptom from the early stages of the disease.

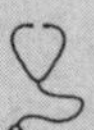

Nursing action point

- Advise the patient to plan activities that include rest periods.

Psychological Aspects

Newly diagnosed people may go through a stage of bereavement as they come to terms with the diagnosis. They may experience feelings of denial and anger, which may be directed at their family or healthcare professionals.

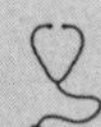

Nursing action points

- Assess the psychological impact of diagnosis upon the patient.
- Recognize signs of denial and anger as reflecting underlying stress and anxiety.

Clinical Signs and Symptoms related to Areas of Dysfunction

Motor Area

Weakness, paralysis, spasticity and abnormal gait.

Sensory Area

Paresthesias, Lhermitte's sign, decreased temperature perception, decreased propioreception.

Cranial Nerve

Blurred central vision, faded colours, blind spots (optic neuritis), diplopia, dysphagia, facial weakness, numbness and pain.

Cerebella

Dysarthria, tremor, inco-ordination, ataxia, vertigo.

Bladder and Bowel

Urinary frequency, urgency, hesitancy, nocturia, retention and incontinence. Faecal urgency, constipation and incontinence.

Cognitive

Decreased short-term memory, difficulty in word finding and learning new information, short attention span, decreased concentration, emotional lability.

Sexual Dysfunction in Women

Decreased libido and genital sensation, decreased ability to experience orgasm.

Sexual Dysfunction in Men

Erectile, orgasmic and ejaculatory dysfunction (Beare and Myers, 1994).

Prognostic Indicators

Prognosis is better when

- Patient is female.
- Onset of disease is before age 35.
- There are few lesions on MRI.
- There is complete recovery after a relapse.
- There is a long period between the onset and progressive phase (15 + years).
- There are early visual and sensory symptoms.
- There are no mobility/cerebral signs five years after onset.

Prognosis is worse when

- Patient is male.
- Onset is at age older than 35 years.
- There is a short time between the onset and start of progressive phase (less than ten years).
- Cerebellar symptoms and signs are present.
- Mobility problems and cerebellar signs are present five years after the onset.
- There are multiple lesions on MRI.
- There are residual deficits.

(Barnes, 1997; Watkiss and Ward, 2001)

Diagnostic Investigations

History

An initial thorough clinical history and neurological examination are essential.

Multiple sclerosis is often difficult to diagnose accurately because the symptoms are so numerous. Diagnosis is essentially clinical as there is no single definitive diagnostic test.

Diagnostic investigations

- Lumbar puncture
- Radiological tests
- Evoked potential tests

Lumbar Puncture

- There may be a mild rise in cell count (Allan and Craig, 1994). There is no particular correlation between the cell count and the duration of the disease, the degree of disability or whether the patient is in relapse or remission (Hopkins, 1993).
- An elevated gamma globulin in the CSF that is not associated with an elevation in the blood is very suggestive of MS; especially if the CSF total protein is low or normal (Clark, 1991).
- In 90 per cent of patients, oligoclonal banding is present. This is a significant property of IgG elevation. These bands are consistent and stable during the course of the illness and their intensity does not correlate with the clinical progress of the disease. Oligoclonal bands may represent an antibody response to an antigen such as a virus but equally may be synthesized in response to an antigen liberated by demyelination caused by a quite separate primary event (Hopkins, 1993).

- Myelin basic protein (MBP) is liberated into the CSF at the time of a relapse and higher levels are found in cases where the disease is running a more aggressive course (Hopkins, 1993). This test involves a radioimmunoassay of CSF for the presence of MBP (Clark, 1991).

Radiological Tests

Computerized Axial Tomography (CT) Scan

This is a radiological technique that produces images of the brain and allows neurologists to identify some lesions present and the generalized catastrophic changes. The accuracy with which CT scans can be interpreted, however, depends upon the density and size of the lesions. This depends upon the contrast they make against the surrounding matter (O'Brien, 1987).

Magnetic Resonance Imaging (MRI)

This is a more sophisticated test and provides more extensive information. Radio frequency radiation is used to excite hydrogen nuclei. Grey matter contains more water than white matter and therefore more hydrogen. Demyelinated plaques have lost much of their lipid content, replaced in part by water, and can thus be detected by MRI (O'Brien, 1987). Gadolinium, a chemical compound, administered during repeated scans, enables old lesions to be distinguished from new lesions (Clark, 1991).

X-rays and Myelograms

These are often used to eliminate other disorders and support a diagnosis of MS.

Evoked Responses

Visual/Auditory/Somatosensory Evoked Response Potential Tests

These tests measure the delay found between the application of a stimulus and the initial response. The visual evoked potential measures the conduction rate between the retina and the occipital lobe of the brain. The auditory evoked potential is used to identify lesions in the brainstem. Conduction in the nerve tracts that are carrying pain and touch sensations are measured by the somatosensory evoked potential.

Probable and Definite Multiple Sclerosis

Diagnostic criteria as suggested by Poser *et al.* (1983) distinguish between two groups of cases, essentially definite and probable MS, each with two clinical and laboratory supported sub-groups. The presence or absence of clinical and/or laboratory findings based on the diagnostic criteria help to clarify the diagnosis.

Potential precipitating factors

- Trauma
- Post-natal period
- Immunization

Trauma

Early claims that there is an increased chance of relapse following trauma have not been substantiated by case control and prospective studies; however, if a new episode begins after trauma, symptoms appear more often in the traumatized limb than would be expected by chance (Hopkins, 1993).

Post-natal Period

There is no increased chance of relapse during pregnancy. There is, however, two to three times the risk of relapse during the first six months after the birth than at any other time. In the months after having a baby, between 20 and 75 per cent of women have some sort of relapse. Such relapses usually make no difference to long-term disability (Graham, 1988). It is not known whether these relapses are due to the hormonal changes taking place during the puerperium or to the extra demands of caring for the newborn infant.

Immunization

Acute demyelinating encephalitis did occur following smallpox vaccination and it was therefore considered unwise to vaccinate MS patients. Although there is no proven ill effect of immunization against other infective agents, many neurologists prefer to avoid immunization unless absolutely necessary (Hopkins, 1993).

Some patients may attribute relapses to factors such as getting cold or wet, physical fatigue and emotional stress. Some neurologists feel that myelography may induce exacerbation (Hopkins, 1993).

Treatment

- Drug therapy
- Modified diet
- Hyperbaric oxygen
- Immunosuppression

Drug Therapy

Corticosteroids (Prednisolone; Methylprednisolone)

In acute episodes intravenous injections of a corticosteroid, typically methylprednisolone, are used to reduce CNS inflammation. This usually produces a faster improvement than intramuscular injections of adrenocorticotrophic hormone (ACTH) or oral prednisolone.

Beta Interferons (Betaferon (beta 1b); Avonex (beta 1a))

These drugs reduce the relapse rate in MS and delay long-term accumulation of disability. Interferon beta 1b has to be given by subcutaneous injection usually on alternate days. Interferon beta 1a is given once a week by intramuscular injection.

Co-polymer 1

This is a synthetic polypeptide with some resemblance to MBP. Its exact mode of action in MS is not known but studies have shown a reduction in the relapse rate similar to that seen with beta interferon. It is given daily by subcutaneous injection (Barnes, 1997).

Baclofen

This works within the CNS and is used to counter spasticity, by depressing the neurotransmitters that cause the spasticity. Physiotherapy can be an effective alternative treatment.

Oxybutin

This drug relaxes smooth muscle and is commonly used to combat bladder problems. Reducing caffeine intake may also help to reduce spasms.

Amytriptiline

This is commonly used as an antidepressant drug but in small doses it may be used to reduce pain experienced by MS patients. It works by reducing the person's perception of pain. The effects may take some time to develop.

Carbamezapine

While this is a commonly used anti-epileptic drug it also helps to relieve pain in MS. The exact action is unknown but it is believed to stop the short-circuiting of the nerves.

Cannabis

The effectiveness of the use of cannabis for people with MS is as yet unproven and the legalization of such use is currently the subject of controversy (Sutton, 1998).

Regimens

A vast number of different regimens have been proposed.

Modification of the Diet

A gluten free diet has been associated with improvement in some cases but is considered coincidental.

Supplementing the Diet with Polyunsaturated Fatty Acids

Patients in some studies have been found to have less linoleic acid in plasma-esterified cholesterol than normal subjects. Unsaturated fatty acids are constituents of oligodendroglial cell membrane and also precursors of prostaglandin and theoretically could influence the course of MS. There is no good evidence, however, that supplements such as sunflower oil or oil of evening primrose significantly alter the course of the disease.

Hyperbaric Oxygen

As plaques of demyelination tend to arise around small vessels it has been suggested that capillary microthrombi might initiate demyelination. Since plaques arise in areas around veins occluded by fat emboli and hyperbaric oxygen was seen as a way of forcing oxygen in. Controlled trials failed to show any benefit.

Immunosuppression

There has been no evidence from trials that immunosuppression is of any great benefit whereas it does carry the risk of significant adverse effects (Hopkins, 1993).

Nursing Interventions

A diagnosis of MS may have a devastating effect upon an individual given the chronic and unpredictable nature of the disease. The psychological impact upon the patient must be assessed along with the physical symptoms. The needs of the patient, and thus the demands made upon health resources are likely to vary considerably during the course of the disease. In many cases there will also be a need to assess the needs of carers, as many people with MS will ultimately be cared for in their own homes by relatives.

Connection

Chapter 2 (Family-centred Care) discusses how adopting a caring role can affect the health of carers. Ways in which nurses can support carers are also explored.

The needs of patients can be met by effectively using the nursing process. Given the range of symptoms a person may experience at different times an accurate assessment is a vital part of the care and should involve the patient in both the planning and decision-making. The nursing diagnoses must focus not only on functional impairment but also on teaching the patient and his or her family (Clark, 1991).

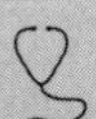

Nursing action points

Assess the patient in relation to the following

- sensory symptoms
- ocular symptoms
- motor symptoms
- vestibular/auditory functions
- mental behaviour symptoms
- hyperactive reflexes
- impotence
- loss of sphincter control
- urine and faecal incontinence
- loss of swallow and gag reflex
- Lhermitte's phenomenon
- Charcot's triad (intentional tremors, nystagmus and staccato speech) with brainstem involvement
- respiratory insufficiency or respiratory failure
- nutritional status

(Thompson *et al.*, 1993)

The overall aim of nursing interventions will be to help keep the symptoms under control and to ensure that patients remain independent for as long as possible and to avoid complications. This may require input from other agencies, such as social services, and part of the role of nurses is to work as members of a multidisciplinary team.

Nursing Interventions and Health Promotion

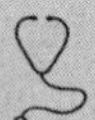

Nursing action points

- Monitor the patient for urinary problems and plan and implement the appropriate management.
- Monitor bowel activity and advise accordingly.
- Plan activities to minimize fatigue and ensure adequate rest periods.
- Assess the degree of spasticity and refer to a physiotherapist.
- Assess the level of pain and plan and implement care to manage pain.
- Ensure a well-balanced diet.
- Maintain skin integrity. Assess the risk of pressure sores and plan care to prevent pressure sore development.
- Maintain mobility according to the individual's capability.
- Maintain a safe environment.
- Adopt a multidisciplinary approach with appropriate referrals to other agencies.

Bladder and Bowel Problems

Continence problems can result from increased urinary frequency or incomplete emptying of the bladder. Incomplete emptying of the bladder may cause repeated urinary tract infections. Problems of urgency are often compounded by poor mobility. Cholinergic drugs, such as bethanechol, may be helpful for patients with atonic bladder while an anticholinergic drug, such as oxybutynin, may relieve the urinary frequency. Intermittent self-catheterization is the most effective way of treating incomplete bladder emptying, and the role of the nurse will be to teach the patient how to carry out the procedure. If the patient is unable to self-catheterize the carer may be taught how to catheterize. The patient should be encouraged to drink adequate fluids. Cranberry juice may be helpful in decreasing urinary tract infections (Schenk, 1993).

Constipation is a common problem and the patient should be advised to have a high roughage diet as well as adequate fluids. The use of prune juice may be helpful, as well as prescribed stool softeners and bulking agents. Patients should be advised to use laxatives judiciously in order to avoid dependence upon them. Abdominal massage can reduce problems (Sparrow, 1998). If faecal incontinence occurs it tends to be secondary to constipation. Assessment of the patient's usual bowel habits is important. A bowel-training programme may be helpful (Schenk, 1993).

Fatigue

This is possibly the most common symptom experienced. Amantadine may be helpful in reducing fatigue and the nurse may help the patient by advising him or her to take brief naps during the day. Also by helping the patient to identify patterns of fatigue the nurse may be able to suggest methods for conserving energy.

Spasticity

Approximately 90 per cent of people with MS will experience spasticity during the course of the disease. The clinical features of spasticity are as follows:

- Increased muscle tone
- Resistance to extending muscles
- Spasms, extensor or flexor
- Brisk tendon reflexes
- Alternating pattern of contraction and relaxation of muscle, in response to a prolonged stretch
- Sudden relaxation of resistance to stretch.

Spasms can be painful and disabling and sleep may be disrupted. Spasticity also affects emotional, social and psychological aspects of the individual's life. Early assessment and intervention can give the person a better quality of life. The role of the nurse involves careful monitoring of the patient's condition and the disease process (Currie, 2001).

Pain

Approximately 50 per cent of MS patients experience some degree of pain that may be associated with depression. Pain may be due to neurological or musculoskeletal impairment and its nature should therefore be identified through careful assessment. Nursing interventions include relaxation and stress reducing exercises (Sparrow, 1998).

Maintaining Adequate Nutrition

A well-balanced diet with plenty of vitamin rich foods is important. Obesity will add to the potential problems of reduced mobility.

Maintaining the Integrity of the Skin

Many people with MS have problems with mobility that prevents them from moving about freely or changing position easily. They may also have sensory losses that affect how they sense pressure. An important task for nurses in such cases is to educate patients and/or their carers, of the need to change position at least every two hours. If appropriate the nurse may arrange for specialist mattresses and other aids.

Promoting Activity and Mobility

A daily routine for rest and activity is important; patients should be advised to avoid exercising to the point of extreme fatigue and during an acute exacerbation are usually advised to rest. Muscle spasm due to nerve damage that increases muscle sensitivity is a common problem and must be treated to ensure that muscle function is not impaired. Medication such as oral baclofen or tizanidine may be prescribed (Sparrow, 1998).

Controlling the Environment

Hot baths can increase weakness and should therefore be avoided. People with MS should also be advised to avoid travelling during the hottest part of the day.

Referrals to other Agencies

Part of the nurse's skill is being able to recognize the need to refer patients for specialist help.

Physiotherapists. Physiotherapy is a vital part of care. A structured programme will help to limit or delay some of the long-term effects of the disease on the muscles and joints that result from the initial nerve damage (Campion, 1997b). Physiotherapists can assist in treating spasticity by the positioning and application of splints. Tremor affecting one in seven people with MS is most common in the head and neck but can be associated with movements such as reaching out to pick up an object. Physiotherapists can teach patients coping strategies (Sparrow, 1998).

Speech Therapists. Patients experiencing dysarthria and dysphagia require referral to speech therapists in order to identify the precise nature of the problem. They can then be taught how to cope with the difficulties of communicating and swallowing.

Occupational Therapists. Occupational therapy can help those with minor disability and those with severe disability. Assessment may identify the need for aids to assist patients to remain independent in feeding and dressing themselves and in the case of the more disabled, use of a wheelchair or the correct seating. If the level of a patient's disability changes or there is a significant change in their weight there must be a reassessment (Campion, 1997b).

Sex Therapists. MS patients, both men and women, may experience a variety of problems from loss of libido to impotence. Erectile impotence can be helped by intracorporeal injections but many patients may be too embarrassed to discuss problems of sexuality. The problems may be caused by cognitive as well as physical changes.

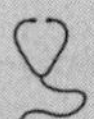

Nursing action points

- Be sensitive to the difficulties sexual problems may pose for both the patient and his or her partner.
- Arrange a referral to other healthcare professionals with specialist knowledge of sexual dysfunction relative to MS (Sparrow, 1998).

Counsellors/Clinical Psychologists/Psychiatrists. The psychological problems of MS may often be ignored (Barnes, 1997). Although only a small percentage of patients experience severe cognitive problems it is estimated that 50 per cent have some cognitive impairment (Sparrow, 1998). People may have slowness in speech and slowness in the ability to respond. They may have sudden explosive emotional outbursts of laughing or crying. Depression is common and early referral to trained counsellors and other healthcare specialists may help alleviate the problems. The effects upon the family should also be assessed as they may find it difficult to cope with the unpredictable behaviour of the patient. The potential stress experienced by carers should not be underestimated.

The Specialist Nurse

A specialist nurse can

- Provide a co-ordinated link between the patient, the family and the multidisciplinary team.
- Offer support and advice on the best management.
- Listen and communicate with all interested parties.
- Develop a sound knowledge of the disorder.
- Keep up to date with current research (Barnes, 1997).
- Be based at designated neurology centres (access to neurology services is important).
- Provide a link between primary and secondary health care teams within the context of local policy.
- Provide counselling support and advice for referred MS patients.
- Provide information and education on MS care to GPs, practice nurses and district nurses.

- Support MS patients during the early stages of new treatment as prescribed by the consultant neurologist.
- Network with appropriate agencies such as physiotherapists, occupational therapists and social services (Pinn, 1997).

Conclusion

Multiple sclerosis is a chronic disease of the CNS and the most common cause of severe disability in young adults. There is no cure at present but recent evidence suggests that it may be possible to influence the progression of the disease. The symptoms experienced by patients vary considerably and change over the course of the disease. Patients with relapsing remitting MS may need intensive nursing during an exacerbation and minimal help at other times. It is important that both healthcare services and social-care agencies are able to respond promptly to these needs. Often the person with MS sees many different healthcare professionals at many different clinics, all with a high degree of expertise but who are only treating one part of the whole. At the moment not many patients can self-refer to a specialist nurse during a relapse. Often they have to wait for a hospital appointment and struggle on with new symptoms. There is a clear need for specialist nurses and the purchasers of healthcare services should recognize the value of the role so that more specialists are employed in the future (Barnes, 1997). There is no cure for MS but good nursing and social care can help to keep the symptoms under control thereby ensuring that patients are able to function independently for as long as possible. Despite recent advances with disease modifying drugs, symptomatic management by a collaborative team of healthcare professionals is still the mainstay of treatment (Watkiss and Ward, 2001). The way forward in the care of people with MS is the development of specialist multidisciplinary teams to liaise and advise patients and their carers (Campion, 1997c). The overall aim of care should be to maximize access to care and other available resources for both patients and those who care for them.

References

Acheson, E. D. 1985, 'The epidemiology of multiple sclerosis' in Matthews, W. B., Acheson, E. D., Batchelor, J. R. and Weller, R. O. (eds), *McAlpine's Multiple Sclerosis.* Edinburgh. Churchill Livingstone.

Allan, D. and Craig, E. 1994, 'The nervous system' in Alexander, M. F., Fawcett, J. N. and Runaman, P. J. (eds), *Nursing Practice, Hospital and Home: The Adult.* Edinburgh. Longman Group UK Ltd, 325–68.

Allen, C. M. C. and Lueck, G. J. 1999, 'Diseases of the nervous system' in Haslett, C., Chilvers, E. R., Hunter, J. A. A. and Boon, N. A. (eds), *Davidson's Principles and Practice of Medicine.* London. Churchill Livingstone.

Barnes, M. and Jones, C. 1996, 'Multiple sclerosis: a new approach'. *Primary Health Care*, 6 (8), 17–24.

Barnes, M. P. 1997, 'Treating and nursing patients with multiple sclerosis'. *Nursing Standard*, 11 (23), 42–4.
Beare, P. and Myers, J. 1994, 'Principles and practice of adult health nursing'. *Mosby Year Book*, 2nd edn. St Louis. Mosby.
Campion, K. 1997a, 'Update: multiple sclerosis'. *Professional Nurse*, 13 (3), 169–71.
Campion, K. 1997b, 'Professional development. Multiple sclerosis – the role of the nurse'. Unit 41, Part 2. *Nursing Times*, 93 (11), 59–62.
Campion, K. 1997c, 'Professional development. Multiple sclerosis – professional issues'. Unit 41, Part 3. *Nursing Times*, 93 (12), 57–60.
Chipp, E., Clanin, N. and Campbell, V. 1992, *Neurological Disorders*. St Louis. Mosby Year Book Inc.
Clark, C. 1991, 'Nursing care for multiple sclerosis'. *Orthopaedic Nursing*, 10 (1), 21–32.
Currie, R. 2001, 'Spasticity: a common symptom of multiple sclerosis'. *Nursing Standard*, 15 (33), 47–52.
Dick, G. 1976, 'The aetiology of multiple sclerosis'. *Proceedings of the Royal Society of Medicine*, 69, 611–15.
Graham, J. 1988, *Multiple Sclerosis, Pregnancy and Parenthood*. Essex. The Multiple Sclerosis Resource Centre Ltd.
Halper, J. and Holland, N. 1998, 'New strategies. New hope. Meeting the challenge of multiple sclerosis'. *American Journal of Neurology*, 98 (10), 26–32.
Hopkins, A. 1993, *Clinical Neurology: A Modern Approach*. Oxford. Oxford University Press.
Jackson, S. M. and Bennett, P. J. 1988, *Physiology with Anatomy for Nurses*. London. Bailliere Tindall.
Kandel, E. R. 1995, 'Nerve cells and behaviour' in Kandel, E. R., Schwartz, J. H. and Jessell, T. M., *Essentials of Neural Science and Behaviour*. London. Appleton and Lange.
Kraft, G. 1986, 'Disability, disease duration and rehabilitation service needs in multiple sclerosis: patient perspectives'. *Archives of Physical Medicine and Rehabilitation*, 67, 164–78.
Lindsay, K. and Bone, I. 1991, *Demyelinating Diseases in Neurology and Neurosurgery Illustrated*. London. Churchill Livingstone.
Marieb, E. N. 2001, *Human Anatomy and Physiology*. 5th edn. New York. Addison Wesley Longman Inc. (an imprint of Benjamin Cummings).
Mattison, Dr. P. 1996, 'Hope for patients with multiple sclerosis'. *Geriatric Medicine*, 26 (2), 19–20.
Mayer, J. 1981, 'Geographic clues about multiple sclerosis'. *Annals of the Association of American Geographers*, 71, 28–39.
O'Brien, B. 1987, *Multiple Sclerosis*. London. Office of Health Economics.
Pinn, S. 1997, 'Multiple sclerosis management'. *Practice Nurse*, 14 (2), 115–8.
Poser, C. M., Patty, D. W., Scheinberg, L. *et al.* 1983, 'New diagnostic criteria for multiple sclerosis: guidelines for research protocols'. *Annals of Neurology*, 13, 227–31.
Revesz, T., Kidd, D., Thompson, A. J. *et al.* 1991, 'A comparison of the pathology of primary and secondary multiple sclerosis'. *Annals of Neurology*, 29, 53–62.
Robinson, I. 1988, *Multiple Sclerosis*. London. Routledge.
Sadovnick, A., Baird, P. and Ward, R. 1988, 'Multiple sclerosis: updated risks for relatives'. *American Journal of Genetics*, 29, 533–4.
Schenk, E. A. 1993, in Long, B. C., Phipps, W. J. and Cassmeyer, V. L., *Medical & Surgical Nursing – A Nursing Process Approach*. St Louis. Mosby Year Book Inc.
Seeley, R. R., Stephens, T. D. and Tate, P. 1989, '*Anatomy and Physiology*'. St Louis. Times Mirror/Mosby College Publishing.

Sparrow, S. 1998, 'The nurse's role in the care of people with MS'. *Nursing Times*, 94 (40), 54–5.
Sutton, L. 1998, 'Multiple sclerosis'. *Nursing Standard*, 12 (16), 48–51.
Swank, R. L. 1950, 'Multiple sclerosis; correlation of its incidence with dietary fat'. *American Journal of the Medical Sciences*, 220, 421–30.
Thompson, J. M., McFarland, G. K., Hirsch, J. E. and Tucker, S. M. 1993, *Clinical Nursing*, 3rd edn. London. Mosby.
Walton, J. N. 1977, *Brain's Diseases of the Nervous System*. 8th edn. Oxford. Oxford University Press.
Watkiss, K. and Ward, N. 2001, 'NT systems and diseases, nervous system part 8'. *Nursing Times*, 97 (14), 41–4.

8

Epilepsy

Norma Whittaker

Hippocrates (460–377 BC) was the first person to recognize epilepsy as an organic process of the brain. Epilepsy is the most common serious neurological disorder (Frost and Laville, 1998), yet no other is as misinterpreted and misunderstood (Royal College of Nursing [RCN], 1995). As well as being a common medical condition it carries a considerable social stigma (Goodridge and Shorvon, 1983). People with epilepsy have to cope with problems in almost every sphere of their lives (RCN, 1995).

Contents

Learning Objectives

By he end of the chapter you should be able to demonstrate knowledge of

- Factors relevant to the epidemiology and aetiology of epilepsy.
- Changes in the transmission of nerve impulses that give rise to a seizure and the different types of seizure.
- The way that epilepsy is diagnosed and treated.

- Nursing interventions that reflect the need to empower the patient while taking into account the chronic nature of the disorder.
- Nursing interventions that reflect the physical, psychological and social effects of epilepsy upon the individual.
- The role of the specialist nurse.

Definition of Epilepsy

The brain consists of a vast network of nerve cells (neurones) (Figure 8.1) with billions of electrical messages passing between them, controlling everything a person thinks, feels and does. The body has a balancing mechanism ensuring that these messages between nerve cells travel in an orderly manner. An altered chemical state in the brain causes messages to become scrambled resulting in excessive electrical activity with neurones firing off faster and in bursts. This disturbed activity triggers off a seizure. (The word epilepsy is from the Greek to 'seize' or to 'attack'.) Epilepsy is not an illness but a symptom. Someone is said to have epilepsy if they have repeated seizures of primary cerebral origin. The terms seizure, convulsion and fit are interchangeable (British Epilepsy Association [BEA], 1997).

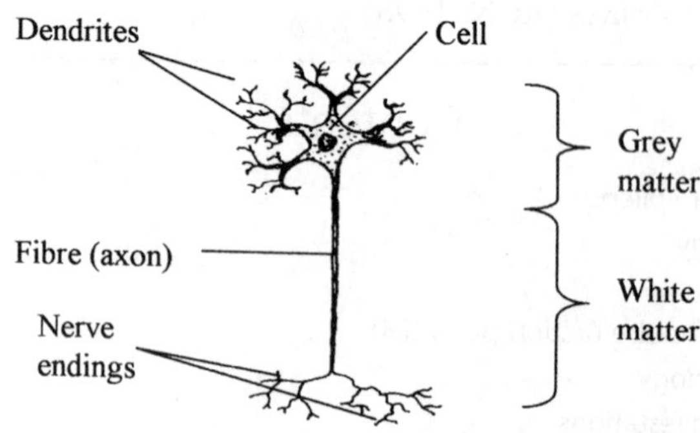

Figure 8.1 A neurone

Epidemiology

Several factors contribute to a lack of accurate data (Griffin, 1991):

- Doctors are not obliged to report diagnosed cases.
- Results of epidemiological data have shown considerable discrepancy due to differences in definitions of epilepsy, measurement methodologies and analytical methods (Holmes, 1987).
- Not all people with epilepsy symptoms report to a doctor.

It is estimated that 1 in 200 people experience recurrent seizures at some time in their life (Nursing Times, 1994). Frost and Laville (1998) suggest that the figure could be 1 in 135 people. Figures calculated on a prevalence rate of 5–10 per 1000 of the population in the United Kingdom (UK) would indicate that approximately 435 000 people in the UK might suffer from epilepsy. Seizures may occur at any age but are more common in the first 20 years of life and in elderly people. It is estimated that more than half of those who develop epilepsy will have had their first attack by the age of 15 years (Russell, 1996). According to a survey carried out by Sander and Thompson (1989) the proportion of elderly people affected is rising. At present 1 in every 100 elderly persons has an epileptic seizure. Epilepsy is the third most common neurological disorder to affect the elderly after strokes and dementia (Duncan, 1997). First seizures are twice as common over the age of 65 as between the ages of 25 and 64.

It is estimated that between 150 000 and 350 000 people have chronic epilepsy, defined as a tendency to have had seizures for more than five years. Of these, around one-third may experience more than one seizure a month (Epilepsy Explained, 1994). Males tend to be slightly more prone to developing epilepsy than females (Hopkins and Appleton, 1996). The prevalence of epilepsy is higher among people with learning disability than the general population. About 30 per cent of people with learning disability have some form of epilepsy and the incidence increases to 80 per cent in cases of severe learning disability (National Society for Epilepsy [NSE], 1995a). The average GP will have an estimated ten patients on active treatment for epilepsy and 15–20 patients who have had a seizure and not been treated or who have stopped treatment (Management Protocol for Epilepsy in General Practice, 1994). The overall mortality for people with epilepsy is between two and three times higher than that of the general population and even higher in the younger age groups. Causes of death include accidents such as drowning and road traffic accidents, status epilepticus and sudden unexpected death (Russell, 1996).

Aetiology

- No cause identified (idiopathic epilepsy)
- Symptomatic of some underlying cerebral pathology (symptomatic epilepsy).

No specific cause may be found in some 60 per cent of people who are said to have idiopathic epilepsy. For the remaining 40 per cent of epilepsy sufferers, epilepsy is a symptom of an underlying problem and can be associated with any form of cerebral pathology that is in part related to age (Buchanan, 1995).

Accident and Illness

Epilepsy related cerebral pathologies

- Head injury
- Brain tumours
- Infections
- Cerebrovascular disease and haemorrhages.

Head Injury

In all age groups, head trauma can produce seizures within a few days of experiencing concussion. The risk of developing epilepsy has been found to be higher if seizures occurred soon after the injury or if a haematoma was present (Jennett, 1962). These seizures do not necessarily predict the development of chronic epilepsy and such acute events should be viewed as reactive seizures, the head injury being the underlying precipitating factor (Griffin, 1991). Post-traumatic amnesia has also been implicated in the development of epilepsy: the longer its duration the greater the chance of the development of later epilepsy (Jennett, 1962).

Brain Tumours

These can cause epileptic seizures by interfering with the surrounding neurones (Scambler, 1989). The incidence of primary brain tumours, however, is low: approximately 10 per 100 000 per annum and, overall, only 35 per cent of patients will experience one or more seizures (Griffin, 1991).

Infections

Bacterial meningitis can damage cortical cells at any age. If antibiotic treatment is delayed or the infecting agent is resistant to the type of antibiotic given, there is the potential for the affected cortical cells to act as a focus for seizures in subsequent years. While viral meningitis is self-limiting and does not cause epilepsy, encephalitis can give rise to seizures. Cytomegalovirus and herpes are two of the more common viruses causing seizures in this way. HIV can also give rise to seizures, either by itself, or by depressing immunity so that other viruses invade the body and give rise to seizures (Hopkins and Appleton, 1996). Bacterial brain abscesses and parasites, *Toxocara* for example, can also cause seizures (Scambler, 1989). Meningitis due to tuberculosis is particularly associated with later epilepsy. Creutzfeldt–Jakob disease (CJD) is a rare disease caused by an infectious agent that is not bacteria or a virus, and affected adults may have seizures as part of the serious neurological disorder (Hopkins and Appleton, 1996).

Connection

Chapter 10 (Infectious Diseases) describes some common types of pathogenic microorganisms.

Cerebrovascular Disease and Haemorrhages

Both conditions can cause destruction of brain tissue and lead to the formation of scar tissue. This will lead to aggravation of the surrounding nerve cells. Of patients suffering a stroke, approximately 10 per cent will subsequently develop epilepsy, usually within a year of the stroke. Pre-senile dementia, Alzheimer's disease, in which the cerebral neurones decrease, may be associated with seizures (Hopkins and Appleton, 1996). A number of degenerative disorders which start in childhood, including Batten's disease, present with frequent seizures. Multiple sclerosis can be complicated by both focal and generalized seizures (Griffin, 1991).

Connection

Chapter 6 (Stroke) details the relationship of these two disorders.

Seizures in the Newborn

Seizures are most likely to develop in new born babies due to

- Birth trauma
- Anoxia
- Hypoglycaemia
- Hypocalcaemia.

Birth Trauma

Seizures that begin after the first week and during the first year of life often reflect brain damage either before or during the birth. Such seizures tend to be relatively severe and difficult to control (Chadwick and Usiskin, 1987). Epilepsy is experienced quite commonly in individuals with learning difficulties (Peattie and Walker, 1995).

Anoxia

This may occur at birth due to

- Prolonged labour (depletion of oxygenated blood to the brain)
- The umbilical cord may become tightly wound around the baby's neck
- Cord prolapse
- Placental separation
- Low Apgar score.

Hypoglycaemia

The pathways of chemical metabolism in the newborn are very unstable. Severe hypoglycaemia resulting in seizures may occur in premature infants and babies born to women suffering from gestational diabetes.

Hypocalcaemia

One cause is early feeding with cow's milk, which is rich in phosphates. This results in increased renal excretion of calcium and subsequent low levels of calcium in the blood (Griffin, 1991). In later life other acquired metabolic disturbances may cause seizures, for example, chronic renal failure (Scambler, 1989). Dialysis has, however, reduced the frequency of seizures due to this cause (Hopkins and Appleton, 1996).

Congenital Malformation

Maldevelopment of blood vessels, known as an angioma, may give rise to seizures (Scambler, 1989). A more common cause of epilepsy is disorders of migration of nerve cells during fetal development. Some cells end up in the wrong place, the wrong layer of the brain or with the wrong connections (Hopkins and Appleton, 1996).

Associated Factors

A few associated factors that are likely to produce seizures are

- Inheritance
- Convulsive threshold
- Alcohol and drugs.

Inheritance

Up until 40 years ago, most doctors believed that inheritance was a major factor in causing epilepsy. While genetic factors contribute, these should be put into perspective. For many individuals the condition was not inherited and the likelihood of passing it on is small. There are, however, some genetic diseases, characterized by seizures, in which inheritance does play a part.

Neurofibromatosis and tuberous sclerosis are genetic diseases affecting the structure of nerve cells and surrounding tissues and inheritance of these diseases is through a dominant gene. The inherited gene may be recessive; examples are the rare disorders of metabolism of the brain, collectively known as the lipidoses (Hopkins, 1993).

There is also evidence that primary generalized epilepsy is inherited. The characteristic electroencephalograph (EEG) is seen in about 40 per cent of the siblings of children with primary generalized epilepsy, even if these siblings have not had any apparent seizures. The abnormality that gives rise to the EEG pattern is inherited but not necessarily expressed in clinically apparent seizures. A smaller proportion of the parents of such children will also show characteristic EEG changes that become much less frequent with age, so the absence of discharges in adult life does not mean that the parent did not have characteristic discharges in childhood. If the parent has primary generalized epilepsy, then about half of his or her children will carry the gene, but only one child in six will have definite seizures (Hopkins and Appleton, 1996).

Convulsive Threshold

Anyone can be made to have a seizure given a strong enough stimulus. In some people seizures may be due to an inherited disposition, those in whom they occur having a lower threshold to seizures and being sensitive to minor electrical disturbances (triggers) (Russell, 1996). The risk of a child inheriting epilepsy from a parent suffering from epilepsy as a result of a severe head injury and resultant cortical scarring is only marginally higher than the risk for the population at large. It is slightly higher due to the inherited convulsive threshold (Hopkins and Appleton, 1996).

Alcohol and Drugs

There is an association between chronic alcohol abuse and the occurrence of seizures, most seizures resulting from the withdrawal of alcohol (Mattson, 1983). Similarly, there is evidence to suggest that continued use of barbiturates over several weeks or months, followed by rapid withdrawal, may precipitate seizures. Antidepressant drugs of the tricyclic group have been found to lower the convulsive threshold and induce seizures in 0.2–4 per cent of patients receiving normal therapeutic doses (Feldman, 1983). It should be noted that many of these patients had been previously diagnosed as suffering from epilepsy or had predisposing risk factors, such as family history, brain damage and electroconvulsive therapy.

Precipitating Factors

> *Nursing action points*
>
> - Consider the following precipitating factors when advising a patient/promoting health:
>   - ☐ lack of sleep
>   - ☐ alcohol
>   - ☐ menstruation
>   - ☐ stress, worry and mood
>   - ☐ photosensitivity.

There are clearly a number of factors that appear to trigger seizures in some people with epilepsy.

Lack of Sleep

The changing electrical activity of the brain during drowsiness and sleep may give rise to seizures. Some individuals have all or virtually all of their seizures while asleep (nocturnal epilepsy), but this does not rule out the possibility of daytime seizures. Sleep deprivation has been shown to alter cerebral electrical activity. In practical terms this means that repeatedly staying up late may precipitate a seizure, particularly in young adults (Hopkins and Appleton, 1996).

Alcohol

Alcohol and sleep deprivation is a particularly bad combination (Buchanan, 1995). Drinking alcohol is said to remove inhibitions in a person's personality and a similar removal of inhibition of an epileptic focus may cause an individual to have a seizure. However, as the seizure often occurs when the blood alcohol is falling or is near to zero, other changes in body chemistry, particularly in the distribution of water within and outside cells, probably play a part in causing such seizures. Large quantities of beer (containing water and alcohol) may therefore be more likely to trigger a seizure than smaller quantities of wine or spirits (Hopkins and Appleton, 1996). Binge drinking is particularly hazardous (Buchanan, 1995).

Menstruation

Some women, particularly those who suffer partial seizures, experience more seizures around the time of their menstrual period. It is not known whether this increase in seizures is linked to the retention of fluid that often precedes menstruation or is the result of hormonal changes.

Stress, Worry and Mood

There is little evidence to suggest that stress causes epilepsy, but ample evidence that stress exacerbates seizures (Betts, 1992). As a general rule increasing anti-epileptic drugs (AEDs) does not bring a good response, indeed the consequential drowsiness and decreasing ability to function normally may increase the stress and fuel the seizures (Buchanan, 1995).

Mothers may claim that they can tell from their child's mood and behaviour that a seizure is imminent and some adults may experience a peculiar feeling of heaviness, depression or in some cases elation prior to having a seizure. It is not possible to tell whether the emotional changes cause the seizure, whether the mood and seizure are caused by a common factor or whether the mood change is in some way caused by a limited paroxysmal discharge that goes on to become an obvious clinically recognizable seizure.

Reflex Epilepsy – Photosensitivity

Some people experience seizures induced by flashing lights, such as in a discotheque, sunlight on water or sunlight filtering through trees. If a light is flashed in the eyes, in most individuals an obvious wave can be recorded in the occipital region of the brain. With repeated flashes, these waves follow the flash frequency. In a young person with photosensitive epilepsy, at a critical frequency, a totally different response of multiple spikes and waves occurs (the photoconvulsive response), and a seizure may be induced. Television epilepsy is encountered most commonly. The bigger the television screen and the nearer the child's proximity the greater the chance of a seizure being induced. If one eye is covered it has been shown that the photoconvulsive response cannot be elicited. Susceptible children should therefore be encouraged to cover one eye when approaching the television set. Video games have also been linked to seizure inducement. Non-specific stimuli, such as a loud noise, or anything that startles, may induce myclonic jerks and in some cases a generalized tonic–clonic seizure (Hopkins and Appleton, 1996). Of the people with epilepsy in the UK only a very small percentage are photosensitive (Russell, 1996).

The Nerve Impulse (Action Potential)

The nervous system is the important control and communication system of the body. There are billions of nerve cells; those nerves, that are carrying nerve impulses towards the CNS, are termed afferent or sensory nerves. Those nerves carrying impulses away from the CNS are called efferent or motor nerves (Rowett, 1988).

Connection

Chapter 7 (Multiple Sclerosis) gives further information on the disorder.

The physiological 'units' of the nervous system are nerve impulses or action potentials, which are like tiny electrical charges. Unlike ordinary electric wires, however, the neurones are actively involved in conducting nerve impulses. The strength of the impulse is maintained throughout the length of the neurone. The cells of some neurones initiate nerve impulses while others act as 'relay stations' passing on impulses or redirecting them (Wilson and Waugh, 1998). Neurones are highly irritable, which means that they are responsive to stimuli. When a neurone is adequately stimulated, an electrical impulse is conducted along the length of its axon. The response, or action potential, is always the same, regardless of the source or type of stimulation, and it underlies virtually all functional activities of the brain (Marieb, 2001).

In order for the nervous system to function, impulses must be transmitted along nerve fibres and passed from neurone to neurone. These nerve impulses can be likened to small electrical charges passing along the nerve fibre. These charges depend upon the concentration of various ions. The concentration of ions inside the nerve fibre is different to the concentration outside.

Inside the fibre: The concentration of potassium ions is high and that of sodium is low.

Outside the fibre: The concentration of potassium ions is low and that of sodium ions is high (Jackson and Bennett, 1988).

Transmission of the impulse, action potential, is due to the movement of ions across the cell membrane. In the resting state the nerve cell is polarized due to differences in the concentrations of ions across the plasma membrane. There is a different electrical charge on each side of the membrane that is called the resting membrane potential. At rest the charge on the outside is positive and inside it is negative (Wilson and Waugh, 1998).

Pumps in the cell membrane maintain this imbalance, potassium ions are pumped in and sodium ions out. Because the membrane is not very permeable to sodium ions, they cannot diffuse in again; however, potassium ions can slowly diffuse out of the nerve fibre. The unequal concentration of ions results in the inside of the fibre being negatively charged compared with the surrounding fluid (Jackson and Bennett, 1988).

When the end of the nerve is stimulated, the difference in charge between the inside and the outside of the fibre is reduced in the adjacent part of the cell. As soon as this difference reaches a certain threshold, the sodium pump stops working and the membrane becomes more permeable to sodium ions (Jackson and Bennett, 1988). Initially sodium ions flood into the neurone from the extracellular fluid and the potassium floods outward, causing depolarization, which creates a nerve impulse or action potential. Depolarization is very rapid, enabling the conduction of a nerve impulse along the entire length of a neurone in a few milliseconds. It passes from the point of stimulation in one direction only, which is away from the stimulation towards the area of resting potential. The direction of transmission is ensured because following depolarization it takes time for repolarization to occur. This period is called the refractory period during which restimulation is not possible. As the neurone returns to its original resting state, the action of the sodium pump expels sodium from the cell in exchange for potassium (Wilson and Waugh, 1998). In myelinated fibres, depolarization only occurs at the nodes of Ranvier. When an impulse occurs at one node, depolarization passes along the myelin sheath to the next node so that the flow of current appears to 'leap' from one node to the next. This is called salatory conduction. This also conserves energy because less repolarization is needed. In spite of differences in the speed of transmission down nerve fibres, ultimately the time taken from original stimulus to response depends mainly upon the number of synapses involved. At these, transmission is chemical and not electrical (Rowett, 1988).

Synapse and Chemical Transmitters

There is always more than one neurone involved in the transmission of a nerve impulse from its origin to its destination, whether it is sensory or motor. There is no anatomical continuity between neurones, and the point at which the nerve impulse passes from one to another is called the synapse (see Figure 8.2). At its

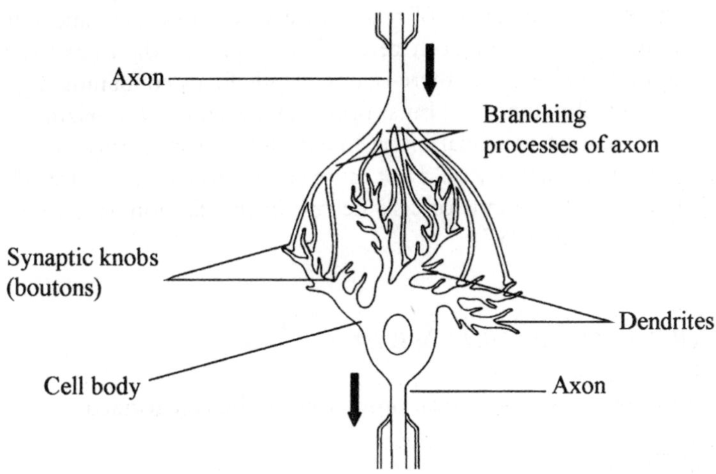

Figure 8.2 A synapse

free end the axon of one neurone breaks up into minute branches that terminate in small swellings called synaptic knobs, which are in close proximity to the dendrites and the cell body of the next neurone. The synaptic cleft is the space between them. At the ends of the synaptic knobs there are spherical synaptic vesicles, containing chemical transmitters, which are released into synaptic clefts. Chemical transmitters are secreted by nerve cells, actively transported along the nerve fibres and stored in the vesicles. They are released by exocytosis, diffuse across the synaptic cleft and act on specific receptor sites on the postsynaptic membranes. Their action is short lived as immediately they have stimulated the next neurone they are either inactivated by enzymes or taken back into the synaptic knob. Usually chemical transmitters have an excitatory effect at the synapse but they are sometimes inhibitory (Wilson and Waugh, 1998).

Pathophysiology

In epilepsy, cortical neurones show abnormalities of membrane potential and firing patterns. The most prominent behaviour of neurones within the epileptic focus is the paroxysmal depolarization shift (PDS). The PDS is characterized by a slow membrane depolarization, which elicits a high frequency burst of action potentials. Epileptiform activity can spread to adjacent neurones so that other neurones may be excited to behave similarly. This occurs in spite of the epileptic focus being surrounded by a zone of strong inhibition (Elger and Lehnertz, 1994). The PDS can result from an imbalance between excitatory neurotransmitters (aspartate and glutamate) and/or inhibitory neurotransmitters (gamma-aminobutyric acid [GABA] related) or abnormalities of voltage-controlled membrane ion channels. (GABA is the main inhibitory transmitter at central synapses.) In primary generalized seizures, spike wave activity is generated in cortical structures with rapid spread of recurrent excitation (spikes) and inhibition (slow waves) to the whole of both cerebral hemispheres via a corticoreticular cortical loop. In partial seizures there is an epileptic focus containing a group of neurones which exhibit abnormal burst firing. The extent of the seizure is determined by the extent of neuronal involvement (Buchanan, 1995). A single cell behaving in an abnormal way would not cause anyone to have a seizure. This only happens when many thousands of cells behave in this fashion at the same time (Chadwick and Usiskin, 1987).

Classification of Epileptic Seizures

Partial or focal seizures have a local onset and can be categorized as

- Simple partial
- Complex partial

Simple Partial

The paroxysmal discharge spreads locally from a focus of abnormal cells. These seizures are almost certainly secondary to some area of cortical scarring or developmental abnormalities.

Consciousness is not impaired. Symptoms will reflect the function of the discharging area of the brain (Figure 8.3). These may involve

- Motor symptoms (formally called Jacksonian epilepsy)
- Sensory/somatosensory symptoms
- Autonomic symptoms
- Psychic symptoms
- Bizarre bilateral movements and behaviour (formally called frontal epilepsy)

Complex Partial Seizures – Impairment of Consciousness

- Simple partial features evolving to complex partial
- Impaired consciousness at onset
- Impairment of consciousness from onset with abnormal behaviour/sensation that includes auras, automatism, chewing, lipsmacking (formally called psychomotor/temporal lobe epilepsy)

Both simple and complex partial seizures may evolve to become secondarily generalized tonic–clonic seizures.

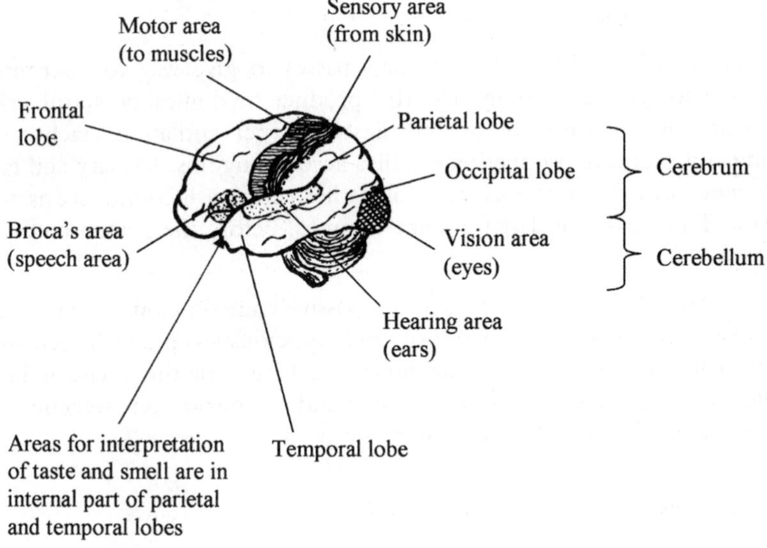

Figure 8.3 The cerebral cortex

Primary Generalized Seizures – Bilaterally Symmetrical, no Focal Onset

- Tonic–clonic (formally called grand mal)
- Tonic
- Atonic
- Clonic
- Myoclonic
- Absence (formally called petit mal)
- Infantile spasms
- Akinetic

Generalized absences must be distinguished from complex partial seizures. Generalized absences have no aura, the onset is abrupt and recovery of consciousness is immediate. The duration is brief and the individual usually has no awareness that a seizure has occurred. There are no automatisms.

Tonic–Clonic Seizures

Aura. The person may experience a warning that a seizure is imminent. This may be a smell, a taste, flashing lights or a particular sensation that the person comes to recognize as a warning. Not all people experience an aura.

Tonic Phase. Consciousness is lost, all the muscles contract and if the person is standing he or she will fall to the ground. The teeth are clenched and the tongue may be bitten. Muscular contraction forces air through the vocal cords causing a cry to be emitted. There is a brief period of apnoea and cyanosis and the person is unresponsive.

Clonic (Convulsive) Phase. The stiffness passes to give way to intermittent contraction and relaxation of muscles that produce rhythmical powerful jerking movements of the face, body and limbs. Hyperventilation, tachycardia, sweating and excessive production of saliva accompany this. Urinary and faecal incontinence can occur at this stage or earlier; urinary incontinence is more common. This phase can last for some minutes, before the person enters the final stage.

Post-ictal Phase(Coma). The person lies passively unconscious, often breathing stertorously. Normal colour returns and consciousness gradually returns to normal. This can last for up to an hour, the length of this phase is highly variable. Some may show signs of confusion and restlessness on awakening and may complain of a headache and wish to sleep.

Tonic Seizures

Sudden muscle rigidity. Short duration. May occasionally occur in patients with multiple sclerosis.

Atonic Seizures

Sudden loss of postural tone and collapse, with alterations of consciousness. Recovery is quick but injuries to the head and face, as a result of falling, are common.

Clonic Seizures

The distinction between these and myoclonic jerks is slight. If the jerks are multiple, the seizures tend to be called clonic.

Myoclonic Seizures

Marked by a brief loss of consciousness accompanied by involuntary muscular jerking of the body or limbs that may be rhythmical.

Absence Seizures

These occur almost exclusively in children and adolescents (Sander and Thompson, 1989), with girls experiencing them more than boys (Wallace, 1996). Characterized by a sudden, transistory loss of awareness and motor activity, the posture is maintained, the child stares blankly into space; the eyes roll upwards and all activity ceases. The impairment is so brief, typically lasting ten seconds, that the child is unaware of it and quickly resumes pre-seizure activity. The presence of clonic movements or automatisms leads to the condition being called 'complex typical absences'. Seizures may occur many times a day and may come to attention due to learning difficulties. Typical absence epilepsy implies absences not associated with the characteristic discharges on EEG. Onset in this case is less abrupt, is usually associated with other problems and is less responsive to AEDs (Buchanan, 1995). Absence seizures may progress to generalized tonic–clonic seizures.

Infantile Spasms

These are relatively uncommon, occurring more often in boys and commencing between 3 and 12 months of age. Aetiology can be defined in about 70 per cent of cases (Buchanan, 1995). Characterized by a brief, sudden flexion of the head, trunk and limbs, the infant may seem to be thrown forward or backwards with outstretched arms. The spasms occur in clusters, up to 40–50 at a time, over a five to ten minute period. The infant may appear distressed afterwards and cry. Spasms are more likely to occur just as the child awakes from sleep or is about to fall asleep (Hopkins and Appleton, 1996).

Akinetic Seizures

Characterized by sudden loss of postural muscle tone (drop attacks).

Unclassified Seizures

Seizures that do not fit easily into the categories described.

Status Epilepticus

This is a state of generalized seizure that occurs without full recovery between attacks and may happen with any type of seizure. In the case of tonic–clonic seizures this is a medical emergency. The lack of normal respiratory movements in conjunction with the extreme muscular contractions during seizures places considerable stress upon the cardiovascular system. Precipitating factors include withdrawal of AEDs, fever and infection. Intervention aims to stop the seizures as quickly as possible and maintain adequate oxygenation.

Epileptic Syndromes

The International League Against Epilepsy proposed a revised classification of epilepsy in 1989. In this classification an epileptic syndrome is characterized by both clinical and EEG findings. On the clinical side, the age at onset of seizures and the family history is taken into consideration. The seizure type(s) and neurological findings are all relevant to the classification, as is the appearance of the EEG between and during seizures. This allows a greater precision of diagnosis and of prognosis than simply classifying seizure types (Hopkins and Appleton, 1996).

Sudden Unexplained Death in Epilepsy (SUDEP)

Until a few years ago there was little known about this and it was considered to be a rare phenomenon. Research, however, now indicates that it is not that rare; there are around 500 cases in the UK each year. Research to date indicates a number of factors that may predipose individuals to SUDEP.

Risk Factors

- Sub-therapeutic levels of AEDs have been noted in a significant number of cases.
- Increasing number of AEDs taken at the same time.
- Frequent changes of drug dose.
- Poor seizure control.
- Seizures occurring during sleep.
- Being alone at the time of the seizure.
- Usually associated with tonic–clonic seizures, both idiopathic and symptomatic in nature. Some studies indicate that in the majority of cases there was pre-existing damage to the brain, for example, structural brain lesions.

- Statistics indicate that it is more likely to occur in young adults, particularly males. However, the fact that epilepsy is more common in males may partially explain this.

Causes

Changes in breathing and heart rate are the most likely causes so far indicated, but further research is needed. Usually breathing starts again as a tonic–clonic seizure ends but in some cases this may not happen. There is evidence that the part of the brain that controls breathing can be stimulated by moving the limbs, which is what happens when an individual is turned into the recovery position. This may possibly explain the risks associated with being alone or having a seizure during sleep.

Feedback from relatives has indicated a strong preference for having information about SUDEP. Complete prevention may not be possible but precautionary measures, based upon current information, may help to reduce the risk of SUDEP (BEA, 2001a).

Investigative Tests

- History
- Observation of attacks
- Electroencephalogram (EEG)
- Ambulatory EEG
- Videotelemetry
- Magnetic resonance imaging (MRI)
- Computerized axial tomography (CT)
- Blood tests
- Cerebral angiography
- Echoencephalogram
- Skull roentgenogram

History and Observation

The unpredictable and transitory nature of epilepsy makes it difficult to diagnose. It is necessary to demonstrate that the person has a tendency to recurrent seizures. Diagnosis may rely on observations of attacks and doctors will want to question the patient and any witnesses in relation to such things as

- The sequence and timing of events. Any unusual circumstances prior to the attack, such as hunger, thirst, tiredness, stress, feeling of nausea, pain or breathlessness
- General health
- Family history
- Past medical history (including problems at birth).

Conditions such as faints, heart disease, cerebrovascular accidents, migraine and psychogenic seizures (pseudo-seizures), are often confused with epilepsy. Of those referred with a diagnosis of epilepsy, 20 per cent have been misdiagnosed (Taylor, 1996).

Electroencephalogram

This is a recording of the miniscule electrical discharges generated by the neurones. It is obtained by placing 20 small electrodes onto the scalp (Oxley and Smith, 1991). It should be noted that a person with seizures may have a normal EEG and a person without seizures may have an abnormal EEG.

Ambulatory EEG

This allows recording over several days. Eight electrodes are attached to a small cassette recorder that is worn at the waist.

Videotelemetry

The person is admitted to a specially equipped unit and is videotaped continuously until sufficient information is collected, usually over a period of one to five days. EEG electrodes are attached to the head, enabling any attack to be recorded on video and simultaneously obtaining an EEG trace of the seizure (Sander and Thompson, 1989).

Magnetic Resonance Imaging (MRI)

This is a scanning technique that produces very clear, detailed images of the brain. The scan can reveal even very small structural abnormalities. In some people it may be possible to remove an abnormal area by surgery.

Computerized Axial Tomography (CT)

In this test a computer produces pictures of the brain at different levels and is useful in determining whether there is any structural abnormality.

Blood Tests

These can establish the general health of a person and exclude other causes of the seizures, such as hypoglycaemia, electrolyte imbalance, increased blood urea nitrogen, blood alcohol levels.

Cerebral Angiography

May identify possible vascular abnormalities; evaluation of subdural haematoma.

Echoencephalogram

May show possible midline shifts of brain structures.

Skull roentgenogram

May show evidence of fractures, shift of calcified pineal gland, bony erosion, separated sutures (Thompson *et al.*, 1993).

Treatment

- AEDs
- Surgery
- Dietary manipulation
- Complementary therapies

Anti-epileptic Drugs (AEDs)

The first major breakthrough in anti-epileptic therapy came about unexpectedly (serendipity). A marked reduction in the number of seizures experienced by patients with sexually transmitted diseases being treated with potassium bromide was noted (Griffin, 1991).

A single seizure does not warrant treatment but recurrent seizures would. A cocktail of drugs (polytherapy) was the most widely used and accepted practice until the 1970s. Monotherapy is now the accepted practice, the choice of AED being based upon accurate diagnosis and assessment of the type of seizure. What is effective in controlling one person's seizures may be totally ineffective in another. A second drug may be introduced and the first one withdrawn if a single AED has not successfully controlled the seizures. About 30 per cent of patients will need to be on more than one AED. However, the majority of patients with epilepsy can be reassured of a good outcome for seizure control, regardless of age or seizure type (Cockerell *et al.*, 1995). A significant reduction in the quality of life may result from attempting to reduce seizures. More than 70 000 school children have epilepsy and many of them may be suffering an unacceptable level of side effect from standard AEDs, which can affect all aspects of their lives (Sadler, 1994). For patients with mental impairment and multiple seizure types who need constant supervision, the occasional seizure may be preferable to levels of AEDs that further compromise the cognitive function or otherwise lower the quality of life (Griffin, 1991).

AEDs are divided into two groups (see Table 8.1):

First line drugs – drugs of choice, highly effective for some types of seizure (Table 8.2).

Second line drugs – used if first line drugs are not satisfactory. Used instead of or in combination with first line drugs (Table 8.3).

The most common cause of treatment failure is not taking the prescribed drug(s). Most seizures are self-limiting. If a seizure is prolonged or in the case of status epilepticus, diazepam is usually given intravenously but can be given rectally. AEDs can make some drugs less effective, for example the oral contraceptive pill, so some women with epilepsy may require a higher oestrogen pill (NSE, 1994). Webber *et al.* (1986) found the fertility of women with epilepsy to be 85 per cent of the expected rate, while the fertility of men with epilepsy was reduced to 80 per cent. Low sex drive in men is possibly due to low levels of testosterone caused by AEDs (Griffin, 1991). During pregnancy medication may be withdrawn or amended. Some AEDs can cause fetal abnormalities such as cleft

Table 8.1 Potential side effects of first and second line AEDs

Side effects	*First line drugs*	*Second line drugs*
Skin rash	Carbamezapine Phenytoin Lamotrigine	Piracetam
Diplopia	Carbamezapine Lamotrigine	
Unsteadiness	Carbamezapine Phenytoin	Primidone
Nausea	Carbamezapine Ethosuximide	Primidone
Drowsiness	Ethosuximide Phenytoin Sodium valproate Lamotrigine	Acetazolamide Clobazam Clonazepam Gabpentin Phenobarbitone Piracetam Primidone Topiramate Vigabatrin
Slurred speech	Phenytoin (dose too high)	
Coarsening of facial features	Phenytoin	
Overgrowth of gums	Phenytoin	
Acne (with prolonged treatment)	Phenytoin	
Tremor and drowsiness (infrequent)	Sodium valproate	
Hair loss (not severe and reversible with reduction of dose)	Sodium valproate	
Liver damage (very uncommon)	Sodium valproate	

Table 8.1 Contd.

Side effects	*First line drugs*	*Second line drugs*
Headache		Gabpentin Acetazolamide Topiramate
Fatigue		Gabpentin Acetazolamide
Sedation and slowing of mental performances		Phenobarbitone Primidone Acetazolamide Clobazam Piracetam Topiramate
Mood changes, psychotic reactions		Vigabatrin
Weight loss		Acetazolamide Topiramate
Weight gain		Piracetam
Depression		Acetazolamide Piracetam
Pins and needles in hands, feet, joint pains		Acetazolamide Topiramate
Increased urine output, thirst, dizziness irritability		Acetazolamide

Table 8.2 First line drug/seizure type

First line drug	*Seizure type*
Carbamezapine	Effective against generalized tonic–clonic and partial seizures Ineffective against absence seizures
Ethosuximide	Only effective against absences
Lamotrigine	Partial and generalized tonic–clonic seizures where previous treatment has been ineffective
Sodium valproate	Generalized tonic–clonic absences and partial seizures
Phenytoin	Generalized tonic–clonic and partial seizures. Ineffective against absences

Table 8.3 Second line drug/treatment

Second line drug	*Treatment*
Acetazolamide	Generalized tonic–clonic, atypical absences and partial seizures
Clobazam	Generalized tonic–clonic
Clonazepam	Generalized tonic–clonic, absences, myoclonic jerks and partial seizures
Gabpentin	Partial seizures, where previous treatment has been ineffective
Phenobarbitone	Generalized tonic–clonic and partial seizures
Piracetam	Myoclonic seizures where previous treatment has been ineffective
Primidone	Generalized tonic–clonic and partial seizures, ineffective against absences
Topiramate	Partial or generalized seizures where previous treatment has been ineffective
Vigabatrin	Partial and secondary generalized seizures where previous treatment has been ineffective

lip, cleft palate, malformation of the heart and neural defects. No AED is entirely safe but a simple regime reduces the risks. As the fetus is exposed to AEDs *in utero*, there is usually no objection to breast-feeding. This should be discontinued, however, if the baby becomes drowsy (Oxley and Smith, 1991).

During Pregnancy

- 20 per cent seizures improved
- 60 per cent remained unchanged
- 20 per cent frequency increased

(Feely, 1990)

Surgery

This will be considered if

- AEDs have been unsuccessful.
- Seizures are arising from one focal point.
- Normal function would not be affected by removal of that part of the brain.
- The focal area is accessible and can be removed without damaging any other part of the brain.
- The area to be removed is not near the areas responsible for speech, sight, movement or hearing.
- The person is fit for surgery and there is a very good chance of being seizure free after surgery.

(Hopkins and Appleton, 1996)

Radiosurgery

In recent years non-invasive radiosurgery has emerged, in which beams of gamma radiation are used to kill the abnormally functioning brain cells. It is not possible to treat all types of epilepsy in this way and more research is required (BEA, 2001b).

Vagal Nerve Stimulation

It is believed that stimulation of the vagus nerve may be able to disrupt epileptic activity. A pulse generator is inserted into an opening in the chest wall, for example, the cavity just below the left collarbone. The generator is linked, via an under-the-skin electrode inserted into an opening at the side of the neck. The electrode is then fitted around the vagus nerve. The generator is then programmed continuously to stimulate the nerve at varying frequencies, typically for 30 seconds every five minutes. The frequency is adjusted to the individual's needs by using a small magnet. Patients who experience an aura can use the magnet to manually activate the generator. This may stop or reduce the severity of the seizure. A relative or companion can also use the magnet if they notice that the person is in the early stages of a seizure. Many patients feel some degree of tingling in the neck and hoarseness when the generator is stimulated but they appear to become accustomed to these sensations.

Vagal nerve stimulation is suitable for people with complex partial seizures or generalized seizures. It is also suitable for people who have epilepsy as a result of head injury and those with photosensitive epilepsy. Some studies suggest that around 15 per cent will stop having seizures and the majority of the remaining patients will experience a 50 per cent reduction in their seizure frequency and less severe seizures. A minority of patients will experience no change and some studies suggest that this treatment may not be as effective as it was hoped (BEA, 2001c).

Dietary Manipulation

Fasting or starvation appear to reduce seizures; in this state metabolism is altered and ketones are found in the blood. It is not known how or why ketones reduce seizures. A diet producing ketones is very rich in fats, which makes it rather unpalatable. Its use is restricted to infants and children with very severe epilepsy (Hopkins and Appleton, 1996).

Complementary Therapies

The most successful appear to be those relieving stress – yoga, hypnosis, reflexology and aromatherapy. Some aromatherapy oils can, however, trigger seizures (Fenwick and Fenwick, 1996). It is advisable for sufferers of epilepsy to avoid the essential oils of rosemary, fennel and sage, as there is a remote possibility that these essences may trigger an attack (Wildwood, 1996). EEG feedback, combined with a behavioural approach has also had some success (Taylor, 1996).

Nursing Interventions

Management of Seizures

Management of seizures has two aims

- Protection from injury
- Observation of the seizure.

First Aid

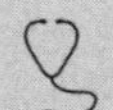

Nursing action points – Non-convulsive seizures

- Speak to the person calmly and reassuringly.
- Stay with the person and ensure a safe environment.

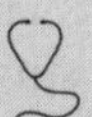

Nursing action points – Convulsive seizures

- If the person is seen to be falling, try to ease their fall.
- Loosen clothing around the neck; if possible cushion the head.
- Do not attempt to put anything between the teeth.
- Do not restrict movement.
- Turn into the recovery position once convulsive movements have ceased.
- Wipe any secretions from around the mouth.
- Stay with the individual until full recovery.
- Maintain privacy and dignity.
- If seizure continues without recovery, or one seizure follows another, seek help.

Observations noted and recorded at the time of a seizure may be important in helping doctors to determine the type of seizure being experienced by the individual.

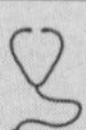

Nursing action points

Note the following observations:

- the time of onset and the duration of the seizure.
- did the patient cry out?
- what was the person doing at commencement of the seizure?
- did the muscular contractions start in one part of the body and if so what was the course of the spread?
- was one side affected more than the other?
- was there a tonic phase?
- was there any cyanosis?
- were the movements symmetrical or asymmetrical?
- was there any incontinence?
- was the person unconscious?
- was the person disoriented after the seizure?
- could the person move their limbs, and was there normal power in them?
- did the patient fall asleep afterwards?
- did any injuries result from the seizure?

A seizure is self-limiting: it cannot be stopped once it has started. During a seizure the patient's safety is a priority. The care for a patient during a seizure while in hospital is essentially the same as when administering first aid. The nurse in the latter situation does, however, have access to oxygen and mechanical suction should these be required.

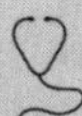

Nursing action points

- If the patient is in bed, remove the pillows and top covers in order to observe the individual.
- If on the floor place a folded blanket or towel under the head to prevent injury during the clonic phase.
- Do not attempt to place anything in the patient's mouth. Any injury to the tongue is likely to have already occurred and such action may result in further damage to the gums and teeth or the nurse's fingers.
- Wipe away any excessive salivary secretions.
- As soon as possible place the patient in the recovery position, loosening any restrictive clothing and clearing the airways as appropriate.
- Stay with the patient and ensure that the patient is not in danger from the immediate environment.
- Screen the patient from other people, so protecting his or her privacy and dignity.
- Administer prescribed oxygen in order to prevent hypoxia.
- Carry out oral hygiene to remove secretions and bleeding.

Health Promotion

The nurse has an important part to play in helping the patient and his or her family to come to terms with a diagnosis of epilepsy, emphasizing the need to avoid being over protective. Education is a prime consideration, which requires the nurse to have an up-to-date knowledge of epilepsy and to ensure that practice is research based. Nurses have a significant role to play in assessing adherence to treatment by careful monitoring of long-term drug therapy, its efficacy and toxicity, and by liaising with doctors. In general, it is important to stress the need to avoid 'over the counter medications' without seeking advice and to attend check-ups as required, in order to monitor general health as well as seizure control. The nurse can assist the patient to identify potential predisposing factors and subsequently offer the appropriate advice to avoid such triggers, thus promoting health and reducing the potential for seizure attacks. The patient should be encouraged to continue with normal routines as far as possible. The safety of the patient will be at the fore of advice given; for example, the patient may be advised to take showers rather than baths. A full driving licence will be issued, providing that the normal criteria have been fulfilled and the applicant has been seizure free for one year. In the case of large/heavy goods vehicles, the applicant must be seizure free for ten years and have no neurological evidence of a continuing liability to seizures. The nurse may be able to offer advice in relation to the types of employment from which the patient would be excluded, but should emphasize that there are very few occupations that people with epilepsy are restricted from undertaking. Advice about stress management and alternative therapies may also be employed as a useful health promotion strategy.

Psychological Needs

The unpredictability of epilepsy may generate anxiety in the sufferer and nurses can do much to reduce this anxiety by ensuring that the patient is fully informed of the condition and what is likely to happen during an attack. Fear of stigma may cause people to be secretive about their epilepsy (Brimacombe, 1985). Studies have shown that people with epilepsy have felt that the condition made it more difficult to obtain employment and restricted their social life when no statistical differences were found between sufferers and non-sufferers (Scambler and Hopkins, 1986). Stigma may be the result of the individual's perception and fear of perceived stigma rather than enacted stigma (Dawkins *et al.*, 1993). Nurses can do much to dispel such fear of stigma by promoting a positive attitude. Education and support is particularly important at the time of diagnosis, when sufferers and their families are likely to be distressed and fearful (Crawford and Nicholson, 1999).

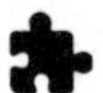 **Connection**

Chapter 2 (Family-centred Care) discusses the potential effects of illness on other family members and potential ways in which nurses can support both the patients and their relatives.

The Role of the Nurse in the Epilepsy Liaison Service

The aim of this service is to encourage an effective, co-ordinated approach to epilepsy. Liaison service has a big part to play in disseminating information across all boundaries, that is, to clients, families, schools, general practitioners, practice nurses and specialists. This will enable all parties to make informed decisions about treatment options and adaptations to lifestyle. An important aim of care is to empower sufferers by providing information and advice that is tailored to their specific needs. Local advice could include information on client organization self-help/support groups and meetings. Good management involves setting standards of care and monitoring performance. Giving clients seizure diaries might reveal what impact seizures have on their lives. Practice nurses are well placed to act as epilepsy support specialists and have an essential role in devising treatment plans and goals; under the guidance of a liaison officer, they may also run a mini-clinic, help audit practice and offer advice and reassurance to those with epilepsy (Smith, 1995). The epilepsy liaison nurse programme provides a free support service for practice nurses nationwide. Specially trained nurses help GPs and practice nurses to develop protocols for the management of epilepsy, liaise on their behalf with hospital departments and specialists, help them to implement systems for recall and review, offer advice on how to audit and how to create an epilepsy register. Primary healthcare is important in the management of epilepsy (Reid, 1994), a community-based team approach is essential and nurses have the appropriate skills to bring to such a team, thus ensuring more effective management of epilepsy.

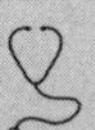

Nursing action points

- Be knowledgeable about all aspects of epilepsy, in order to act effectively as health educators and health promoters.
- Support the patient and family as this is an essential goal of practice.
- Have knowledge of family-centred care as this is important in assessing the needs of the family as a unit.
- Liaise with patients, their families and other agencies as this is a vital component of the overall nursing care.
- Where specialist practitioners are available make early referrals and seek advice where appropriate.
- Advice to patients should be tailored to individual needs.
- Empower individuals as a goal of care.

Connection

Chapter 2 (Family-centred care) explores the theoretical concept of family-centred care.

Conclusion

Nurses can play a significant role in restoring optimal functioning and thus have a positive effect on epilepsy sufferers' well-being and quality of life (Walker, 1999). Concern with communication between patient and professional was highlighted in a survey of BEA members and a sample of clients and supporters carried out in 1995. It revealed that 63 per cent felt that information about epilepsy from health professionals had been inadequate. There is evidence from the BEA survey that people with epilepsy want more say in treatment and more of a cooperative relationship with health professionals. In order for people with epilepsy to take some control over their position, they need to be armed with accurate information if they are to have any impact upon policy makers and services, otherwise they will simply not be heard (Collings, 2001).

The BEA survey found that fear of discrimination or prejudice is still widespread among epilepsy sufferers whether or not such fears are borne out by actual instances. There is a need for further strategies to combat actual discriminatory practice as well as proper counselling and education for people with epilepsy themselves to help gain immunity from prejudicial forces (Collings, 2001).

Perhaps one of the most helpful functions that a nurse has is to promote a positive attitude, not only in those who suffer seizures but also in their family, friends and the general public. It is a disorder that crosses the boundaries of all branches of nursing and also midwifery. It can affect all age groups and there will be specific needs to be taken into account, not only for the various age groups but also relating to the various underlying causes. The diversity of epilepsy poses a challenge for nurses to provide the right sort of support in terms of the immediate care of patients experiencing seizures, as well as in meeting the challenge of ongoing care and, importantly, in empowering patients to make their own decisions about management and treatment. The role of the specialist nurse is a step nearer to making care more effective and improving the quality of life for those who suffer from epilepsy.

References

Betts, T. 1992, 'Epilepsy & Stress'. *British Medical Journal*, 305, 378–9.

Brimacombe, M. 1985, 'The Stigma of Epilepsy'. *New Society*. May, 202–3.

British Epilepsy Association (BEA) 1997, *Epilepsy and Everyone*. Leeds. British Epilepsy Association.

British Epilepsy Association (BEA) 2001a, 'Sudden Unexplained Death in Epilepsy'. http://www.epilepsy.org.uk/info/sudepfrm.html

British Epilepsy Association (BEA) 2001b, 'Epilepsy and Medical Management'. http://www.epilepsy.org.uk/info/mmintfrm.html

British Epilepsy Association (BEA) 2001c, 'Vagal Nerve Stimulation'. http://www.epilepsy.org.uk/info/vagalfrm.html

Buchanan, N. 1995, *Epilepsy: A Handbook*. London. W. B. Saunders Company Ltd.

Chadwick, D. and Usiskin, S. 1987, *Living with Epilepsy*. London. Macdonald & Co. (Publishers) Ltd.

Cockerell, O. C., Johnson, A. L., Sander, J. W. A. S., Hart, Y. M. and Shorvon, S. D. 1995, 'Remission of Epilepsy: Results from the National General Practice Study of Epilepsy'. *The Lancet*, 344 (8968), 140–4.

Collings, J. A. 2001, 'Perceptions of Epilepsy and Attitudes towards Services and Advice'. http://www.epilepsy.org.uk/medical/restrict/gme2.asp

Crawford, P. and Nicholson, C. 1999, 'Epilepsy Management'. *Professional Nurse*, 14 (8), 565–9.

Dawkins, J. L., Crawford, P. M. and Stammers, T. G. 1993, 'Epilepsy: A General Practice Study of Knowledge and Attitudes Among Sufferers and Non-sufferers'. *British Journal of General Practice*, 43, 453–7.

Duncan, J. S. 1997, 'Epilepsy: Matching Drugs to Patients'. *Geriatric Medicine*, 27 (5), 13–14.

Elger, C. E. and Lehnertz, K. 1994, in Wolf, P. (ed.), *Epilepsy Seizures and Syndromes*, 541–6. London. Libby & Company Ltd.

Epilepsy Explained 1994, *Patient Information*. London. Shire Hall Communications.

Feely, M. 1990, 'Epilepsy no bar to motherhood'. *Doctor*, 2 August.

Feldman, R. G. 1983, 'Management of Underlying Causes Precipitating Factors', in Browne, T. R. and Feldman, R. G. (eds), *Epilepsy: Diagnosis and Management*. Boston. Little, Brown & Co.

Fenwick, P. and Fenwick, E. 1996, *Living with Epilepsy: A Guide to Taking Control.* London. Bloomsbury

Frost, S. and Laville, L. 1998, 'RCN Nursing Update. Learning Unit 085. Epilepsy: A Journey'. *Nursing Standard*, 13, 6.

Goodridge, D. H. G. and Shorvon, S. D. 1983, 'Epileptic Seizures in a Population of 6000'. *British Medical Journal*, 287, 641–7.

Griffin, J. 1991, *Epilepsy Towards Tomorrow*. London. Office of Health Economics.

Holmes, G. L. 1987, *Diagnosis and Management of Seizures in Children*. W. B. Saunders. Philadelphia.

Hopkins, A. 1993, *Clinical Neurology. A Modern Approach.* New York. Oxford University Press Inc.

Hopkins, A. and Appleton, R. 1996, *Epilepsy: the Facts.* 2nd edn. New York. Oxford University Press Inc.

Jackson, S. M. and Bennett, P. J. 1988, *Physiology with Anatomy for Nurses.* London. Bailliere Tindall.

Jennett, W. B. 1962, *Epilepsy after Blunt Head Injuries.* London. Heinemann Medical Books Ltd.

Management Protocol for Epilepsy in General Practice 1994, London. Shire Hall Communications.

Marieb, E. N. 2001, *Human Anatomy and Physiology.* 5th edn. London. Benjamin Cummings, an imprint of Wesley Longman Inc.

Mattson, R. G. 1983, 'Seizures Associated with Alcohol Use and Withdrawal' in Browne, T. R. and Feldman, R. G. (eds), *Epilepsy: Diagnosis and Management.* Boston. Little, Brown & Co.

National Society for Epilepsy 1994, *Drug Treatment of Epilepsy.* London. National Society for Epilepsy.

National Society for Epilepsy 1995, *Epilepsy and Learning Disabilities.* London. National Society for Epilepsy.

Nursing Times 1994, 'Professional Development'. Unit 4. *Nursing Times*, 90 (18), 1–12.

Oxley, J. and Smith, J. 1991, *The Epilepsy Reference Book.* London. Faber.

Peattie, P. L. and Walker, S. 1995, *Understanding Nursing Care.* 4th edn. New York. Churchill Livingstone. Pearson Professional Limited.

Reid, T. 1994, 'Helpful Liaisons'. *Nursing Times*, 90 (1), 18.

Rowett, H. G. Q. 1988, *Basic Anatomy and Physiology.* 3rd edn. London. John Murray (Publishers) Ltd.

Royal College of Nursing (RCN) 1995, 'Epilepsy CE'. Article 302. *Nursing Standard*, 10 (3), 33–9.

Russell, A. 1996, 'Epilepsy'. *Nursing Standard*, 10 (32), 49–54.

Sadler, C. 1994, 'Seen But Not Heard'. *Nursing Times*, 90 (21), 23.

Sander, L. and Thompson, P. 1989, *Epilepsy: A Practical Guide to Coping*. Wilts. Crowood Press.

Scambler, G. 1989, *Epilepsy*. London. Routledge.

Scambler, G. and Hopkins, A. 1986, 'Being Epileptic: Coming to Terms With the Stigma'. *Social Health Illness*, 8, 26–43.

Smith, K. 1995, 'Bringing Epilepsy Care into the 1990s'. *The Epilepsy Liaison Service Profession Nurse*, 10 (4), 255–8.

Taylor, M. 1996, *Managing Epilepsy in Primary Care*. Oxford. Blackwell Science.

Thompson, J. M., McFarland, G. R., Hirsch, J. E. and Tucker, S. M. 1993. *Mosby's Clinical Nursing*. 3rd edn. St Louis. Mosby-Year Book Inc.

Walker, C. 1999, 'Helping People with Epilepsy'. *Professional Nurse*, 14 (8), 525.

Wallace, S. 1996, *Epilepsy in Children*. London. Chapman and Hall Medical.

Wildwood, C. 1996, *Aromatherapy*. London. Bloomsbury Publishing Plc.

Wilson, K. J. W. and Waugh, A. 1998, *Ross and Wilson Anatomy and Physiology in Health and Illness*. London. Harcourt Brace and Company Limited.

Webber, M., Hauser, W., Ottman, R. and Annegees, J., 1986, 'Fertility in Persons with Epilepsy 1935–47'. *Epilepsia*, 27, 746–52.

Chronic Obstructive Pulmonary Disease (COPD)

9

NORMA WHITTAKER

Chronic obstructive pulmonary disease (COPD) is a major cause of morbidity and mortality. It is now the third most common cause of death in the European Union, after cancer and heart disease, and the fifth leading cause of death worldwide according to a World Health Organization Report (WHO) (1997). As COPD affects people at the height of their productive years, it places a heavy burden on society, industry and health services. The direct costs of COPD include inpatient and outpatient treatment, domiciliary and home-nursing care and the costs of medication. In the United Kingdom (UK) COPD costs the economy 360 million pounds per year and is responsible for the loss of 22 million working days (Jones, 2000). Indirect costs include loss of finance due to absences from work and premature retirement due to disablement (Madden, 1999). Despite these grim statistics, COPD remains under diagnosed and under-treated, possibly because of its strong links with smoking and with increasing age (Jones, 2000).

Contents

- Definition of chronic obstructive pulmonary disease
- Definition of chronic bronchitis
- Definition of pulmonary emphysema
- Epidemiology
- Aetiology
- Anatomy and physiology of the bronchi, smaller air passages and the lungs
- Pathophysiology
- Clinical manifestations
- Investigative tests
- Treatment
- Nursing interventions

Learning Objectives

By the end of the chapter you should be able to demonstrate knowledge of

- Factors associated with the epidemiology and aetiology of COPD.
- Differences between the pathophysiology of chronic bronchitis and pulmonary emphysema.
- The effects that changes in respiratory function have upon the individual.
- How COPD is diagnosed and treated.
- Nursing interventions that reflect the chronic nature of the disorder and which take account of the physical, psychological and social effects that chronic pulmonary disease has upon the individual.

Definition of Chronic Obstructive Pulmonary Disease

Chronic obstructive pulmonary disease is a chronic, slowly progressive disorder that is characterized by reduced maximal expiratory flow and slow forced emptying of the lungs, features that do not change markedly over several months and may be accompanied by airway hyper-reactivity. The impairment of lung function in COPD is largely fixed, but may be partially reversible by bronchodilator or other therapy (Crompton *et al.*, 1999).

Chronic obstructive pulmonary disease is an umbrella term used to describe closely related disorders of the respiratory system, including chronic bronchitis and emphysema, Although pure forms of these two conditions do exist, there is considerable overlap in the majority of cases, one rarely occurring without a degree of the other. Chronic bronchitis and emphysema differ from COPD in that they may occur in the absence of airflow obstruction. As the mortality and morbidity of COPD are due to airflow obstruction, this is an important differentiation to make. In contrast, asthma is an inflammatory disease producing limitation to expiratory airflow that is generally reversible with the administration of inhaled and/or oral corticosteroids. Rarely, patients with asthma may develop airflow obstruction that does not improve with steroid treatment, becoming indistinguishable from COPD. Differentiation between asthma and COPD may be difficult in this case (Raashed and Allen, 1998a).

Definition of Chronic Bronchitis

Chronic bronchitis is defined as a clinical disorder characterized by excessive mucus secretion in the bronchi; manifested by chronic or recurring cough. The cough is present for a minimum of three months per year for at least two consecutive years, and other causes of productive cough have been excluded (Ames and Kneisl, 1988).

Definition of Pulmonary Emphysema

Pulmonary emphysema is a chronic destructive disease of the respiratory bronchioles, alveolar ducts and alveoli. Emphysema is abnormal permanent enlargement of gas-exchange airways accompanied by destruction of alveolar walls. In emphysema, obstruction results from changes in lung tissues, rather than mucus production, as is the case in chronic bronchitis (Davey *et al.*, 1994). There are two main types of pulmonary emphysema which may coexist and which are exacerbated by severe and persistent coughing. These are centrilobular and panlobular emphysema (Edmond, 1994).

Epidemiology

The exact figures for prevalence are difficult to determine because some patients with mild to moderate COPD may not be diagnosed. It is estimated, however, that in the UK around 18 per cent of men and 14 per cent of women aged 40 to 68 may have features associated with COPD (Mak, 1997). By 1997 the annual prevalence rate of diagnosed COPD in women had risen from 0.8 per cent to 1.36 per cent, the same rate seen in men in 1990. During a seven-year study of the prevalence and mortality rates for COPD between 1990 and 1997, researchers found that the rate of increase in women was 68 per cent, compared with 25 per cent in men. COPD rates reached a plateau in men in the mid 1990s but in women aged 45 to 65 they continue to increase, approaching the rates of men. In the 20 to 40 years age group there were low rates of COPD, but by 1997 the prevalence in women had overtaken that in men. Researchers suggest that on current trends, the annual number of deaths attributable to cigarette smoking in women should exceed that for men (The Pharmaceutical Journal, 2000).

The UK has the world's highest prevalence of COPD, where it is the largest single cause of absence from work (Stobart, 1999). Approximately 600 000 people in the UK are affected by COPD and it causes more than 25 000 deaths each year (Postma and Siafakas, 1998). This is over ten times higher than deaths from asthma (Crompton *et al.*, 1999). An average group practice of 5000 patients can expect to have 75 to 100 patients with COPD (Madden, 1999). Acute exacerbations of COPD are a common cause of hospital admissions, assessment of an average health district of 250 000 people found that 25 per cent of all medical admissions were due to respiratory disease and over half of these were individuals with COPD (Anderson *et al.*, 1994).

Chinese and Afro-Caribbean races seem to have a reduced susceptibility to developing COPD (Mak, 1997). It is more common in middle-aged men than women and is more prevalent among cigarette smokers than non-smokers. Morbidity and mortality rates rise with increasing age and with decreasing economic status. Socio-economic status is strongly linked to the incidence, prevalence and mortality of COPD (Stobart, 1999). Prevalence in social class V is over three times that of class I, correlating strongly with the prevalence of cigarette smoking (Social Trends, 1995). There is considerable geographical variation in the prevalence of COPD with a higher prevalence, particularly among men, in areas such as Durham, Yorkshire, Lancashire, North Wales and London. These high rates are thought to be due to the predominantly working-class population (Hart, 1998). This may relate to poorer housing and nutrition and the use of fossil fuels for heating without adequate ventilation and there is also more likelihood of employment in jobs where there is a higher risk of occupational exposure (Stobart, 1999).

Aetiology

Atmospheric pollution and occupational dust exposure are minor aetiological factors in chronic bronchitis; the dominant causal agent is cigarette smoke. Smoking also causes emphysema, probably damaging the lung by the release of proteolytic enzymes. Individual susceptibility to smoking is, however, very wide, with only 15 per cent of smokers likely to develop clinically significant COPD (Crompton *et al.*, 1999). It is not known why some smokers develop bronchitis and others develop emphysema (Phipps and Brucia, 1991). By the time subjects are symptomatic with breathlessness, severe impairment of lung function will be present and stopping smoking at this stage may extend life expectancy but may not improve the symptoms (Stobart, 1999).

Primary Risk Factors for COPD

- Tobacco exposure of more than 20 pack years. Pack years are estimated by dividing the number of cigarettes smoked per day by 20 and multiplying by the number of years of smoking (British Thoracic Society, 1997).
- Deficiency of alpha-1-antitrypsin, an inherited autosomal recessive disorder (Madden, 1999). Alpha-1-antitrypsin is contained within lung secretions and protects tissues against digestion by proteolytic enzymes released from neutrophils, macrophages and microorganisms in the course of the response to infection. Alpha-1-antitrypsin deficiency results in the breakdown of the structures of the alveoli (Stobart, 1999), causing severe, disabling emphysema early in life. It affects one in 5000 people and it is equally common in men and women (Moxham and Costello, 1997). Alpha-1-antitrypsin deficiency accounts for probably less than 5 per cent of all cases of COPD (Mak, 1997). A more common variant of this trait, where protease inhibitors are around 35 to 60 per cent of normal, will also increase the risk of developing COPD, especially if there is an interaction with another risk factor, such as cigarette smoke (Madden, 1999).

Associated risk factors for COPD

- Environmental pollution, for example, dusty work environment. Occupational exposure to irritants, for example, silica, cadmium
- Low social class
- Diet deficient in vitamin C
- Low birth weight
- Pre-existing bronchial hyper-responsiveness
- Childhood respiratory infection
- Gastroesophogeal dysfunction (mainly gastric reflux)
- Obesity
- Passive smoking

(Fehrenbach, 1998; Madden, 1999; Mak, 1997)

Air Pollution and Occupational Exposure

Studies in the UK have shown a relationship between levels of atmospheric pollution and respiratory problems, particularly cough and sputum production, in both adults and children. Acidic gases and particulates have been implicated. As with smoking some people will be more susceptible than others. Any occupation polluted with the aforementioned gases and particulates increases the risk of developing COPD, especially if the subject smokes.

Occupations at risk include:

- Coal miners
- Construction workers who handle cement
- Metal workers
- Grain handlers
- Cotton workers
- Paper mill workers.

(The effects of smoking far outweigh any influences from the environment.)

Infections

The role of viral infections of the upper and lower respiratory tract remains unclear. Viral infections in the lung enhance inflammation and predispose to bronchial hypersensitivity. There is increasing evidence linking early childhood infections with an increase in respiratory problems in adulthood. Implicated viruses are adenovirus and respiratory syncitial virus. Once COPD is established, repeated infective exacerbations of airflow obstruction by viral or bacterial agents, may speed up the decline in lung function.

Passive Smoking

Smoke coming from the burning end of a cigarette (side stream smoke) is actually higher in concentration of toxic substances than exhaled smoke. Recent evidence, based upon measuring levels of nicotine metabolite in the blood, urine or saliva of children from smoking and non-smoking families suggests that respiratory infections and respiratory symptoms are more common in households where one or both parents smoke. There is also a small but significant difference in the prevalence of respiratory symptoms and lung function in adults and children who are regularly exposed to passive smoking. Whether these differences are clinically significant is yet to be resolved (Mak, 1997).

Anatomy and Physiology of the Bronchi, Smaller Air Passages and the Lungs

The Bronchi

The two bronchi commence at the bifurcation of the trachea and one leads into each lung (Figure 9.1). The left main bronchus is narrower, longer and more

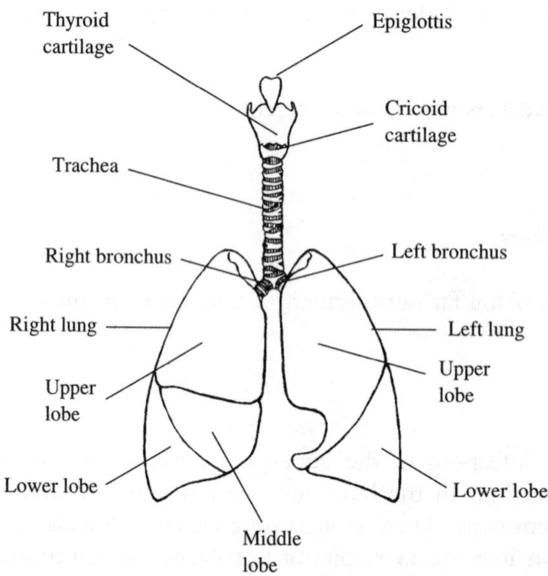

Figure 9.1 Lungs and respiratory passages

horizontal than the right main bronchus because of the position of the heart. Each main bronchus divides into branches, one for each lobe of the lungs (Jackson and Bennett, 1988). The bronchi are lined with ciliated columnar epithelium. The bronchi progressively subdivide into bronchioles, terminal bronchioles, respiratory bronchioles, alveolar ducts and finally alveoli (Figure 9.2). Towards the distal end of the bronchi the cartilages become irregular in shape and are absent at the bronchiole level. The smooth muscle in the walls of the bronchi becomes thicker and is responsive to autonomic nerve stimulation and irritation. Ciliated mucous membrane changes gradually to cuboidal shaped cells in the distal bronchioles (Wilson and Waugh, 1998).

The Alveoli

The terminal bronchioles branch repeatedly to form minute passages called alveolar ducts from which alveolar sacs and alveoli open (Jackson and Bennett, 1988). The walls of the alveoli are composed primarily of a single layer of squamous epithelial cells, surrounded by a flimsy basal laminar. The external surfaces of the alveoli are covered with a very fine network of pulmonary capillaries (see Figure 9.3). Together, the alveolar and capillary walls and their fused basal lamina form the respiratory membrane, which has gas on one side and blood flowing past on the other. Gas exchange occurs readily by simple diffusion across the respiratory membrane. Deoxygenated blood enters the capillary network from the pulmonary artery and oxygenated blood leaves it to enter the pulmonary veins. The 300 million or so gas filled alveoli in the lungs account for most of the lung volume and provides a tremendous surface area for gaseous exchange (Marieb, 2001).

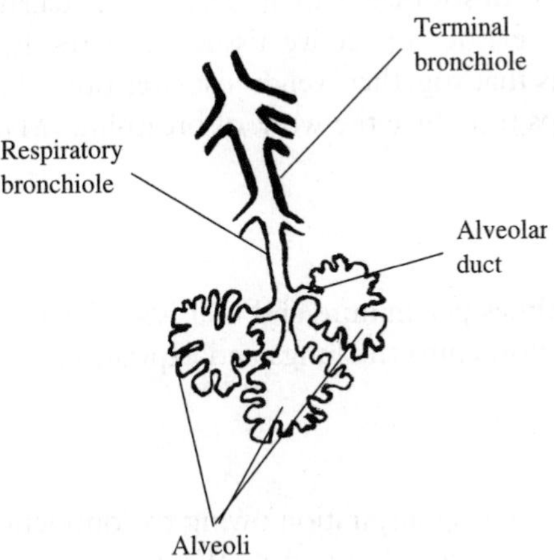

Figure 9.2 Lung lobule

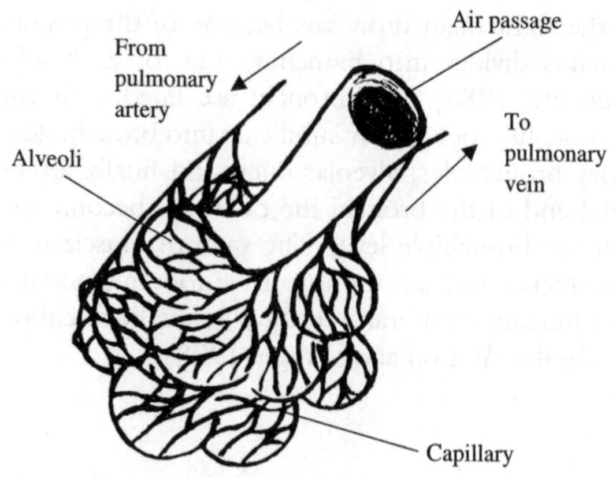

Figure 9.3 The alveoli

The Lungs

The lungs are the principal organs of respiration and on a volume basis they are one of the largest organs in the body. Each lung is conical in shape, with its base resting on the diaphragm and its apex extending above to a point approximately 2.5 centimetres superior to each clavicle. The right lung is larger than the left and has three lobes as compared to the left lung, which has only two. Deep, prominent fissures separate the lobes on the surface of the lung. Each lobe is further divided into lobules separated from each other by connective tissue, but the separations are not visible on the surface of the lung. There are nine lobules on the left lung and ten in the right lung. Because major blood vessels and bronchi do not cross the connective tissue, individual diseased lobules can be removed, leaving the rest of the lung relatively intact (Seeley *et al.*, 1989). As previously mentioned, the lungs consist mainly of air spaces. The balance of lung tissue, or its stroma, is mostly elastic connective tissue. As a result, the lungs are soft, spongy elastic organs that together weigh just over one kilogram. The elasticity of healthy lungs helps to reduce the work of breathing (Marieb, 2001).

Respiration

This occurs 15–20 times per minute and consists of two phases: inspiration is the period when air flows into the lungs and expiration, the period when gases exit the lungs.

- *Inspiration*
  The chest expands during inspiration owing to contraction of the diaphragm and the external intercostal muscles. When the diaphragm contracts it is flattened and lowered and the thoracic cavity is increased in length.

The external intercostal muscles lift the ribs and draw them outwards, increasing the width of the thoracic cavity. Together, these actions increase the volume of the thoracic cavity. As the chest wall moves up and out, the closely attached parietal pleura, lining the chest wall, moves with it. The visceral pleura, which are firmly attached to the lungs, follow the parietal pleura, the lungs expand to fill the space and air is sucked into the bronchial tree (Jackson and Bennett, 1988).

- *Expiration*
  Expiration in healthy adults is a passive process that depends more on the natural elasticity of the lungs than on muscle contraction (Marieb, 2001). The diaphragm relaxes and assumes its original domed shape, the intercostal muscles relax and the ribs return to their original position. The lungs recoil and air is forced out of the bronchial tree. During deep or forced breathing, for example when the airway is obstructed, the accessory muscles of respiration may be brought into use (Jackson and Bennett, 1988).

Physiological Variables Affecting Respiration

- Elasticity
- Airflow resistance
- Compliance

Elasticity

Loss of elasticity of the connective tissue in the lungs necessitates forced expiration and increased effort on inspiration.

Airflow Resistance

When this is increased, for example, in bronchoconstriction, more respiratory effort is required to inflate the lungs (Wilson and Waugh, 1998).

Compliance

The ease with which the lungs can be expanded, in other words, their distensibility, is referred to as lung compliance. It is a measure of the effort required to inflate the alveoli. Lung compliance is determined mainly by the distensibility of the lung tissue and the surrounding thoracic cage and the surface tension of the alveoli. In healthy people compliance tends to be high, which favours efficient ventilation. This is because lung and thoracic distensibility is generally high and alveolar surface tension is kept low by surfactant, a phosolipid fluid that prevents the alveoli from drying out (Marieb, 2001). When compliance is low, for example where elasticity is reduced or there is inadequate surfactant, the effort to inflate the lungs is greater than normal, thus more energy is needed just to breathe (Wilson and Waugh, 1998).

Factors that diminish compliance

- Reduction of the natural resilience of the lungs, such as fibrosis
- Blockage of the smaller respiratory passages, for example with thick mucous
- Reduced production of surfactant
- Decreased flexibility of the thoracic cage

(Marieb, 2001)

Pathophysiology

Pathophysiology of Pulmonary Emphysema

Loss of elastic recoil is the major mechanism of airflow limitation. The main defect underlying emphysema is the derangement of lung elastin by the neutral proteases. Elastase is the most important of these; it is made and released by polymorphonuclear leukocytes and alveolar macrophages. Under normal conditions, proteases become fused with bacteria present in the alveoli. A fraction of the total protease produced is liberated in the lung in response to inhaling particles and following cell death. A supply of the protease inhibitor alpha-1-antitrypsin normally acts as a counterbalance to the protease liberation. Recurrent infections, environmental irritants and cigarette smoking, along with alpha-1-antitrypsin deficiency, probably lead to a degrading of elastin in the distal airways and alveoli. Cigarette smoking alone may also depress the activity of alpha-1-antitrypsin. The imbalance in this elastase/antielastase system allows for the destruction of the basic elastin structure of the distal airways and alveoli (Thompson *et al.*, 1993).

The destruction of the alveoli walls will be accelerated by repeated infections. The obstruction in emphysema typically begins in the small, peripheral bronchioles, due to inflammation, infection, retained secretions and oedema. The narrowing of the airways traps air in the alveoli. As the disease progresses, alveolar walls become disrupted by hyperinflation and some alveolar septa are destroyed (Ames and Kneisl, 1988). As the walls of the alveoli are destroyed, the alveolar surface area that comes into direct contact with the pulmonary capillaries continually decreases, causing an increase in dead space (the lung area where no gas exchange can occur). This results in impaired oxygen diffusion, which in turn results in hypoxaemia. In the later stages of the disease, carbon dioxide elimination is impaired, resulting in increased carbon dioxide tension in arterial blood (hypercapnia) and causing respiratory acidosis (Smeltzer and Bare, 1994). If not reversed, hypoxaemia leads to pulmonary hypertension and eventually leads to cor pulmonale (right-sided heart failure) and congestive heart failure (Davey *et al.*, 1994).

The loss of elasticity of the lung tissue leads to the premature collapse of the minute respiratory and terminal bronchioles during exhalation. This causes increased airway resistance and a slowing of expiratory airflow, making exhalation of air from the lungs more difficult. Since the alveolar and vascular changes are not uniform throughout the lungs, ventilation–perfusion abnormalities occur. Some alveoli will be ventilated but not perfused and others will be perfused but under ventilated (Ames and Kneisl, 1988). Secretions are increased and retained because the person is unable to generate a forceful cough to expel them, and chronic and acute infections will persist, further adding to the problem.

Changes in Respiration

The person with emphysema has a chronic obstruction (marked increase in airway resistance) to the inflow and outflow of air from the lungs, which are in a state of chronic hyper expansion. In order to move air in and out of the lungs, negative pressure is required during inspiration and an adequate level of positive pressure must be attained and maintained during expiration. The resting position is one of inflation. Expiration becomes active rather than passive, requiring muscular effort. The person becomes increasingly breathless. The chest becomes rigid and the ribs fixed at their joints. The 'barrel chest' is due to loss of lung elasticity in conjunction with the continued tendency of the chest wall to expand. In some cases the spine may become curved leading to a barrel chest. Patients may lean forward to breathe and use accessory muscles of respiration and retraction of the superclavicular fossa causes the shoulders to heave upward (Smeltzer and Bare, 1994).

Normal exhalation becomes increasingly difficult and finally impossible. Pulmonary function tests demonstrate an increased residual volume (RV), functional residual capacity (FRC), and total lung capacity (TLC). Diffusing capacity is significantly reduced because of lung tissue destruction. Diminished respiratory airflow is demonstrated by a decreased forced expiratory volume (FEV) and maximal midexpiratory flow rate (MMFR). The vital capacity (VC) may be normal or only slightly reduced until late in the disease progression, so the ratio of forced expiratory volume in one second to the vital capacity is decreased ($FEV_1 : VC$). This is due to the loss of elasticity. The ability to adapt to changing oxygen needs is greatly compromised. The degree of respiratory impairment may be estimated on the basis of the ratio of FEV to forced vital capacity (FCV). A significant finding that differentiates emphysema from other obstructive airway pathologies is the failure of bronchodilators to improve pulmonary function tests (Phipps and Brucia, 1991).

There are two types of pulmonary emphysema, which are classified on the basis of lung changes as follows

Panlobular Emphysema

In panlobular emphysema the whole acinus (the unit of the lung distal to the terminal bronchii) is involved (Davey *et al.*, 1994). There is destruction of the respiratory bronchiole, alveolar duct and alveoli (see Figure 9.4). All air spaces

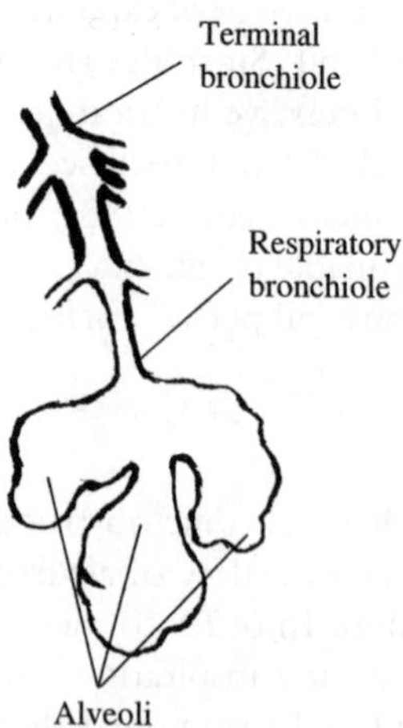

Figure 9.4 Panlobular emphysema

within the lobule are more or less enlarged, with little inflammatory disease. A hyper inflated chest is typical with marked dyspnoea on exertion and weight loss. As the patient usually remains 'pink' or well oxygenated until the terminal stages of the disease, the term 'pink puffer' has sometimes been used in describing this patient (Smeltzer and Bare, 1994). This type of emphysema is usually more diffuse and is more severe in the lower lung. It is found in elderly people who have no evidence of chronic bronchitis or impairment of lung function. It occurs just as frequently in women as in men, but is less common than centrilobular emphysema. It is a characteristic finding of homozygous alpha-1-antitrypsin deficiency (Phipps and Brucia, 1991).

Centrilobular Emphysema

Septal destruction occurs in the respiratory bronchioles, and alveolar ducts. Inflammation develops in the bronchioles, but the alveolar sac (alveoli distal to respiratory bronchiole) remains intact (Davey *et al.*, 1994). There is distention and damage of the respiratory bronchioles selectively. Openings develop in the walls of the bronchioles; they become enlarged and confluent and tend to form a single space as the walls enlarge (see Figure 9.5). This type of emphysema tends to be unevenly distributed throughout the lung but is usually more severe in the upper portions (Phipps and Brucia, 1991). Frequently there is a derangement of ventilation–perfusion ratios, producing chronic hypoxia, hypercapnia, polycaethemia and episodes of right-sided heart failure. This leads to cyanosis, peripheral oedema and respiratory failure. The term 'blue bloater' has sometimes been used to describe this patient (Smeltzer and Bare, 1994). Smokers tend to develop centrilobular emphysema and it tends to occur with chronic bronchitis (Davey *et al.*, 1994).

Both types of emphysema very often occur in the same patient.

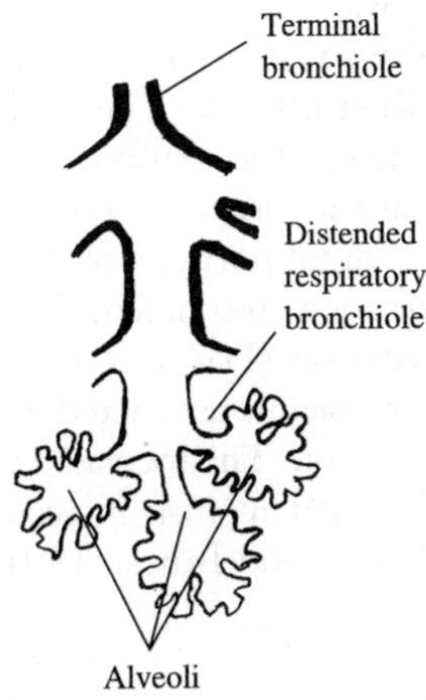

Figure 9.5 Centrilobular emphysema

Pathophysiology of Chronic Bronchitis

One of the earliest changes in chronic bronchitis appears in the secretory glands. Hypertrophy and hyper secretion occur in the goblet cells and bronchial mucus glands. The goblet cells and mucous gland cells increase in both size and number. The goblet cells extend distally into the terminal bronchioles, where they are not normally found. The overall result is increased amounts of sputum, bronchial congestion and narrowing of bronchioles and small bronchi. In time, bacteria colonize the normally sterile lower respiratory tract. The resulting increase in polymorphonuclear neutrophil leukocytes probably stimulate further bronchial swelling and eventual tissue destruction. Granulated and squamous epithelium replaces the normal ciliated epithelium. Stenosis and airway obstruction occur (Thompson *et al.*, 1993).

The mucus produced is thicker and more tenacious than normal and the impaired function of the cilia further reduce the mucus clearance, compromising the lung's defence mechanisms and increasing susceptibility to pulmonary infection and injury. Bacteria proliferate in the mucus secretions in the lumen of the bronchi. The most common infectious agents are streptococcus pneumoniae and haemophilus influenzae. As bacteria multiply, they exert a neutrophilic chemotaxis and pus cells migrate from between bronchial epithelial cells to produce a mucopurulent exudate in the lumen, or the disease may progress to ulceration and destruction of the bronchial wall. The presence of peribronchial fibrosis results in stenosis and airway obstruction. Small airways may be completely obliterated, and others become dilated. There is some evidence that the pathological changes occur initially in the small airways and move to larger bronchi (Phipps and Brucia, 1991).

As infection and injury increase mucus production further, the bronchial walls become inflamed and thickened from oedema and accumulated inflammatory cells resulting in increased airway resistance. Excess mucus in the airways not only obstructs airflow but also causes bronchospasm, which further increases airway resistance (Ames and Kneisl, 1988). The thick mucus and hypertrophied bronchial smooth muscle obstructs the airways and leads to closure, especially during expiration, when the airways are narrowed. The airways collapse early in expiration, trapping gas in the distal portions of the lung. Obstruction eventually leads to ventilation–perfusion mismatch, hypoventilation, hypercapnia, hypoxaemia and respiratory acidosis (Davey *et al.*, 1994). Cor pulmonale may result; the hypercapnia and hypoxaemia associated with chronic bronchitis cause pulmonary vascular vasoconstriction. The increased vascular resistance results in pulmonary vessel hypertension that in turn increases vascular pressure in the right ventricle of the heart (Phipps and Brucia, 1991).

The Effects of Smoking

Cigarette smoke is composed of various irritants that stimulate mucus production and impair ciliary function and increase the number of goblet cells in the peripheral airways. These changes increase vulnerability to respiratory tract infections and interfere with recovery from infections. Furthermore, cigarette smoking causes bronchospasm, which increases airways resistance. Smokers also experience a steeper decline in lung function with age than non-smokers, and this cannot be regained (Stobart, 1999).

Smoking is also thought to have the effect of inducing persisting airway inflammation and causing a direct imbalance in oxidant/antioxidant capacity and proteinase/antiproteinase load in the lungs. The imbalance allows proteolytic enzymes to attack lung tissue. Smoke-affected pulmonary alveolar macrophages, present in greater numbers than usual, release neutrophil chemotactic factor and the attracted neutrophils are damaged by smoke and release proteolytic enzymes, especially elastase, capable of lysing elastin, collagen and basement membranes. The effectiveness of alpha-1-antitrypsin is impaired by smoking and the unchecked proteolysis results in centrilobular emphysema (Moxham and Costello, 1997).

Low levels of alpha-1-antitrypsin allow the uninhibited action of elastase on the lung parenchyma, giving rise to destruction of the alveoli and the eventual development of emphysema rather than bronchitis. The pattern of emphysema in anti-1-antitrypsin deficiency differs slightly from that of smoking-induced pure emphysema in that it results in panlobular emphysema affecting predominantly the lower lung fields, whereas smoking induced emphysema is usually centrilobular, affecting the upper lung fields initially. Lung destruction will be accelerated by cigarette smoking (Moxham and Costello, 1997).

Complications of COPD

Pulmonary bullae are thin walled air spaces created by rupture of alveolar walls. They may be single or multiple, large or small and tend to be situated subpleurally. Rupture of subpleural bullae may cause pneumothorax. Occasionally bullae increase in size and compress lung tissue, thus further compromising pulmonary ventilation. Respiratory failure and cor pulmonale are generally late complications in COPD patients whose main problem is emphysema (Crompton *et al.*, 1999).

Clinical Manifestations

Symptoms of COPD

- Few symptoms in the early stages of the disease, even when there has been significant loss of lung function
- Dyspnoea on exertion is of insidious onset and worsens gradually over many years, gradually compromising the activities of living
- Chronic cough
- Increased sputum production. Sputum tends to be freely expectorated, with the volume and purulence changing during exacerbations
- Wheeze
- Weight loss

The clinical state is dictated by the severity of the disease. Chronic bronchitis and emphysema develop over many years and patients are rarely symptomatic before middle age. Symptoms are initially minor, perhaps a morning cough productive of a little sputum (Moxham and Costello, 1997). In patients with predominantly chronic bronchitis the main symptoms are cough and sputum, which precede dyspnoea. A chronic productive cough, usually after colds, in the winter months is the earliest sign of chronic bronchitis. Cold weather, dampness and pulmonary irritants may exacerbate the cough. There is a steady increase in the severity and duration with successive years until the cough is present all the year round. Patients suffer recurrent infections, exertional breathlessness, regular morning cough, wheeze and occasional chest tightness. Sputum may be scanty, mucoid and tenacious and occasionally streaked with blood during infective exacerbations. Frankly purulent sputum is indicative of bacterial infection, which is common in these patients (Crompton *et al.*, 1999). The patient usually has a history of cigarette smoking (Smeltzer and Bare, 1994). When emphysema is dominant, patients present with dyspnoea on effort, inexorably progressive over several years (Laszlo and Catterall, 1998). The onset of emphysema is insidious and symptoms may not appear until about one third of the lung parenchyma is affected. In advanced cases the slightest activity can cause severe respiratory distress and cyanosis. As the disease progresses the patient must work harder and harder at breathing especially exhalation. Patients often breathe through pursed lips to prolong expiration and reduce the tendency of the airways to collapse, thus removing more air from the lungs. Accessory muscles are used to breathe and patients often sit with their hands firmly supported. The chest is barrel shaped. Anorexia and weight loss are common, causing an emaciated appearance and concomitant muscle wasting. Cough and sputum are not common unless infection is present, which is a frequent occurrence during winter months (Ames and Kneisl, 1988).

Clinical Patterns

Some patients with severe chronic airflow obstruction are able to maintain relatively normal oxygenation by hyperventilating. These patients are constantly breathless and tend to lose weight but are not cyanosed; do not develop cor pulmonale or secondary polycaethemia. In contrast other patients develop central cyanosis, hypoxaemia, carbon dioxide retention, secondary polycaethemia and cor pulmonale with elevation of the jugular venous pressure and peripheral oedema. The reasons for these different clinical patterns are poorly understood and most patients lie within these two extremes (Laszlo and Catterall, 1998).

Psychological Aspects of COPD

Recurrent chest infections further compromise lung function with a resultant spiralling of disability. Travelling, shopping, driving, holidays and leisure pursuits become increasingly difficult for the patient. Persistent symptoms may cause the patient embarrassment and eventual withdrawal from social interactions. As the disease progresses the individual has to rely more and more upon others and the loss of independence may lead to feelings of frustration, irritability, anxiety and depression. The constant exhaustion and the knowledge that the breathlessness cannot improve with time only add to feelings of being a burden upon others (Crawford, 1997).

Investigative Tests

It is estimated that many individuals with COPD are misdiagnosed, and that up to one in three of those aged 40 and over who are diagnosed as suffering from asthma, are in fact suffering from COPD. Many people who suffer symptoms do not visit their doctor (Hart, 1998). As COPD shares some symptoms with asthma, it is important to make a proper diagnosis. Clinical features that favour a diagnosis of COPD include a history of smoking and little response to steroids (Madden, 1997).

Diagnostic features of COPD

- History of chronic progressive breathlessness with little variability
- Smoking history of over 20 pack years
- Evidence of airflow obstruction on lung function testing
- No significant response to steroid treatment

Investigations and Assessment

- History
- Radiology
- Basic observations
- Lung function testing

History

The patient's medical/nursing history will establish the amount smoked and the progression and nature of the symptoms. The finding on examination depends upon the stage of the disease.

Radiology

A chest x-ray can be useful in excluding other causes of symptoms such as bronchial carcinoma. Although hyperinflation can be seen on chest x-ray, this could also be the case in uncontrolled asthma. X-ray cannot differentiate between asthma and COPD (Tutt and Jennings, 1999). It can be used to diagnose emphysematous bullae in severe COPD (Fehrenbach, 1998). CAT can indicate the extent of thick walled bronchi and macroscopic lesions of emphysema (Laszlo and Catterall, 1998).

Basic Observations

- Blood pressure and pulse.
- Electrocardiogram and echocardiogram may be undertaken to exclude ischaemic heart disease, but is insensitive for assessing right ventricular hypertrophy, which is an indication of cor pulmonale (Fehrenbach, 1998).
- A full blood count, especially in the advanced stage, is necessary to identify polycythemia secondary to chronic hypoxaemia. The correction of unsuspected anaemia is also helpful. In advanced disease, arterial blood gas analysis is necessary to identify patients with hypoxaemia who should be considered for long-term oxygen therapy. If pulse oximetry measures more than 92 per cent, this will reduce the need to monitor blood gases if the patient remains stable. In younger patients serum alpha-1-antitrypsin should be measured (Raashed and Allen, 1998a).

Lung Function Testing

An objective measure of airflow obstruction is necessary, as it cannot be predicted from symptoms. Spirometry allows COPD to be accurately diagnosed, assessed and monitored. Spirometry measures the volume of air a patient can blow out from full inspiration to full expiration. This measurement shows how well the small airways are functioning. Research has shown that there

Table 9.1 Stages of COPD

Mild	*Moderate*	*Severe*
FEV_1 is between 60 and 79% of normally expected lung function. ■ Few symptoms; history of morning cough, recurrent respiratory infections. ■ The patient experiences shortness of breath when hurrying on the level or walking up a slight hill.	FEV_1 is 49–59% of normally expected lung function. ■ Wide range of symptoms; cough, production of sputum, acute worsening of symptoms on infection, wheeze, over-inflation of the lungs. ■ The patent walks more slowly on the level than contemporaries because of breathlessness, or has to stop for breath when walking at his/her own pace.	FEV_1 is below 40% of normally expected lung function. ■ Breathless on minimal exertion, cough, wheeze, loss of weight, central cyanosis, peripheral oedema, pulmonary hypertension, over-inflation of the lungs. ■ The patient is breathless while dressing or undressing and may be too breathless to leave the house.

Madden, 1999; Fehrenbach, 1998.

is a tendency for GPs and nurses to under-diagnose COPD and many health professionals are still ignorant about the role of spirometry in diagnosing COPD. Training is vital for all members of the healthcare team. Those competent in using spirometers in general practice will be able to diagnose COPD correctly and then give treatment and advice that might halt its progression (Kilgarriff and Pascoe, 1999) (see Table 9.1).

The care and diagnosis of COPD is not the same as asthma. COPD diagnosis relies upon spirometry. Surveys suggest that only about one quarter of practices have a spirometer and many in the practice may be inexperienced in its use (Harrison, 2000).

- *Relaxed vital capacity (RVC)*
  This is the volume of air that can be blown out from maximum inspiration to maximum expiration, but the air is blown out in a relaxed manner, like a heavy sigh. The result is recorded on a volume/time graph. Usually two RVC blows are performed.
- *Forced vital capacity (FVC)*
  This measures the volume of air a patient can blow out forcibly from full inspiration to full expiration, using maximum effort. The volume of air exhaled is measured against the time taken to perform the manoeuvre.
- *Forced expiratory volume in one second (FEV_1)*
  This is the volume of air blown out in the first second of a forced expiration from maximum inspiration. The result is obtained from the FVC manoeuvre as shown on the volume/time graph.

- *FEV_1/FVC ratio*
  This is the amount blown out in the first second as a percentage of the total volume of air that has been exhaled. This is calculated by dividing the measured FEV_1 by the measured FVC multiplied by 100.

In healthy lungs the total volume of air is exhaled in four seconds, whereas in severe obstruction, this may take up to 15 seconds before a plateau is reached. In healthy lungs the RVC should produce the same result as the FVC, but in patients with emphysema the RVC may be higher. This is because in the forced manoeuvre the airways collapse due to a rise in the inter-pleural pressure and cause air trapping. The highest measurements of RVC or FVC should be used in assessing results. There are predicted normals for spirometric measurements that vary according to the patient's age, sex and height. An FEV_1 and FVC of more than 80 per cent of predicted normals is considered to be acceptable. The FEV_1/FVC ratio should be above 70 per cent. Spirometry will give four patterns of results: normal, obstructive, restrictive and combined. If airway obstruction is present FVC will be within normal limits but it will take longer for the air to be expelled. The patient will have an FVC_1 of less than 80 per cent and an FEV_1/FVC ratio of less than 70 per cent. Airway obstruction is then diagnosed, but the cause of the obstruction still needs to be established (Tutt and Jennings, 1999; Booker, 1998).

Reversibility Testing

This is carried out in order to demonstrate any reversibility in spirometry and/or exercise tolerance following the administration of drugs such as, steroids or bronchodilators (Matthews, 1999).

Peak flow measurements are likely to be normal in mild to moderate disease and may underestimate the severity of airflow obstruction in severe disease. FEV_1 is the measurement of choice. It is objective, reproducible over time and can help determine appropriate treatment by assessing the degree of reversibility or improvement in obstruction after a bronchodilator trial (Raisbeck, 2000).

Treatment

Aims of treatment

- Early and accurate diagnosis
- Prevention of deterioration
- Prevention of complications
- Improved quality of life

(British Thoracic Society [BTS], 1997)

Smoking Cessation

This is the single most important way of influencing the outcome in patients at all stages of COPD as this can slow lung function deterioration.

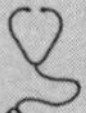

Nursing action points

- Counsel patients on the benefits of stopping smoking.
- Advise patients on the use of nicotine patches, nicotine gum, inhalers and transdermal patches that can alleviate withdrawal symptoms and are useful adjuncts to behavioural modification.
- Advise patients that sudden cessation has the best outcome in the short term.
- Offer continued support and nicotine replacement therapy. A sustained cessation rate of up to 30 per cent can be achieved.

(Raashed and Allen, 1998b)

Vaccination

Influenza vaccine has been shown to reduce serious illness and mortality by 50 per cent and is therefore recommended every autumn. Pneumococcal vaccine is also recommended, although there are little data on its efficacy (Raashed and Allen, 1998b).

Oxygen Therapy

Oxygen therapy is an important part of the management of patients with COPD.

Acute Exacerbations

Oxygen is administered at rates sufficient to maintain arterial oxygen between 50 and 60 mm Hg, usually by nasal cannulae. The use of a controlled percentage face mask allows more precise oxygen administration. In some cases mechanical ventilation may be necessary (Thompson *et al.*, 1993).

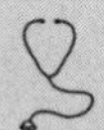

Nursing action point

- Monitor oxygen administration closely, as patients with chronic hypercapnia are considered sensitive to increased alveolar oxygen. Their borderline or diminished respiratory drive may be further suppressed by increasing PaO_2.

Long-term Therapy

Some patients with severe COPD will benefit from long-term low concentration oxygen therapy (two litres per minute by nasal cannulae). Without it the prognosis is poor, only 30 per cent will survive for more than three years. The three-year survival rate could improve to 70 per cent when oxygen is given for 15 hours a day or more (Roberts, 1999). Long-term oxygen therapy decreases pulmonary hypertension, reduces secondary polycaethemia, improves neuropsychological health and prolongs life in hypoxaemic COPD patients (Crompton *et al.*, 1999). Oxygen therapy can also improve exercise tolerance and the quality of life in general. Patients with severe disease, low lung function, cyanosis and episodic ankle oedema, despite optimum drug therapy, should be referred. Short periods of oxygen via a face mask are widely prescribed to relieve breathlessness after periods of exertion. There may be some relief from this but the benefits of long-term oxygen therapy in terms of increased life expectancy will be absent. Many patients using this therapy would meet the criteria for long-term oxygen therapy (Roberts, 1999). Long-term oxygen therapy defined as the administration of oxygen for more than 15 hours in every 24 hours, is required for severe hypoxaemia. To avoid the need for large numbers of oxygen cylinders, oxygen is best administered by a concentrator. This is usually on the recommendation of a hospital consultant. Concentrators work by atmospheric air passing either through a molecular sieve or a semi-permeable membrane. This removes nitrogen and other low concentration gases, leaving oxygen-enriched flow. A back-up cylinder should be available in the event of the concentrator failing (Harman, 1999).

Carbon Dioxide Narcosis

In healthy people when CO_2 levels rise, the respiratory rate increases and excess CO_2 is blown off by the lungs. In COPD where chronic ventilatory problems result in constantly high levels of arterial CO_2, this mechanism becomes blunted and eventually has no effect on the respiratory centre in the brain. With severe CO_2 retention the respiratory drive is created by the low arterial oxygen (hypoxic drive). A high concentration of oxygen will suppress the hypoxic drive, breathing will become shallow, even if arterial oxygen is raised to normal, and more and more CO_2 is retained, further depressing the respiratory centre. This is characterized by increasing drowsiness and eventual death.

The hypoxic drive must always be considered when O_2 is prescribed for patients with COPD. Usually this is not more than 24 per cent of O_2, slightly more than room air. This is enough to improve oxygenation without eliminating the hypoxic drive (Ames and Kneisl, 1988).

Drug Therapy

Bronchodilator drugs relax smooth muscle in the airways and are the mainstay of treatment for mild to moderate COPD (Raisbeck, 2000). Inflammation in

COPD is predominantly neutrophilic and not resolved by steroids, and airway narrowing is fixed and irreversible.

The British Thoracic Society (BTS) Guidelines for Treatment

Mild COPD: Short acting beta-agonists or inhaled anticholinergic as required, depending upon symptomatic response.

Moderate COPD: May also be treated with a short acting beta2-agonist or anticholinergic. A combination of the two drugs may be more effective than either drug alone.

Severe COPD: Combination therapy with beta2-agonist and anticholinergic (Hart, 1998) (see Table 9.2).

Venesection for Secondary Polycythaemia

Venesection can reduce the symptoms of polycythaemia, including somnolence, lethargy, poor concentration and headache. The first-line therapy for secondary polycythaemia, whenever possible, should be to improve lung function (Moxham and Costello, 1997).

Table 9.2 Drug treatment

Drugs	*Therapy*
Short-acting bronchodilators	They are usually given by inhalation and produce bronchodilation within a few minutes, peaking at 15 to 30 minutes. The effects last three to four hours so dosage may have to be repeated three to four times a day.
Long-acting bronchodilators	These are useful for patients with nocturnal and early morning symptoms. At present, salmeterol (Serevent) is the only long acting bronchodilator to be licensed in the UK.
Anticholinergics	The onset of action is slower than beta-agonists, reaching a maximum in 30 to 90 minutes and lasting for four to eight hours.
Methylxanthines	Theophylline and aminophylline may improve symptoms in some patients. Regular blood monitoring is necessary to prevent side effects.
Oral steroids	Some patients with COPD experience improved lung function with oral steroids. The ratio of risk to benefit of long-term treatment, however, needs careful assessment.
Inhaled steroids	A large number of studies are currently underway to assess the effects of inhaled steroids. Results from the recent study (Inhaled Steroids in Obstructive Lung Disease in Europe), look promising. Results showed that fluticasone reduced the absolute decline in lung function by nearly a third over three years. Patients suffered fewer exacerbations and had a better quality of life than those on placebo (Madden, 1999).

Pulmonary Rehabilitation

A pulmonary rehabilitation programme is of proven efficacy in improving exercise tolerance and quality of life in cases of moderate to severe COPD. The programme includes tailored exercise and education (Raashed and Allen, 1998b). Pulmonary rehabilitation aims to help people with COPD to attain as normal a life as possible by helping them to cope more effectively with their respiratory dysfunction (Stobart, 1999).

The main problem is getting access to a programme as they are mainly hospital based and are not widely available (Roberts, 1999).

The components of the programme are

- Clinical assessment
- Education
- Nutritional advice
- Tailored exercise programmes
- Social assessment and support
- Psychological support and coping strategies
- Optimal drug treatment and improved compliance

(Raashed and Allen, 1998b)

Surgical Options

Surgical procedures, such as lung volume reduction, resection of compressive bullae and single or double lung transplant are increasingly considered, and often provide significant improvement in pulmonary function and symptoms (Raashed and Allen, 1998b).

Physiotherapy

No benefit has been proven in patients with chronic bronchitis and emphysema. During acute exacerbations of bronchitis and pneumonia several studies have shown no benefit from physiotherapy. In the absence of excessive secretions physiotherapy is not justified (Moxham and Costello, 1997).

Nursing Interventions

Nurses have a multidimensional role in the management of COPD.

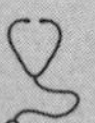

Nursing interventions

- Health promotion
- Health education
- Psychological support
- Respiratory rehabilitation
- Support during an acute exacerbation
- Respiratory assessment
- Empowering patients

Health Promotion

Cigarette smoking is the single most important factor in the aetiology of COPD. Prevention is the key to bringing the incidence of COPD under control. Women stop smoking more slowly than men and, along with 11 to 15 year olds, require specific targeting for help and support.

Measures to reduce the prevalence of cigarette smoking include

- Stopping tobacco advertising and promotion
- Restricting smoking in public places and work environments
- Prohibition of sale of cigarettes to children
- Educating the public
- Raising the cost of cigarettes

(Stobart, 1999)

Smoking cessation is the prime factor in preserving lung function and is just as important in severe COPD as in the earlier stages. Many patients who continue to smoke are long-term heavy smokers who may have little confidence in their ability to stop. The nurse has an important role to play, in discussing intervention methods, assisting with a plan to stop, advising on nicotine replacement therapy and sustained support, all of which are significant factors in success or failure (Crawford, 1997). Patients should be given information on the benefits of not smoking and unequivocal but non-judgemental advice and encouragement to stop. Nurses should learn to identify when patients are ready to change and be positive and supportive throughout the process of managing this change (Stobart, 1999).

Health Education

Recognizing worsening symptoms is important for the patient who should be made aware of what action to take.

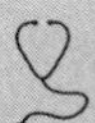

Nursing action points

- Advise patients of the need to seek medical help in the case of increased breathlessness and thick purulent sputum as a result of an infective exacerbation.
- Advise patients about the use of a reserve course of antibiotics, which in some cases are kept in the patient's home, to reduce any delay in treatment.
- Remind patients to inform the GP.
- Explain that headaches and drowsiness may signal the insidious onset of respiratory failure.
- Advise patients to report ankle oedema. This is suggestive of hypoxemia and cardiac failure, both of which require hospital admission.
- Encourage patients to have protective vaccination each autumn.

(Crawford, 1997)

Patients and their carers also need to be given information about the disease and the prescribed regimens of treatment. The nurse also has an important part to play in teaching the patient the correct way to use inhalers and nebulizers where this is appropriate. Patients may not divulge information and may choose to stop taking medication (Jordan and White, 2001). Nurses need to take account of this when monitoring response to medication and where there appears to be a lack of expected progress.

Nutrition

Breathlessness, anorexia and sputum production may contribute to malnutrition. Malnutrition may result in obesity or emaciation and body mass index should be assessed. Weight reduction in obese patients will reduce oxygen demands imposed by exercise and improve the individual's coping ability. Steroid-induced obesity is more problematic.

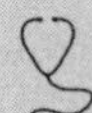

Nursing action points

- Advise patients to take bronchodilators prior to meals.
- Advise the patient about good oral hygiene (especially if sputum is purulent or to combat the dry mouth side effect of drug therapy).
- Recommend an ample fluid intake, to keep sputum loose.
- Encourage sputum clearance. Teach the patient how to effectively remove sputum.

- Suggest small amounts of food.
- Inform the patient about high-energy foods such as butter, cream and sugar, which should be included in the diet.

(Fehrenbach, 1998)

Exercise

A pulmonary rehabilitation programme is designed to improve peripheral and respiratory muscle strength and can be run in either primary or secondary care environments and usually consists of twice-weekly group sessions. Breathing exercises can be used to gain an element of control over breathlessness and slow the respiratory rate. Relaxation techniques can also be useful (Fehrenbach, 1998).

Psychological Support

COPD patients frequently feel angry, depressed and anxious over their condition. Patients have to adapt not only to the loss of physical well-being, but also to loss of independence and a place within the wider society. COPD can be isolating not only for the individual but also for the carers, and nurses have an important role to play in recognizing the physical and emotional needs of the patient and the primary carer. This is particularly essential during the terminal stages of the disease. It is important that nurses acknowledge this and answer their questions honestly (Ames and Kneisl, 1988).

 **Connection**

Chapter 2 (Family-centred Care) explores the concept of family nursing in situations where the burden of caring has the potential to affect the health and well-being of the carer.

Drugs such as theophyllines can increase anxiety and long-term oral steroids may contribute to mood swings. Many patients may have a fear of death that is heightened during nights of disturbed sleep (Fehrenbach, 1998). There is also the knowledge for both patient and carer that there is no cure for the disease. Referral to self-help groups can be helpful (Crawford, 1997). Because of the fear of breathlessness, many patients with COPD maladapt by becoming inactive and sedentary. They often become more limited by the deconditioning than by the disease itself (Ryan, 2000).

Breathlessness is not merely a symptom of disordered breathing but a complex interplay of physical, psychological and emotional factors. The nurse who is thinking primarily of the biological implications of breathlessness may overlook how the person affected is thinking and feeling. Knowledge of the patient's own perceptions of the experience is vital as there is a distinction between the phenomena of breathlessness as the onlooker perceives it and by the person experiencing it. By exploring the psychological dimensions of breathlessness the nurse is able to gain insight, and be guided towards the right level of intervention. Some situations may merely require the use of non-verbal language, such as touch. Others may warrant the provision of an environment conducive to solitude that allows the individual to concentrate all his or her efforts into the act of breathing or the support of the nurse in aiding the patient to use recommended breathing techniques (Morgan, 2000).

Respiratory Rehabilitation

Lost lung function can never be fully restored in patients with COPD and the progressive nature of the disease eventually leads to disability. By using spirometry the extent of COPD can be the classified, but two sufferers can have the same lung function results and have very different experiences of breathlessness and how it affects their health (Ryan, 2000). In attempting to evaluate the full effect of COPD on individual patients, there may be a need to move beyond purely physiological measures such as FEV_1, important though this is in confirming the diagnosis. Health status instruments can be used to gather information about overall health status and can be incorporated into routine clinical practice, alongside FEV_1 measurements. In this way the well-being of patients and the true benefit of medical interventions can be assessed more accurately (Jones, 2000).

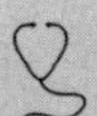

Nursing action points

- Assess the patient's perception of his or her breathlessness.
- Support the patient in times of breathlessness by encouraging learned breathing techniques.

Acute Exacerbation

One of the important aspects of the shift from secondary care to primary care is that diagnosis and treatment in both sectors should become more accurate (Harrison, 2000). Both GPs and hospital physicians are often unsure whether hospital admission is necessary during an acute exacerbation. An acute deterioration in the patient's condition usually results in a hospital admission.

It is possible that some admissions could be avoided if patients are assessed in the accident and emergency department, by a specialist team of nurses and doctors. Angus (2001) describes an initiative that allows nurses to manage patients in their own homes. This is a nurse-led service. The nurses perform a full clinical examination, organize investigations and analyse the results. Following assessment a team determines whether with suitable medication, nursing and social support the patient may be safely cared for at home. If the patient meets the criteria for homecare a member of the respiratory medical team reviews the case in order to support the nurse's decision. Where homecare is more appropriate full support for the patient can be arranged. A nurse then visits the patient at home every day until the condition has stabilized, after which care is transferred to the primary care team.

Respiratory Assessment

The acute respiratory assessment service provides rapid assessment and homecare for patients with acute uncomplicated exacerbation of their condition. The service is predominantly nurse-led, with respiratory nurses trained in the management of COPD. These specialist nurses are responsible for the initial assessment and ongoing community care of patients during an exacerbation (Flanigan *et al.*, 1999).

The role of the nurse during an acute exacerbation will be to assist the patient in maintaining the activities of living and in symptom control. This may include the administration of drugs, effective bronchial secretion clearance and preventing the complications of reduced mobility. Encouraging compliance with medication is of paramount importance during an acute exacerbation and in long-term treatment.

Models of homecare

- Homecare teams
- Acute respiratory assessment services (offer rapid access to specialist assessment and treatment)
- Schemes providing an alternative to admission
- Rapid discharge schemes

(Angus, 2001)

Empowering Patients

The development of improved partnerships between healthcare professionals and patients is necessary to ensure greater flexibility in patient-centred care. Pulmonary rehabilitation provides the framework for such initiatives. While information leaflets can be helpful, the role of the practice nurse in providing effective education and promoting a positive attitude and behavioural change is paramount. Regardless of formal rehabilitation programmes, practice nurses can be pivotal in encouraging patients in the initial development and long-term maintenance of an active lifestyle (Meighan-Davies and Parnell, 1999). Patients with COPD experience ongoing challenges in preserving a sense of wholeness as they face physical changes that interfere with their daily activities according to a study by Leidy and Haase (1999). Patients in the study wanted to maintain personal integrity, which was described as having a sense of effectiveness and connectedness, that is a sense of 'being with other people' through their daily activities.

Loss of Sexual Activity

Relationships can suffer through lack of sexual activity, as 30 per cent of men with COPD are impotent (Fehrenbach, 1998). While studies examining sexual arousal in women with respiratory disease are rare, there is anecdotal evidence to suggest that the psychogenic problems described in male studies also affect women and their potential sexual arousal. People with COPD experience a wide range of symptoms, each of which may have an impact on the sexual health of the individual from both a physical and psychological perspective. There are a variety of positions for sexual intercourse, which limit energy expenditure for the breathless patient. Nurses should recognize that they often need to take the first steps in initiating this avenue of discussion and give the patient permission to raise areas of concern, albeit this is not always easy in a busy ward or clinic (Law, 2001).

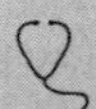
Nursing action points

- Make time to talk to patents.
- Be prepared to initiate discussion relative to the loss of sexual activity.
- Refer to an experienced counsellor, if appropriate and acceptable to the patient and the partner.

Conclusion

Chronic obstructive pulmonary disease, which encompasses chronic bronchitis and emphysema, is a major medical and social problem that causes physical, psychological and social problems to sufferers and their families. It is a major and growing cause of mortality and morbidity worldwide (Jones, 2000). The BTS guidelines advocate a specific quantitative indicator of airway function. The FEV_1 measurement, using a spirometer, distinguishes COPD from asthma and other lung conditions and classifies the disease into 'mild', 'moderate', and 'severe' on the basis of residual lung function. However, the effects upon patients' daily lives extend far beyond the experience of breathlessness and other respiratory symptoms. Normal activities may be severely curtailed, independence and confidence lost and social isolation experienced (Jones, 2000).

Even though there is no national service framework for respiratory disease, it still takes a high priority in public health strategies (McIntyre, 2002). COPD can have a profound impact upon an individual's life and all of the actual or potential problems are most effectively managed by a collaborative multidisciplinary team approach. Nurses play a key role in COPD management by helping the patient to identify the difficulties experienced as a consequence of the disease, mobilizing services, maintaining good communication with all disciplines and by offering patients continuing practical help and support (Crawford, 1997). One of the most exciting advances in patient care has been the development of specialist nursing teams to address the needs of specific client groups. Training nurses to treat patients with COPD at home has improved the ability of health services to deal with patients' exacerbations. Home care schemes have the potential to free medical beds, with logistical and financial benefits, while providing excellent patient care (Angus, 2001). The self-management techniques taught by respiratory nurses are fundamental in improving the morbidity rates for respiratory disease (McIntyre, 2002).

Patients with COPD represent a heavy burden on both doctors and practice nurses (Madden, 1999). The costs associated with smoking related illness justify more help being made available to people trying to give up smoking and for the promotion of non-smoking. Research has shown that there is a great potential for influencing behaviour through a variety of settings. This has major implications for respiratory nurses, as helping patients to give up smoking may be the most important intervention that can be made on his or her health. The implications for the future of respiratory nursing include setting up pulmonary rehabilitation programmes aimed at reducing symptoms and improving exercise performance. Respiratory nurses fulfil a key role in planning care and providing support for this vulnerable group and can educate, advise and support other health professionals. COPD will remain one of the greatest causes of disease, misery and death in future decades and a more positive attitude towards people with advanced COPD is needed, backed up by appropriate and speedy hospital evaluation and treatment. The need for services should be established, services evaluated and a more expansive view to prevention implemented (Stobart, 1999).

References

Ames, S. W. and Kneisl, C. R. 1988, *Essentials of Adult Nursing*. Menlo-Park California. Addison-Wesley Publishing Company.

Anderson, H. R., Esmail, A., Hollowell, J. *et al.*, 1994, *Epidemiologically Based Needs Assessment: Lower Respiratory Disease*. London. HMSO.

Angus, R. 2001, 'Managing chronic obstructive pulmonary disease at home'. *Nursing Times*, 97 (12), Supplement VI–VII, *NT Plus: Respiratory.*

Booker, R. 1998, 'Using spirometers: taking a blow for good health'. *Community Nurse*, 4 (4), 19–21.

British Thoracic Society (BTS) 1997, 'Guidelines for the management of COPD'. *Thorax*, 52 (5).

Crawford, A. 1997, 'Chronic lung disease: an invisible disability'. *Community Nurse*, 3 (2), 18–21.

Crompton, G. K., Haslett, C. and Chilvers, E. R. 1999, 'Diseases of the respiratory system' in Haslett, C., Chilvers, E. R., Hunter, J. A. A. and Boon, N. A. (eds), *Davidson's Principles and Practice of Medicine.* 18th edn. London. Churchill. Livingstone.

Davey, S. S., McCance, K. L. and Budd, M. C. 1994, 'Alterations of pulmonary function' in McCance, H. L. and Huether, S. E. *Pathophysiology: The Biologic Basis for Disease in Adults and Children.* 2nd edn. London. Mosby-Year Book Inc.

Edmond, C. 1994, 'The respiratory system' in Alexander, M. F., Fawcett, J. N. and Runciman, P. J. (eds) *Nursing Practice and Home: The Adult.* London. Churchill Livingstone.

Fehrenbach, 1998, 'Chronic obstructive pulmonary disease'. *Professional Nurse*, 14 (11), 771–7.

Flanigan, B. A., Irwin, A. and Dagg, K. 1999, 'An acute respiratory assessment service'. *Professional Nurse*, 14 (2), 839–42.

Harman, R. 1999, 'Management of COPD with oxygen therapy at home'. *Community Nurse*, 5 (7), 25–6.

Harrison, G. 2000, 'COPD TaskForce'. *Nursing Management*, 7 (4), 30–2.

Hart, M. 1998, 'Learning to recognise the signs and symptoms of COPD'. *Community Nurse*, 4 (8), 18–19.

Jackson, S. M. and Bennett, P. J. 1988, *Physiology with Anatomy for Nurses.* London. Bailliere Tindall.

Jones, P. W. 2000, 'Measuring health status in COPD'. *Geriatric Medicine*, 30 (1), 51–3.

Jordan, S. and White, J. 2001, 'Bronchodilators: implications for nursing practice'. *Nursing Standard*, 15 (27), 45–52.

Kilgarriff, J. and Pascoe, M. 1999, 'An education programme on diagnosing COPD'. *Community Nurse*, 5 (11), 15–16.

Laszlo, G. and Catterall, J. R. 1998, 'Respiratory medicine' in Jones, J.V. and Tomson, C. R. V. (eds), *Essential Medicine.* 2nd edn. London. Churchill Livingstone.

Law, C. 2001, 'Sexual health and the respiratory patient'. *Nursing Times*, 97 (12), Supplement XI–XII, *NT Plus: Respiratory.*

Leidy, N. K. and Haase, J. E. 1999, 'Functional status from the patient's perspective: the challenge of preserving personal integrity'. *Evidence-Based Nursing*, 2 (4), 135.

McIntyre, P. 2002, 'Breathing space'. *Nursing Standard*, 16 (28), 61.

Madden, V. 1999, 'Quality of life and COPD'. *Practice Nursing*, 10 (11), 17–20.

Mak, V. 1997, 'The causes of COPD and who is at risk'. Priory Lodge Education Ltd. http://www.priory.com/cmol/causesof.htm.

Marieb, E. N. 2001, *Human Anatomy & Physiology.* 5th edn. London. Benjamin Cummings, an imprint of Wesley Longman Inc.

Matthews, H. 1999, 'Helping Mary: a case study in COPD'. *Practice Nursing*, 10 (3), 31–4.

Mead, M. 1998, 'Drugs for COPD'. *Practice Nurse*, 16 (8), 516–18.

Meighan-Davies, J. and Parnell, H. 1999, 'Empower patients to take control of COPD'. *Practice Nurse*, 17 (9), 622–6.

Morgan, C. 2000, 'Chronic obstructive pulmonary disease and it's psychological impact on the individual'. *Assignment*, 6 (4), 18–27.

Moxham, J. and Costello, J. 1997, 'Respiratory disease' in Souhami, R. L. and Moxham, J. (eds), *The Textbook of Medicine.* 3rd edn. London. Churchill Livingstone.

The Pharmaceutical Journal 2000, 'COPD death rate in women might soon exceed that of men'. *The Pharmaceutical Journal*, August, 265, 289.

Phipps, W. J. and Brucia, J. J. 1991, 'Management of persons with problems of the lower airway' in Phipps, W. J., Cassmeyer, V. L., Sands, J. K. and Lehman, M. K. (eds), *Medical–Surgical Nursing: Concepts and Clinical Practice.* 5th edn. London. Mosby-Year Book.

Postma, D. S. and Siafakas, N. M. (eds) 1998, 'European respiratory monograph'. *Monograph*, 3 (7), May, 250.

Raashed, M. and Allen, M. B. 1998a, 'COPD clinical features and diagnosis'. *Geriatric Medicine*, 28, 31–3.

Raashed, M. and Allen, M. B. 1998b, 'COPD guidelines for management'. *Geriatric Medicine*, 57–60.

Raisbeck, E. 2000, 'The role of bronchodilators in controlling COPD symptoms'. *Community Nurse*, 6 (5), 19–20.

Renwick, D. S. and Connolly, M. J. 1996, 'Prevalence and treatment of chronic airways obstruction in adults over the age of 45'. *Thorax*, 51, 164–8.

Roberts, J. 1999, 'Management of COPD'. *Practice Nursing*, 10 (3), 27–30.

Ryan, S. 2000, 'Chronic obstructive pulmonary disease: boosting quality of life'. *Community Nurse*, 6 (3), 31–2.

Seeley, R. R., Stephens, T. D. and Tate, P. 1989, *Anatomy and Physiology.* St Louis. Times Mirror/Mosby College Publishing.

Smeltzer, S. C. and Bare, B. G. (eds) 1994, *Brunner and Suddarth's Textbook of Medical & Surgical Nursing.* 8th edn. Philadelphia. Lippincott-Raven Publishers.

Social Trends 1995, London. HMSO.

Stobart, M. J. 1999, 'Prevention and management of COPD'. *Professional Nurse*, 14 (4), 241–4.

Thompson, J. M., McFarland, G. K. and Hirsch, J. E. 1993, *Mosby's Clinical Nursing.* London. Mosby-Year Book.

Tutt, C. and Jennings, J. 1999, 'Presentation and assessment of COPD'. *Practice Nursing*, 10 (3), 23–6.

Wilson, K. J. W. and Waugh, A. 1998, *Ross and Wilson Anatomy and Physiology in Health and Illness.* London. Harcourt Brace and Company Limited.

World Health Organization (WHO) 1997, *Report. Conquering Suffering, Enriching Humanity.* 19. Geneva. WHO.

10

Infectious Diseases

NORMA WHITTAKER

The relationship between humans and microorganisms is usually one of balanced conflicts. Encounters with microorganisms in the first months of life are both a threat and a stimulus to the development of complex immune responses (Wansbrough-Jones and Wright, 1997). Humans are constantly exposed to potentially pathogenic microorganisms yet clinical infections are rare events and fatal infections even rarer (Greenwood, 2000). To become infected a person must be exposed to an infective dose of a microorganism to which he or she is susceptible and the host and microorganism must be brought together by environmental factors. Considering the ubiquity of many pathogens, severe infections are relatively uncommon, but pathogens survive better if the host is not incapacitated or killed (Mayon-White, 2000).

Contents

Learning Objectives

By the end of the chapter you should be able to demonstrate knowledge of

- Infectious agents and the potential for transmitting infection from one individual to another.
- Factors that increase a client's susceptibility to infection.
- The clinical manifestations of an infection and potential nursing interventions.
- Nursing care based upon measures to prevent the spread of infection from one person to another.

Epidemiology

In many parts of the world microorganisms appear to have the upper hand. Infectious gastroenteritis, for example, is the most common cause of death among children under one year of age. The frequency of some infections varies in different parts of the world. These differences may be attributed to climate, for example malaria, standards of hygiene, for example typhoid and immunizations, for example measles, diphtheria and poliomyelitis. The higher mortality associated with these diseases in under-developed countries is due to the poor nutritional state of individuals at the onset of illness and the lack of medical facilities (Wansbrough-Jones and Wright, 1997).

Epidemics occur when the incidence of disease is abnormally high. The term outbreak is used to describe small, confined epidemics, two or more associated cases of any disease. Seasonal variation in incidence is predictable, for example in respiratory infections such as influenza. This occurs more often in the winter in both the Northern and Southern hemispheres and results in increased deaths and hospital admissions from pneumonia. Interactions between different organisms also play a part in seasonal variations. Influenza is associated with the increase of meningococcal disease in winter. Viral damage to the pharyngeal mucosa caused by the influenza virus may facilitate the invasion of meningococcal disease, resulting in bacteraemia and meningitis. The arrival of a new infection in a susceptible population or a fault in normal control mechanisms may result in unexpected fluctuations (Mayon-White, 2000).

The Pattern of Infections

The pattern of infections is constantly changing. As the standard of living improves infectious diseases become less important as a cause of death. Improvements in hygiene, nutrition, sanitation and immunization account for changes in regard to many infectious diseases, but sometimes the pathogen itself changes in virulence. Scarlet fever (scarletina) is less of a threat today than it was 50 years ago due to the erythrogenic toxin-producing streptococci becoming less virulent. Most changes in the pattern of infections are gradual. Demographic and social changes have been reflected in increased prevalence among otherwise healthy young people, for example infection with the human immunodeficiency virus (HIV) (The Scottish Office, 1998). New infections are rare but can have an enormous impact as in the case of HIV, which is the cause of the acquired immune deficiency syndrome (AIDS). All of the infections found in temperate and developed areas of the world will also be found in tropical regions but some infections are found only in the tropics. This is due to the climate and the presence of animal reservoirs and insect vectors (Wansbrough-Jones and Wright, 1997).

Common Terms and Definitions in Relation to Infectious Diseases

- Pathogen
- Infection
- Colonization
- Communicable diseases
- Incubation period

Pathogen

Rice and Eckstein (1995) have defined this as a microorganism or substance capable of causing disease (see Figure 10.1).

Infection

This is the presence in the body of a pathogen that multiplies and produces effects that are injurious to the host (Rice and Eckstein, 1995). It is important to recognize the difference between infection and disease. Infectious disease is where the host displays a decline in health due to the infection. Often an infection is present in which the host interacts immunologically with the pathogen but remains symptom free (Donegan, 2000).

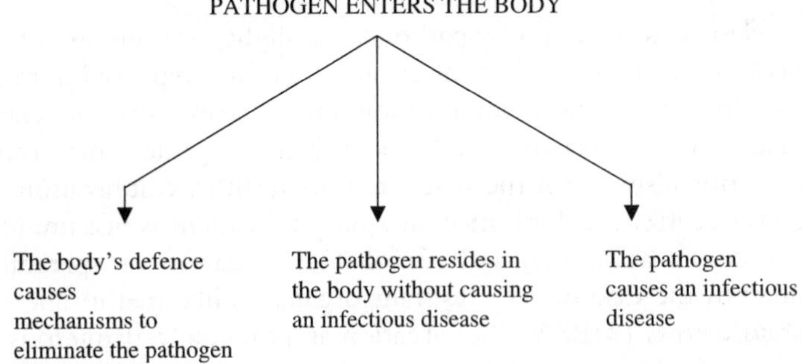

Figure 10.1 Potential outcomes following exposure to pathogens

Stages of infection

The course of infection has four stages (Taylor *et al.*, 1993).

1. Incubation period
2. Prodromal period
3. Full stage of illness period
4. Convalescent period

Incubation Period. The incubation period, is the time between the organism's entry to the host and the onset of symptoms.

Prodromal Period. The prodromal period is the time from the onset of non-specific signs and symptoms to the specific symptoms of the infection (Gormley, 1995). A person is most infectious during the prodromal stage. Early signs and symptoms of the disease are present but are vague, ranging from fatigue and malaise to low-grade fever. This period lasts from hours to days (Taylor *et al.*, 1993).

Full Stage of Illness Period. The third stage is the illness period, when the local specific signs and symptoms combine with a generalized feeling of being unwell (Gormley, 1995). The presence of specific signs and symptoms indicates the full stage of illness. The type of infection determines the length of the illness and the severity of the manifestations. Localized symptoms are limited or restricted to a discrete area whereas systemic symptoms are manifested throughout the entire body.

Convalescent Period. The convalescent period represents recovery from the infection and may vary according to the severity of the infection and the general condition of the affected person (Taylor *et al.*, 1993).

Colonization

When the response to invasion by pathogens is slight, or even absent, there is said to be colonization rather than infection. Organisms reported in microbiology test results often reflect colonization rather than infection (Donegan, 2000). A laboratory report of a swab taken from a leg ulcer may record the growth of an organism but if the tissue appears healthy, colonization and not infection, has occurred. Colonization in a hospital patient is not unimportant, however, as colonization may indicate that an organism is spreading in a ward or unit. In the case of very resistant organisms like methilcillin-resistant *Staphylococcus aureus* (MRSA) the situation is potentially dangerous, as the organism can spread from the colonized patients and cause infection in others (Thomlinson, 1989a).

Communicable Disease

This is an illness caused by a specific infectious agent or its toxic products that is transmitted directly or indirectly from an infected person or animal to a susceptible host.

Incubation Period

Once a pathogen gains entrance to a host a time known as the incubation period elapses before the clinical symptoms of the disease appear. During the incubation period the organism is establishing itself, spreading to target organs or tissues and proliferating within various body sites. The incubation period varies depending upon the condition of the host but is often predictable and diagnostically significant (Rice and Eckstein, 1995). The incubation period for the common cold is one to two days, whereas the incubation period for tetanus ranges from two to 21 days (Taylor *et al.*, 1993). In tuberculosis the incubation period may be difficult to determine because months or years may elapse between the time of the primary tubercular infection and the development of tuberculosis and other factors in the host determine the actual development of disease.

 **Connection**

Chapter 11 (Tuberculosis) provides detailed information about the pathophysiology of this disease.

Agents of Infection

Some of the more prevalent agents that are capable of causing infection include the following:

- Bacteria
- Viruses
- Rikettsia
- Protozoa
- Mycoplasmas
- Fungi
- Parasitic worms (helminths)

Bacteria

Bacteria are the most significant and most commonly observed infection-causing agents in health care settings. Bacteria can be categorized in various ways. According to shape they are classified as spherical (cocci), rod-shaped (bacilli), or corkscrew (spirochetes). Based on their reaction to the Gram stain, bacteria may be categorized as Gram-positive or Gram-negative. Gram-positive bacteria have a thick cell wall that is resistant to loss of colour and are stained violet. Gram-negative bacteria have chemically more complex cell walls and can be decolourized by alcohol. This difference is an important aid in choosing the appropriate antibiotic as antibiotics may be either specifically effective against only Gram-positive organisms or may be broad-spectrum antibiotics that are effective against several groups of microorganisms (Taylor *et al.*, 1993).

Viruses

Viruses are small infectious agents and differ from other living organisms in that they are not cells but simply a piece of either DNA (deoxyribonucleic acid) or RNA (ribonucleic acid) surrounded by a protein coat, and sometimes a lipid envelope. Viruses are unable to reproduce themselves but are obligate parasites of living cells in plants, animals and even bacteria. Once inside the cell they direct the host's metabolic machinery to reproduce themselves. New viruses are released from the cell by budding out of the membrane or by causing the cell to rupture. The host's symptoms are caused by the damage to the cells. Some viruses can become integrated within the host cell genome and become established indefinitely. While the initial symptoms of the invasion may disappear the virus remains dormant, to reactivate and produce symptoms at later intervals, as in herpes simplex infection (Wilson, 1997).

Rickettsia

Rickettsia and chlamydia are prokaryotes that are unable to grow outside a host cell. They are referred to as obligate intracellular parasites. Both rickettsia and chlamydia require factors from the host cell to support their growth (Thomlinson, 1989b). These microorganisms bridge the gap between bacteria and viruses (Gould and Brooker, 2000). Rikettsiae are natural inhabitants of the intestinal canal of arthropods and spread, for example, typhus fever. Infection is usually passed to humans through the skin from excreta of the arthropods but the saliva of some infected vectors is infected. Transmission to humans is by fleas, ticks, lice and mites; there is no recognized person-to-person spread (Stucke, 1993). Chlamydiae are round, slightly smaller than rickettsia and are responsible for a number of diseases such as the sexually acquired inflammatory pelvic disease and non-specific urethritis (Thomlinson, 1989b).

Protozoa

Protozoa are single celled organisms that belong to the animal kingdom and are more complex in structure and activity than bacteria. Diseases that are caused by protozoa include malaria, amoebic dysentery and trichomoniasis (Wilson, 1997).

Mycoplasmas

Mycoplasmas can be thought of as defective bacteria. They are single celled with no cell wall; they therefore have no fixed shape but are capable of complete metabolic activity (Thomlinson, 1989b). They primarily infect surface linings, affecting the respiratory, genitourinary and gastrointestinal tracts. *Mycoplasma pneumoniae* is the commonest cause of atypical pneumonia, especially in children and young adults, and some minor respiratory diseases (Stucke, 1993).

Fungi

Fungi are plant-like organisms such as moulds and yeasts that can cause infection. They are present in the air, soil and water and many are resistant to infection (Taylor *et al.*, 1993). Fungi have more complex, eukaryotic cells. The cell wall or membrane forms the outer boundary of the eukaryotic cell. There is rarely any extra coating equivalent to the prokaryotes (Stucke, 1993). Some fungi (for example, yeast) form a simple structure and exist as single cells, but complex forms exist with filamentous hyphae branching out to form an extensive interwoven mesh called a mycelium (Gould and Brooker, 2000). A disease caused by a fungus is called a mycosis, or it may be indicated by the suffix -osis, preceded by the name of the causative fungus (Wilson, 1997).

Fungal infections in humans are classified as follows:

1. Deep or systemic mycoses involving internal organs, for example, histoplasmosis infection
2. Superficial or subcutaneous mycoses growing in the deeper layers of the skin or outer layers of the hair, skin and nails. These include athlete's foot, ringworm and thrush (candida) infections (Thomlinson, 1989b).

Parasitic Worms

Parasitic worms or helminths can also cause infection. The most common infections are those caused by the roundworm, pinworm (threadworm) and tapeworm (Wilson, 1997).

Factors that Influence the Development of an Infection

- The numbers present (dose) and the duration of the exposure
- The source of the agent and the mode of transmission

- The susceptibility of the host
- The nature of the infectious agent in relation to the following
  - □ Infectivity
  - □ Pathogenicity
  - □ Virulence
  - □ Antigenicity
  - □ Toxigenicity

Dose

The importance of the infecting dose as a determinant of the outcome of infection has probably been underestimated. Studies of animals and in human volunteers have clearly shown the importance of dose in determining the severity of gastrointestinal infections. Thus infection from drinking contaminated water is likely to be greater than cleaning the teeth in contaminated water. Infective dose is likely to be an important factor in determining the outcome of infections spread by droplets (Greenwood, 2000).

Infectivity

Infectivity of the organism is its ability to invade and multiply within the host. It is affected by

- Host defensive mechanisms
- Pathogen-produced enzymes that facilitate its invasiveness

Most bacteria have to adhere to some sort of surface; when they interact with humans these organisms usually initially colonize a mucosal surface. Some streptococci are specifically adapted to colonize the oropharynx and adhere to epithelial cells in the mouth. Some strains of *Escherichia coli* produce surface antigens that allow specific adhesion to urothelial cells rather than colonic epithelium, increasing the risk of urinary tract infection. Many antigens expressed by bacteria to promote adherence are encoded by plasmids and may thus be transferred to other bacteria (Conlon and Syndman, 2000). Once the organisms have become adherent to an epithelial surface and established colonization they need to invade the host in order to cause disease. Some Gram-negative bacteria have a protective cell wall that makes them relatively resistant to lysis by the host. The outer membrane proteins of these organisms may form a layer that blocks the attachment of antibody or complement so that the bacteria can invade the immune system. Gram-positive organisms, such as *Streptococcus pneumoniae*, have a thick polysaccharide capsule that is antigenically variable and often quite resistant to phagocytosis by the host cells. Mycobacteria can be phagocytosed but can evade intracellular destruction by remaining inside the phagosome and inhibiting fusion between the phagosome and the lysosome (Conlon and Syndman, 2000).

Pathogenicity

Pathogenicity is the ability of an organism to produce disease. This is determined by its ability to enter the host and colonize, to penetrate tissues, to evade host defences and to damage tissues (Wansbrough-Jones and Wright, 1997). Pathogenicity depends upon

- The speed of reproduction
- The extent of tissue damage caused
- The production of a toxin

(Gould and Brooker, 2000)

Virulence

The virulence of an organism is its degree of pathogenicity. The virulence or potency of a pathogen determines the severity of disease that it produces. An organism is described as highly virulent if a small number of microbes can cause severe disease (Wansbrough-Jones and Wright, 1997).

Characteristics that contribute to an organism's virulence include its ability to

- Adhere to receptor surfaces
- Resist inactivation in nature
- Establish a safe residence outside the host
- Proliferate and create local tissue damage
- Invade and disseminate and alter its cell wall or membrane
- Transform its surface to a different antigenic structure to resist attachment by host antibodies

(Murphy and McMahon, 2000)

Antigenicity

Antigenicity is the ability of microorganisms and their products to induce an immune response in the host and this varies considerably (Gould and Brooker, 2000). Some pathogens have intrinsic antigens such as proteins, polypeptides or polysaccharides that stimulate antibody production against the antigen. Others lack antigenetic structures and may be able to evade destruction within the host for some time (Scherer, 1991).

Toxigenicity

Toxigenicity is an important factor in determining a pathogen's virulence. Most pathogenic organisms traverse the epithelium and their further success depends upon their ability to avoid host defence mechanisms but some pathogenic organisms cause disease at the site of colonization by producing toxins (Wansbrough-Jones and Wright, 1997). Numerous bacteria elaborate a variety of toxins that may either facilitate invasion by the bacteria or damage the host in some way. Bacterial toxins can be classified into different groups according to their localization in the growing microorganisms. Endocellular toxins are associated with the bacterial body and are only released with the death of the microorganism. Extracellular toxins are proteinaceous and are secreted by bacteria during their growth phase (Sansonetti, 1996).

- *Exotoxins*, which are distributed rapidly by the blood, cause potentially severe systemic and neurological manifestation. Gram-positive exotoxins are released outside the cell into the surrounding extracellular fluid, where they dissolve and are carried throughout the tissues. Exotoxins destroy host cells or inhibit specific metabolic functions. The exotoxin secreted by *Clostridium botulinum*, which causes botulism, interrupts the transmission of nervous impulses, paralysing the victim. The exotoxins released by *Staphylococcus aureus* and *Bacillus cereus* result in food poisoning (Gould and Brooker, 2000). Cholera toxin specifically affects enzymes in the small bowel mucosa that are responsible for ion and water transport, leading to profuse diarrhoea. *Staphylococcus aureus* produces a variety of toxins, one of which is toxic shock syndrome toxin-1 (TSST-1). This toxin can act as a superantigen, leading to T-lymphocyte proliferation. The resulting release of cytokine can lead to a multitude of problems (Conlon and Syndman, 2000).
- *Endotoxin*, or lipopolysaccharide, is a constituent of the bacterial cell wall of Gram-negative organisms (Conlon and Syndman, 2000). The release of endotoxins corresponds with symptoms experienced by the host. Examples include meningococcal meningitis and typhoid (Gould and Brooker, 2000). Irrespective of the organism from which the exotoxin came the symptoms produced in the host are similar and range from fever, malaise and leucopenia to shock, intravascular coagulation and death. The severity of the effect depends on the dose of endotoxins and the host's sensitivity to it (Stucke, 1993).

The Chain of Infection

An infection occurs as a result of inter-related factors. An infection will not result if the sequence is interrupted (see Figure 10.2). Hence efforts to control infections are directed toward interrupting the sequence (Taylor *et al.*, 1993).

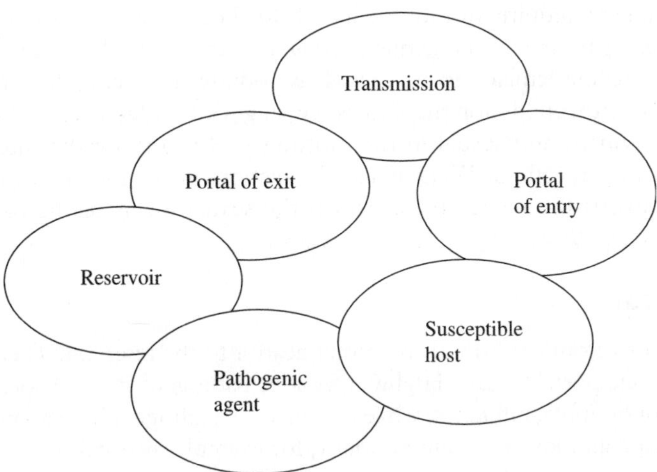

Figure 10.2 Chain of infection

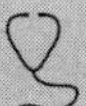

Nursing action points

Understand the characteristics of each link of the chain of infection. This provides the nurse with

- methods to support vulnerable patients
- ways to prevent the spread of infection
- knowledge of methods of self-protection.

(Truman College, 2001)

Pathogen

This is the causative agent. The pathogen is removed by cleaning, disinfection, sterilization and drug therapy, such as antibiotics and antimicrobials (Waugh, 1995).

Reservoir

The reservoir for growth and multiplication of the microorganisms is the natural habitat of the organism. Food, water, milk, inanimate objects, animals and other humans are potential reservoirs that support organisms pathogenic to humans (Taylor *et al.*, 1993). The pathogen depends upon the reservoir for reproduction and consequent survival. Humans may be the only reservoir and may be critically ill, subclinically ill or carriers. An individual who is a 'carrier' may exhibit no signs of illness but can pass on the infection to others.

Some pathogens require an intermediate host. For example, malaria is caused by protozoan parasites of the genus *Plasmodium* transmitted to humans by the bite of anopheline female mosquitoes. Plasmodium has a complex cycle using humans and arthropods for the successive stages of its life cycle. The cycle is asexual in humans and sexual in the mosquito. Humans are the intermediate host in malarial infections. While malarial infections are confined to humans the definitive host is the mosquito, in which the sexual forms of the parasite are found (Stucke, 1993).

Portal of Exit

Pathogens exit from the host at the portal nearest to the reservoir. There may be more than one portal of exit. Highly infectious pathogens have a short duration of escape for example, influenza; while less infective pathogens have a longer duration of escape and lower communicability, for example tuberculosis. The organism cannot extend its influence unless it moves away from its original source. In humans common escape routes include the respiratory, gastrointestinal and genitourinary tracts as well as breaks in the integrity of the skin. The blood and tissue can also serve as a portal of exit for pathogens (Taylor *et al.*, 1993).

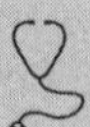

Nursing action points

- Contain infectious microorganisms, for example, educate patients to cover the mouth and nose with a tissue when coughing or sneezing.
- Use gloves when in contact with body fluids, moist body surfaces and areas of non-intact skin.
- Wear aprons when in contact with body secretions.
- Wear facial masks when in potential contact with respiratory droplet secretions.

(Truman College, 2001)

Transmission

An organism may be transmitted from its reservoir by various means and routes (see Figure 10.2). Some organisms can be transmitted by more than one route.

- *Direct*
  Involves transmitting the microorganisms directly from the reservoir to the person. This involves close proximity between the susceptible host and the infected person or a carrier, such as occurs in touching, kissing and sexual intercourse (Taylor *et al.*, 1993).
- *Indirect*
  Indirect spread requires an intermediary such as food, airborne particles, contaminated instruments or hands to pass the infection on (Wilson, 1997).

Contaminated blood, food and water or other inanimate objects (fomites) are vehicle routes of transmission. Vectors such as mosquitoes, ticks and lice, are non-human carriers that transmit organisms from one host to another. Organisms can be spread by means of the airborne route by droplet nuclei when coughing, sneezing and laughing and becoming attached to dust particles (Taylor *et al.*, 1993). The transmission of many diseases is multifactorial in that variables must act together to produce the disease (Murphy and McMahon, 2000).

Nursing action points

- Identify the source of infection.
- Isolate infectious patients when appropriate.
- Disrupt the direct contact of transmission by washing hands. Hand washing is the single most important measure, which all staff must carry out after patient contact. This is because the hands not only carry resident flora but may also have acquired other microorganisms, referred to as transient flora. These are frequently pathogenic but are removed more easily by hand washing than resident microorganisms (Murphy and McMahon, 2000).
- Facilitate hand washing practice for those patients who are confined to bed and also for those individuals who are unlikely to carry this out voluntarily. For example, children, individuals with learning difficulties and some people with mental health problems (Waugh, 1995).
- Eliminate pathogens from contaminated equipment by thorough sterilization or the use of disposable equipment.
- Interrupt indirect contact by using bags and covered containers for isolating contaminated materials.
- Prevent contamination of common vehicles of infection, such as, adequately refrigerating food in hospitals, and other healthcare settings.
- Educate clients in the basic principles of the prevention of infection transmission.

(Murphy and McMahon, 2000)

Portal of Entry

A portal of entry is needed because the organism must gain access to the host. The portal of entry often corresponds to the portal of exit in the human reservoir (Taylor *et al.*, 1993) (see Table 10.1). *Mycobacterium tuberculosis* does not cause disease if it settles on the skin of an exposed host. The only entry route of significance is through the respiratory system (Donegan, 2000). In pregnancy the placenta normally acts as a barrier, preventing microorganisms from reaching the fetus; however, some pathogens are able to cross the placental barrier to cause infection in the fetus (Wilson, 1997).

Invasive diagnostic and therapeutic devices that bypass the patient's normal defence mechanisms provide a portal of entry into the body and therefore increase the risk of infection (Rice and Eckstein, 1995).

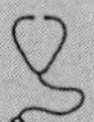

Nursing action points

- Keep the door closed in respiratory-isolated patients.
- Use facial masks, for example, when caring for people with tuberculosis (Murphy and McMahon, 2000).
- Be aware of the increased susceptibility to infection associated with the use of indwelling catheters, monitoring devices, intravenous catheters and respiratory assistance devices (Rice and Eckstein, 1995).

Host Susceptibility

Human beings differ in their susceptibility to infectious diseases and in many cases the reasons why some people are more prone to certain infections than the majority of the population are unknown. They may have subtle deficiencies in their defence mechanisms (Conlon and Syndman, 2000). Susceptibility to an infectious disease depends upon the individual's degree of resistance to pathogens. Although everyone is constantly exposed to large numbers of microorganisms, an infection does not develop until an individual becomes susceptible to the strength and numbers of those microorganisms (Long and Miller, 1995).

Host susceptibility is influenced by a number of factors. Age, sex, ethnicity, heredity, cultural behaviour, geographical and environmental factors, previous exposure, immune competence and the health and nutritional status of the

Table 10.1 Portals of exit/entry

Portals of exit	*Portals of entry*
Expiration of droplets especially when coughing or sneezing	Inhalation of contaminated air or droplets
Excretion in faeces	Ingestion of contaminated food or fluid.
Leakage from broken skin, for example, serous fluid, blood	Inoculation of broken skin, for example, abrasions, lacerations, wound drainage, intravenous infusion, open sores
Discharge from mucous membranes.	Inoculation
Penis or vagina during sexual intercourse	Penis or vagina during sexual intercourse
Excretion in urine	Poor genital hygiene Urinary catheter instrumentation

individual, all contribute to a greater or lesser susceptibility to a particular infectious disease. Children and the elderly are more susceptible to bacterial pneumonia and intestinal infections. The incidence of the carrier state of hepatitis B is greater in males than females and is also more frequent among people with Down's syndrome and those receiving haemodialysis (Conlon and Syndman, 2000).

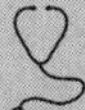

Nursing action points

- Ensure that personal vaccination, for example with the hepatitis B vaccine, is up to date.
- Encourage vaccination in high risk groups, for example influenza vaccine for the elderly and those with chronic respiratory problems.
- Support public health interventions that address areas such as nutrition and vector control.

(Murphy and McMahon, 2000)

Factors Predisposing to Infection

- Age
- Nutritional imbalance
- Gender and hormonal factors
- Stress
- Trauma
- Infections and other underlying conditions
- Drugs
- Invasive procedures and devices
- Local factors
- Genetics
- Inadequate defences

Age

Immunological maturity steadily develops during the first years of life while both cellular and humoral immunity is compromised in infants. The elderly are more susceptible to and have a diminished capacity to combat infection. The thymus gland begins to atrophy at about 45 years of age resulting in a decreased production of its hormones, which play a part in the differentiation of lymphocytes. The response to foreign antigens decreases with ageing and the elderly are not able to sustain resistance against infection (Wilson, 1997). Age influences not only the susceptibility to infection but also its clinical severity (Greenwood, 2000).

Nutritional Imbalances

Lymphoid tissue is vulnerable to excesses and deficiencies of many nutrients because of its rapid rate of proliferation. Protein and calorie deficiency can cause impaired cell-mediated immunity. Humoral immunity and phagocytosis are less affected. The components of the immune system are affected by inadequate intake of vitamins A, B and folic acid and of minerals such as zinc and iron (Wilson, 1997). Iron deficiency has been shown to increase susceptibility to certain bacterial infections and deficiency in vitamin A predisposes to infection at epithelial surfaces and increases the severity of measles (Greenwood, 1996). Without the required nutrients and energy the production of antibodies, lymphocytes and the chemical mediators of the immune response is impaired (Wilson, 1997).

Gender and Hormonal Factors

Young women are more susceptible to tuberculosis than young men, although the reason is not known and some diseases are more severe when they occur during pregnancy, for example, hepatitis.

An excess of glucocorticoids, resulting from adrenal hyperplasia, an adrenal tumour or steroid therapy, increases susceptibility to many infections and also their severity. Patients with diabetes show an increased susceptibility to boils, abscesses and urinary tract infections (Greenwood, 2000).

Exposure to Cold

A lowering of the body temperature below normal is thought to decrease the ciliary movement in the respiratory tract and it reduces the blood supply to superficial tissues.

Stress

It has been shown that white blood cell counts and lymphocyte cytoxicity correlate negatively with lifestyle change stress. Naturally occurring, persistent stress accompanied by poor coping alters the body's immunocompetence (Wilson, 1997).

Trauma

Damage to the surface defences, for example by a severe burn, opens the way for systemic invasion by organisms usually confined to the surface of the body. Severe burns also have a depressive effect upon the immune system (Greenwood, 2000).

Infections and Other Underlying Conditions

Some infections decrease the individual's resistance to a secondary infection. The human immunodeficiency virus depresses cell-mediated immunity and leaves the individual open to many opportunistic pathogens that take advantage of the deficient immune response. Underlying conditions such as leukaemia and liver and renal disease increase the individual's susceptibility to infection (Wilson, 1997). Patients with widespread malignant disease have an increased risk of infection, sometimes with organisms of low virulence. The risk of infection may be further increased by extensive radiotherapy or by treatment with cytotoxic drugs (Greenwood, 2000). Diseases of the immune system, such as AIDS and lymphoma weaken defences against infection; chronic diseases such as diabetes cause general debilitation and nutritional impairment (Long and Miller, 1995).

Drugs

Immunosuppressive drugs are used to treat autoimmune disorders such as rheumatoid arthritis and inflammatory bowel disease and also to prevent rejection of transplanted tissue and to treat cancers. The action of these drugs is to increase the individual's susceptibility to infection. Some antibiotics also increase susceptibility to infection by disrupting the normal flora (Wilson, 1997). Alcohol in excess increases susceptibility to many infections, particularly when cirrhosis of the liver is present. Septicaemia is a common terminal event in intravenous drug addicts who neglect basic hygienic precautions. Smoking predisposes to respiratory infections by damaging the epithelium (Greenwood, 2000).

Invasive Procedures and Indwelling Medical Devices

These increase susceptibility by bypassing defence mechanisms particularly in individuals already weakened by disease (Taylor *et al.*, 1993)

Local Factors

Tissue that is poorly perfused by blood, as is the case following injury, embolus or necrosis, becomes anoxic and more susceptible to invasion by microorganisms. Pressure sores and burns provide an exposed, moist area of tissue in which pathogens can multiply (Wilson, 1997).

Genetic Factors

These are known to play a role but the data are inconclusive. The importance is often difficult to establish given the myriad of socio-economic factors contributing to the state of health and nutrition of individuals. The role of genetics has been established in certain diseases, for example the decreased susceptibility to malaria of persons with the sickle cell trait (Conlon and Syndman, 2000).

Racial differences in the pattern of individual infectious diseases, for example the tendency of patients with tuberculosis, from India, to show bone involvement and the severity of yellow fever in Europeans, suggest that genetic factors have influence on the course of an infection. It is difficult, however, to differentiate between the influence of genetic and environmental factors. Studies of identical twins have shown that the twin of a patient with tuberculosis or leprosy has a higher risk of contracting the infection than a control, even when the twin is brought up in a different environment from his or her sibling. Susceptibility to a variety of diseases, most of which involve some kind of immunological abnormality, is associated with the possession of specific HLA (human leucocyte antigens). Immune responsiveness is related to the possession of certain genetically determined allotypes of immunoglobulin molecules and possession of specific blood-group antigens also influences susceptibility to some infections (Greenwood, 1996).

Genetic factors can influence susceptibility to infection in at least three ways:

1. Influence on surface receptors – the presence or absence of a suitable membrane receptor may be under genetic control.
2. Influence on host cell constituents – an intracellular parasite depends on the constituents of the host cell for nutrition.
3. Influence on the specific immune response – a number of clearly defined, genetically determined, primary immunodeficiency syndromes have been described that are associated with an increased susceptibility to infection. These are responsible for only a small fraction of severe infections. It is possible that subtler genetically determined defects of the immune system contribute to the pathogenesis of a much larger proportion of cases of infectious diseases as yet undefined (Greenwood, 2000).

Inadequate Defences

Inadequate defences such as broken skin, decreased ciliary action, suppressed inflammatory response and low white blood cell count can also increase an individual's susceptibility to infection (Long and Miller, 1995).

Mechanical and Physiological Defence Mechanisms

Skin and Mucosa

These provide an important mechanical barrier to invasion by many pathogenic organisms. The protective properties of the skin are increased by the secretion on to its surface of bactericidal fatty acids (Greenwood, 1996).

The Mouth

An intact multi-layered mucosa provides a mechanical barrier to microorganisms. Saliva washes away particles containing microorganisms and also contains lysozyme, which is a microbial inhibitor (Long and Miller, 1995).

Gastrointestinal Tract

The mechanical barrier to infection provided by the gastric epithelium is enhanced by the acid pH of the stomach contents. This chemically destroys microorganisms incapable of surviving low pH. The pH of 2.0 is lethal to most bacteria but if large numbers are ingested they may be protected by the bulk of the food eaten (Wilson, 1997). People with achlorhydria, common among malnourished people and those who smoke marijuana, have an increased susceptibility to infection (Greenwood, 1996). Rapid peristalsis in the small intestine prevents the retention of bacterial contents (Long and Miller, 1995).

The Respiratory System

A sticky mucous blanket coats cilia lining the upper airways. This traps inhaled microbes and sweeps them outward in the mucus to be expectorated or swallowed. Macrophages engulf and destroy microorganisms that reach lung alveoli.

Urinary Tract

The flushing act of urinary flow washes away microorganisms on the lining of the bladder and urethra. An intact multi-layered epithelium provides a barrier to microorganisms.

Vagina

At puberty, normal flora cause secretions to become acidic and this inhibits the growth of many microorganisms (Long and Miller, 1995).

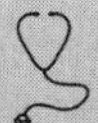

Nursing action points

Consideration should be given to factors that may alter the body's defence mechanisms thus increasing an individual's susceptibility to infection.

- Take great care to maintain the integrity of the patient's skin. Damage to the skin may make the individual susceptible to systemic infection by an organism that would not normally be pathogenic (Greenwood, 1996).

- Ensure good hygiene practice as this is important in helping to remove organisms that adhere to the skin's outer layer.
- Avoid excessive bathing.
- Be aware that trauma to the mouth and poor oral hygiene may alter the body's defence mechanisms.
- Be aware that high concentrations of oxygen and carbon dioxide and cold air can adversely affect defence mechanisms.
- Be aware that obstruction of urinary flow compromises body defence and the introduction of a urinary catheter and the continued movement of the catheter in the urethra can damage the epithelium.
- Be aware that the administration of antacids affects the pH of gastrointestinal contents, and that delayed motility of faecal material, due to faecal impaction or obstruction by tumours can also alter defence mechanisms.
- Be aware that the administration of antibiotics and contraceptive pills disrupts the normal flora increasing the risk of infection.

(Long and Miller, 1995)

Normal Body Flora

The blood, heart and vascular system and the fluids from these sites are usually sterile, whereas most other human tissues have microorganisms present. Most bacteria and some other organisms are neither harmful nor beneficial. Some however, provide beneficial normal flora to compete with pathogens, to facilitate digestion or to work in other ways symbiotically with the host (Donegan, 2000).

Phagocytosis

This is the engulfment, killing and digestion of microorganisms by polymorphonuclear leucocytes, monocytes and the macrophages that originate from the bone marrow (Wilson, 1997).

Polymorphonuclear Leucocytes or Neutrophils

These account for most of the circulating white cells in the blood. They move in an amoeboid fashion along the surface of vessels and can change shape, moving between endothelial cells and into the tissues. These phagocytes are attracted to sites of inflammation by chemotactic signals from other cells and become activated. The infecting organism is engulfed by the neutrophil pseudopod and a phagosome is formed. Granules within the neutrophil fuse with the phagosome, releasing various microbicidal proteins, such as, lysozyme. Neutrophils can also produce large quantities of hydrogen peroxide and other oxidases that act to damage bacteria. Reduction in the number of circulating neutrophils, for example, following chemotherapy can lead to infection (Conlon and Syndman, 2000).

Monocytes

These circulate in the blood and then migrate to the tissues, where they develop into macrophages. They are found in connective tissues in the lungs, liver, spleen, brain and lymph nodes.

Macrophages

These play an important role in both the non-specific and the specific defence mechanisms of the body. They get rid of cell debris, such as microorganisms and worn out cells and play a vital role in immune responses and the development of inflammation (Wilson, 1997).

Complement System

This is an important component of host defences and consists of a group of highly regulated proteins and cell membrane receptors. The complement system consists of numerous enzymes and co-factors that interact with each other in an orderly sequence, called an enzyme cascade (Stucke, 1993). The key elements in the defence against infection are the third component (C_3) and the terminal components (C_5–C_9). Complement can be activated by the 'classical pathway' when antigen–antibody complexes bind to and activate the first complement component (C_1). On the other hand, C_3 can be activated via the 'alternative pathway', which does not depend on the presence of an antibody. The activation of complement leads to a variety of inflammatory responses, including increased vascular permeability and neutrophil chemotaxis. When bound to microorganisms, activated C_3 acts as a potent opsonin (an antibody present in the blood, that renders bacteria more easily destroyed by phagocytosis) (Conlon and Syndman, 2000).

The organisms become coated with derivatives of C_3, which causes the microorganisms to adhere strongly to the membranes of phagocytic cells that have a binding site or receptor for C_3. The efficiency with which the microorganisms are engulfed is increased greatly by this attachment. Other components are then modified enzymically and become active as chemotaxins, attracting more phagocytes to the site of infection. The lytic pathway can kill some bacteria and viruses, but this is not as important as the binding to membranes via C_3. Congenital absence of C_3 leads rapidly to death from infection (Stucke, 1993).

The Inflammatory Response

Inflammation is the response of tissues to trauma, whether the injury involves cuts, chemical damage, and extremes of temperature or pathogenic invasion. The capillary walls vasodilate and become more permeable. This is triggered by the release of prostaglandins from platelets and other locally acting hormones, particularly histamine and bradykinin, the latter being responsible for the pain experienced during inflammation. Leakage of plasma into the intracellular space leads to swelling, which contributes further to pain by exerting pressure on the nerves. The erythema and sensation of heat are due to the increased blood supply, which is beneficial as it boosts the local availability of neutrophils and microphages to combat infection, while the greater volume of fluid helps to dilute the toxins (Gould and Brooker, 2000). Polymorphonuclear leucocytes migrate to the area and phagocytose the pathogens and in so doing they die. Macrophages appear later to mop up the debris, which consists of dead leucocytes, microorganisms and necrotic tissue. Pus is formed if the infection is severe enough. The process can be recognized by local swelling, redness, heat and pain (Wilson, 1997).

Interferon

When certain body cells, leucocytes, fibroblasts and T-lymphocytes are infected by some viruses, they respond by producing interferon. This is a group of small proteins that inhibit virus multiplication within the cells. These proteins will only work in the species that produced them. Interleukins are types of interferons that help to stimulate an immune response (Wilson, 1997).

Natural Killer Cells

These non-specific lymphocytes rid the body of what they perceive as foreign or non-self cells without having to recognize a specific antigen. They migrate from the lymphoid tissue to the site of inflammation or tumour growth where they destroy the pathogens, tumour cells or virus infected cells. Whereas T-lymphocyte cells need to be sensitized before they can react to a foreign cell, a killer cell does not (Thomlinson, 1989a).

Specific Defences

The specific host defence system involves the response of antigen-specific lymphocytes to an antigen, including the development of an immunological memory. The two major subsystems are the humoral immune system and cell-mediated immunity (Murphy and McMahon, 2000).

Cell-mediated Immunity

T-lymphocytes are the cells responsible for cell-mediated immunity, which protects an individual from intracellular bacterial infections, viral and some fungal infections. It is the major element of defence against parasites and tumours. T-lymphocytes are also involved in transplant rejection (Stucke, 1993).

When bacteria enter the body they are first ingested by macrophages. The bacterial antigen then appears on the surface of the macrophage where it is recognized by a corresponding T-cell, which binds with the antigen–macrophage complex (Wilson, 1997). Antigens need to be processed by antigen-presenting cells and presented to the T-lymphocyte receptor in association with major histocompatability complex (MHC) molecules on the cell surface (Conlon and Syndman, 2000).

Binding to the T-lymphocyte receptor can trigger a series of events depending on the T-lymphocyte type. The T-cell produces a range of chemical mediators called lymphokines that include interferons and interleukins (Wilson, 1997). The release of interferon-γ and interleukin-2 can help to recruit macrophages and promote phagocytosis (Conlon and Syndman, 2000). Such activated macrophages show enhanced activity against organisms other than the one, which induced the cell-mediated immune reaction that led to their formation (Greenwood, 1996). Cytotoxic T-lymphocytes recognize and kill cells expressing foreign antigen in association with MHC Class 1 molecules. This is an important means of defence against viruses (Conlon and Syndman, 2000). Direct contact between the T-lymphocyte and the target cell is required and the effector cell must be metabolically active. Neither antibody nor complement is required. Killing is only achieved when the effector cell and the target cell share the same class 1 histocompatability antigens (HLA), the effector cell recognizing a peptide HLA complex on the surface of the target cell (Greenwood, 1996).

Humoral Immunity

Antibodies, in the form of immunoglobulins, form the basis of the humoral immune system. B-lymphocytes differentiate into antibody secreting plasma cells when they are stimulated by the presence of an antigen. B-lymphocytes bind with the antigen that fits their receptors; they then multiply, producing identical clone cells that then differentiate into plasma cells (Wilson, 1997). Antigen binds to the B-lymphocytes via the cell surface immunoglobulin that acts as the B-lymphocyte receptor. The B-lymphocyte differentiates into an antibody-producing cell when stimulated by cytokines, which are released from type 1 T-helper lymphocytes. Recurrent pyogenic infections may occur as a result of deficiencies of immunoglobulin (Conlon and Syndman, 2000). The plasma cells produce large quantities of antibodies specific to the antigen for several days before they die. The antibodies are released into the circulation where they interlock with matching antigens to form antibody–antigen complexes. These complexes stimulate phagocytic activity and activate complement to destroy the bacterial cell or toxin. The antibody production declines as the infection is overcome, plasma cells die and the suppressor T cells exert their control. Some activated B cells are not converted to plasma cells but become memory cells, which are stored and respond at a later date when stimulated by exposure to the same antigen. On first exposure to an antigen there is a time lapse of a few days or weeks. This is called the primary response. On second exposure to the same antigen, months or even years later, antibodies are produced rapidly and this is called the secondary response.

Immunoglobulins

Antibodies are immunoglobulin molecules.

The five major immunoglobulins are

- Immunoglobulin A (IgA) – is found in tears, saliva, respiratory, gastrointestinal secretions, colostrum and the blood. It protects the external openings of the body against invasion.
- Immunoglobulin E (IgE) – is associated with the symptoms of allergic responses.
- Immunoglobulin D (IgD) – functions are unclear but maximum levels are present in childhood.
- Immunoglobulin G (IgG) – the most common antibody in the blood. It is able to enter the tissues. It crosses the placenta to afford protection to the fetus.
- Immunoglobulin M (IgM) – is large and tends to remain in the bloodstream where it produces an early line of attack against bacteria.

(Wilson, 1997)

Harmful Immune Responses to Infection

The value of the immune response in achieving recovery and preventing reinfection is evident when considering the effects on the individual when immunity is impaired. However, destruction of an intracellular parasite can also result in destruction of the host cell. Where cell regeneration is rapid, such as in the liver, damaged cells are easily replaced, whereas immunologically mediated recovery from infections in the nervous system may result in irreversible tissue damage.

- Immediate and delayed hypersensitivity reactions result from the release of histamines and other vasoactive amines. In some infections, for example, leprosy, tuberculosis and salmonellosis, tissue damage produced in this way is more important than that produced by the causative microorganism.

- Antibody-mediated tissue damage occurs as a result of sensitization of host cells by microbial antigens that can render them susceptible to immune attack.
- Immune complex-mediated tissue damage occurs as a result of immune complex deposition. Immune complexes can cause a variety of clinical syndromes, depending on the site where they are formed and ranging in severity from a mild rash to peripheral circulatory collapse and associated intravascular coagulation.

Types of infection

- Local infection is confined to one area.
- Systemic infection is one in which the organisms are disseminated throughout the body.
- Primary infection is the initial infection.
- Secondary infection occurs when during the course of an infection, the individual becomes infected by another type of organism.
- Acute infection is an intense illness of short duration.
- Chronic infection describes a protracted course of illness due to the infection.
- Bacteraemia describes the presence of bacteria in the bloodstream.
- Septicaemia is a condition where bacteraemia is accompanied by symptoms, such as fever and rigors.
- Toxaemia implies a concentration of bacterial toxins in the blood.

(Wilson, 1997)

Clinical Characteristics of Infection

The Clinical Manifestations of Localized Infection

Symptoms are due to the inflammatory response. Inflammation is always present with infection unless the person's immune system is severely impaired, but infection is not always present with inflammation. Symptoms of localized infection are as follows:

- Redness and heat due to vasodilation
- Swelling (oedema) due to increased vascular permeability
- Pain or tenderness caused by the release of chemical mediators and pressure from increased tissue fluid

Table 10.2 Allergic reactions to infection

Infection	*Allergic reaction leading to*
Meningococcal	Pericarditis
Measles	Encephalitis
Post-infective polyneuritis	Peripheral neuropathy
Infectious mononucleosis	Haemolytic anaemia
Streptococcal infection	Nephritis
Reiter's syndrome	Arthritis

- Restricted movement of a body part
- Possible drainage from open lesions or wounds

The Clinical Manifestations of Acute Infection

- Fatigue
- Malaise
- Lymph node enlargement
- Nausea and vomiting
- Headache
- Tachycardia
- Tachypnoea
- Fever associated with anorexia, protein catabolism, negative nitrogen balance, acute-phase protein response, hypoalbuminaemia, low serum iron, sequestration of iron, anaemia and neutrophilia (Griffin *et al.*, 1999). Fever is due to a resetting of the thermostat in the anterior hypothalamus, to a higher setting. This is a purposeful reaction, potentiating the immune and inflammatory responses to infection (Murphy, 2000)
- Inflammation; pain, dysfunction, tissue damage
- Convulsions, especially in children
- Haemorrhage, haemolytic anaemia and intravascular coagulation
- Organ failure; for example, heart, brain, lungs, liver and necrosis of the skin
- Shock: sustained fall in circulating blood volume associated with lowered systemic resistance

(Griffin *et al.*, 1999)

In addition to the common signs and symptoms of infection, certain characteristics of a specific infection may be present, for example, certain infections cause a rash (Wilson, 1997) (see Table 10.2).

Rashes

Rashes are common features of many systemic infectious diseases.

Classification of rashes

- Maculopapular – discrete or sometimes confluent red spots that can be elevated. A mixture of macules (flat lesions) and papules (raised lesions). For example, in measles
- Vesicular – fluid filled sacs, as in chickenpox
- Haemorrhagic – petechiae, which are small, or the larger ecchymoses. The rapid onset of a haemorrhagic rash is associated with meningococcal infection
- Punctiform – pinpoint-like, for example, rubella (Rudd and Nicoll, 1991)
- Nodular, as in erythema nodosum, found in tuberculosis and leprosy
- Erythematous – a diffuse red eruption that blanches on finger pressure, for example, as in scarlet fever
- Urticarial (nettle rash), for example as in toxocariasis
- Chancres are ulcerating nodules, found, for example, in syphilis

(Griffin *et al.*, 1999)

The Clinical Manifestations of Chronic Infection

- Weight loss and muscle wasting
- Malnutrition, especially associated with diarrhoea
- Retardation of growth and intellect in children
- Tissue destruction
- Anaemia
- Post-infective syndromes, such as lactose intolerance, irritable colon

Diagnostic Investigations

The principles of diagnosis are to

1. Establish if the disease is caused by infection and identify the site.
2. Identify the causative microorganism.

(Wansbrough-Jones and Wright, 1997)

History

A number of factors relative to the history of the illness may be significant when the nature of the illness is suspected to be infectious:

- Translating the patient's account of the illness. One problem encountered in history taking, is to reach agreement on the meaning ascribed to various words and phrases in common use. For example, 'gastroenteritis' used to equate with diarrhoea may lead the unwary practitioner to assume an infective illness, whereas diarrhoea and vomiting can have a number of non-infective causes (Lambert, 1996).

- The pattern of the illness.
- A history of contact with patients with a similar illness.
- Behaviour that confers a risk of infection.
- A history of travel to places where particular infections are known to be endemic (Wansbrough-Jones and Wright, 1997).
- Occupation occasionally provides important information relative to diagnosis, for example, psittacosis in bird-handlers and tuberculosis in abattoir workers (Lambert, 1996).

Examination

In addition to the common signs and symptoms of infectious diseases, certain characteristics of a specific infection may be present and play an important role in diagnosis (Wilson, 1997). Examples are the rash of chickenpox or measles, the neck stiffness caused by acute meningitis and the characteristic cough of whooping cough. A combination of signs is common, for example, infectious mononucleosis is suggested by exudative tonsillitis, generalized lymphadenopathy and splenomegaly. Physical signs, such as consolidation in the lungs may indicate the site of the infection (Wansbrough-Jones and Wright, 1997).

Diagnostic Procedures Used in Infection

Leucocyte Count and Differential

Some infections cause an increase in the number of white blood cells well above normal, while in others there may be a fall below normal.

Erythrocyte Sedimentation Rate

This is a non-specific test that measures the rate at which the red blood cells settle, which is increased in infection and inflammation.

Microscopic Examination

Specimens of blood, sputum, urine, faeces, cerebrospinal fluid, discharge or scrapings from a lesion, are examined. These are stained and examined under a microscope for microorganisms. Appearance, shape and certain staining characteristics help to identify different microorganisms.

Culturing the Causative Microorganism

This is achieved by inoculation of the specimen into a nutrient media and allowing time for the microorganisms to multiply. A pure growth of the causative microorganism that is isolated is tested for susceptibility to appropriate antimicrobial drugs. The results of these tests form the basis for the selection of the most effective and appropriate drug treatment.

Antibody Tests

A blood test to determine the concentration of antibodies is referred to as an antibody titre. Antibody titres rise as the infection progresses (Wilson, 1997).

Skin Tests

The Mantoux tuberculin skin test is used to determine whether an individual is immune to *Mycobacterium tuberculosis.*

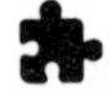 **Connection**

Chapter 11 (Tuberculosis) explains the use of skin testing as a means of determining if an individual has been infected by *Mycobacterium tuberculosis*.

Data may also be obtained from radiological tests, computerized axial tomography (CT), magnetic resonance imaging (MRI) and ultrasound (Rice and Eckstein, 1995).

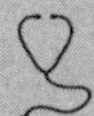 *Nursing action points*

Collection of specimens

- Remember that specimens should be fresh.
- If it is necessary to store specimens, store them in a designated refrigerator at 4°C
- Always put swabs into the appropriate media.
- Obtain swabs from skin lesions from a damp area or exudate. Take throat swabs from the tonsils or any other area where an exudate or lesion can be seen. Insert rectal swabs just inside the anus. Collect vaginal swabs from the vestibular fossa.

(Rudd and Nicoll, 1991)

- Be aware that swabs in transport medium need not be refrigerated or incubated and should be plated out in the laboratory within 24 hours of being obtained (Thomlinson, 1989c).

- Include the following information on specimen labels:
  - □ patient's name
  - □ date and time of the collection
  - □ test requested
  - □ type of specimen
  - □ how the specimen was obtained (for example, clean void or catheter, expectorated sputum or tracheal aspirate)
  - □ where the results are to be sent.

(Rice and Eckstein, 1995)

Treatment

Antimicrobial Drugs

A wide range of antimicrobial drugs is now available; these drugs have revolutionized the management of bacterial, fungal and protozoal infections (Wilson, 1997). The term antibiotic describes substances that are produced by microorganisms and which are antagonistic to the growth of others in high dilution. Improved molecular techniques have led to the synthesis of drugs that have been specifically designed to attack identified targets in microorganisms. Strictly speaking, synthetic antimicrobial drugs are not antibiotics (Davey, 2000). The key to the management of infection is the early recognition of symptoms and identification of the causative microorganism. The correct drug can then be administered before the microorganism is able to overwhelm the host's immune defence. Viruses exist within the host cells and there are very few antimicrobial agents that are effective against them. Treatment mostly involves symptom control and supporting the patient through the acute phase of the illness, which in most cases is self-limiting (Wilson, 1997).

Nursing Interventions

The potential for infection or the presence of an infection in a client suggests possible nursing diagnoses. The focus of nursing care depends upon a nursing diagnosis that accurately reflects the client's condition.

For example:

- High risk of infection related to
  - □ an altered immune response
  - □ chronic disease
  - □ the effects of medication
  - □ altered skin integrity
  - □ malnutrition

  - the presence of an invasive or indwelling medical device
  - lack of proper immunization
- Altered oral mucous membrane related to ineffective dental hygiene or trauma
- High risk of altered body temperature (Taylor *et al.*, 1993)
- Body image disturbance (Long and Miller, 1995)
- Social isolation related to the presence of a communicable disease. Many principles of infection control limit contact between the nurse and patient and impose visiting restrictions

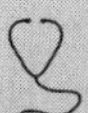

Nursing action points

- Take account of the psychological impact of isolation upon an individual.
- Be aware that wearing gloves prevents direct contact through touch and may cause the individual to feel dirty or contaminated.
- Offer emotional support to the isolated patient. Isolation can result in feelings of loneliness and interferes in needed emotional support.
- Balance the principles of asepsis, standard precautions and psychological support of the patient.
- Be knowledgeable of the infectious agent. This allows the nurse to use protective measures without isolating the patient beyond what is necessary. The appropriate use of gloves when handling body fluids, does not in most cases, exclude holding a hand, without a barrier glove, in order to provide important psychological comfort.
- Allow the patient to express feelings about the constraints of isolation.
- Educate the patient of the need for barrier techniques. This is an important consideration in the development and maintenance of an effective nurse/patient relationship.

(Truman College, 2001)

Nursing interventions when an infection has occurred depend upon the nature of the infection. There are a number of general principles related to the monitoring of complications of infection and symptom control.

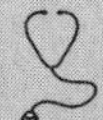

Nursing action points

- Record body temperature and respiration rate – aim to maintain body temperature and normal respiration.
- Record fluid balance – aim to maintain fluid balance.

- Record bowel function – aim to maintain normal bowel function.
- Ensure that nutritional requirements are met.
- Administer prescribed antimicrobial agents.

(Wilson, 1997)

Nosocomial Infection (Hospital-acquired Infection)

This is an infection acquired by patients while they are in hospital or by staff that are working in the hospital. If patients acquire an infection more than 72 hours after admission, it is considered to be hospital-acquired, rather than community-acquired infection (Caddow, 1989). Infections may be endogenous, that is, caused by microorganisms (normal flora) that colonize the body entering another site to establish infection, or exogenous, caused by the transmission of microorganisms from the environment to another person. Bacteria encountered in hospital are frequently resistant to antibiotics because the widespread use of antibiotics encourages the selection and survival of more resistant microorganisms (Wilson, 1997).

Most nosocomial infections are readily recognized because they develop while the patient is in hospital, but infections that have a long incubation period, such as hepatitis B, may not become clinically apparent until months after the patient has been discharged. On a national scale, the number, severity and cost of nosocomial infections have been difficult to measure. Rates of between 5.7 and 8.2 per 100 admissions have been reported. The most common site for nosocomial infection is the urinary tract, followed by surgical wounds and the lower respiratory tract (Bowler and Crook, 2000).

Pathogens with nosocomial infection potential include

- ***Clostridium difficile***
  This is a bacterium with significant nosocomial potential. Spore formation facilitates the microorganism's ability to be spread by environmental sources and personnel. After antibiotic treatment an individual's normal intestinal flora is often disrupted, and *Clostridium difficile* is often resistant to antimicrobial therapy and therefore is able to proliferate relatively unimpeded in this setting. Large areas of intestinal epithelium become necrotic, with the individual experiencing profuse, watery diarrhoea. The nosocomial potential is compounded by the fact that the spore is relatively resistant to cleaning and hand washing agents and can be spread by the hands of healthcare workers and by contaminated equipment (Donegan, 2000).
- ***Staphylococcus aureus***
  Asymptomatic carriage of this microorganism is clinically significant because the bacteria can be carried to susceptible sites, for example from the nose to a wound, or from an asymptomatic person to someone less healthy who will succumb to infection. In hospital *Staphylococcus aureus* causes serious wound infections, bronchopneumonia, endocarditis and osteomyelitis.

- **Methicillin-resistant staphylococcal infection (MRSA)**
  MRSA has become a cause for concern because it is extremely difficult to eradicate. Since the introduction of antibiotics in the 1940s there has been concern about antibiotic-resistant *S. aureus.* In the late 1970s *S. aureus* showed resistance to the synthetic penicillin, methicillin. At that time MRSA was seen infrequently but since the late 1970s *S. aureus* has become increasingly resistant to methicillin and transmission in hospitals and nursing homes has been well documented. Vancomycin is usually the preferred alternative treatment for serious MRSA but the concern is that this too will lose its effectiveness (Donegan, 2000).

  MRSA causes the same range of infections as methicillin-sensitive *S. aureus*; it is disseminated in the same way and is no more virulent. Most people become asymptomatic carriers and never develop clinical infection, especially if they are healthy. However, they act as reservoirs, and have the potential to pass on the infection, especially to seriously ill people. Skin lesions such as chronic wounds and cannula sites can become heavily colonized and so are particularly likely to operate as reservoirs and healthcare workers can easily transmit MRSA to patients. Epidemic methicillin-resistant *S. aureus* (EMRSA) spreads more easily than other strains of MRSA and appears to colonize skin and mucous membranes more readily (Gould and Brooker, 2000).

Guidelines for Controlling MRSA

- Reduce transmission by detecting, treating and isolating all colonized patients.
- Avoid the unnecessary use of antibiotics.
- Implement infection control precautions, especially hand washing, patient isolation and adequate cleaning.
- Develop programmes for community control that involve treating MRSA positive patients discharged from hospital.
- Implement protocols for screening patients, new staff and staff with positive nasal swabs.

(Gould and Brooker, 2000)

Risk Assessment and Flexible Management of MRSA

In the light of limited resources, consideration of other single room priorities and staff shortages, a rational policy should be based upon risk assessment and flexible management. Although isolation in a single room is an important tool in preventing cross-infection the decision should be evidence based. Placement of patients infected with MRSA should be undertaken following a risk assessment based on the knowledge of source of the microorganism, route of transmission and risk factors. As long as effective basic infection control measures are in place and staff and visitors comply, it is appropriate to nurse some infected patients in an ordinary bay. Ultimately it is not always necessary to isolate all patients with MRSA in single rooms (Makoni, 2002).

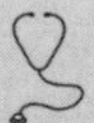

Nursing action points

- Be aware that patients who are only colonized in the nose, throat and groin may be nursed in a bay occupied by patients with indwelling catheters or wounds.
- Be aware that it should not be necessary to isolate a person with a wound infection if other patients have no damaged skin or invasive devices.

(Makoni, 2002)

Streptococcal Infection

Group A beta-haemolytic *Streptococcus* is responsible for serious infections, such as pharyngitis and skin infections. The bacteria can spread through the tissues by releasing toxins, and so generalized infection may result. Group A haemolytic streptococci can be carried in the nasopharynx of 6 to 8 per cent of the general population and can be spread by coughing and sneezing. The elderly and those people with serious underlying medical conditions are most at risk and there appears to be a substantial risk of transmission in hospitals as well as the community, as the incidence of infection with this organism is rising in both hospitals as well as the community. Screening staff to exclude carriers, isolating infected people until antibiotic therapy is effective are recommended (Gould and Brooker, 2000).

The Role of the Nurse in Infection Control

The nurse prevents the onset and spread of infection and promotes measures for the treatment of infection. Nurses maintain the immediate healthcare environment and because they provide care for a variety of patients, there is an increased risk of contamination from pathogenic microorganisms. The practice of medical asepsis and standard precautions provides nurses with techniques for the destruction and containment of pathogens and for the prevention of contamination to other people or to bedside materials and equipment. Medical asepsis helps to contain infectious microorganisms and to maintain an environment free from contamination. It includes hand washing, wearing gowns, gloves and facial masks when appropriate and separating clean from contaminated or potentially contaminated materials.

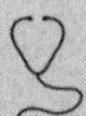

Nursing action points

Universal precautions

- Wash hands before and after patient contact and if the skin is contaminated with body fluid.
- Cover cuts and abrasions with a waterproof dressing.
- Wear gloves for direct contact with body fluids and mucous membranes.
- Wear eye protection and mask where there is a risk of body fluid splashing into the face.
- Wear a plastic apron to protect clothing from contamination with body fluid.
- Use sharps safely, place directly into sharps containers, never resheathe, do not overfill container and close securely before disposal.
- Discard contaminated waste safely either directly into the drainage system or into a clinical waste bag.
- Decontaminate equipment safely between patients.
- Disinfect spills of blood with sodium hypochlorite and clear up using gloves and plastic apron.

(Wilson, 1997)

Universal precautions help control contamination from blood-borne viruses, such as the HIV or the hepatitis viruses (Truman College, 2001). Universal precautions are aimed at avoiding direct contact with body fluids from all patients at all times.

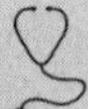

Nursing action points

Infection control

- Identify individuals at risk of acquiring an infection.
- Avoid actions that transmit microorganisms, in order to prevent an infection from developing or spreading.
- Follow universal precautions.
- Select the appropriate method of decontamination depending upon how the equipment is used and the risk of transmission associated with it.
- Practice good hand washing technique. Research has shown that some areas are commonly missed during hand washing. Include the thumbs, nails, fingertips and areas between the fingers. Ensure that the hands are thoroughly dried (Waugh, 1995). Wash hands
  - ☐ prior to manipulation of invasive devices.
  - ☐ before contact with susceptible sites, such as wounds.

- before handling food.
- after contact with contaminated items, such as soiled linen or dressings.
- after using the lavatory.
- before leaving the ward.

- Use alcohol scrubs as an alternative to washing with soap and water, but remember that they may not be effective if hands are soiled and should not be used if hands are visibly contaminated.
- Strengthen the potential host's defences against infection by nutritional support, rest and maintenance of physiological protective mechanisms and appropriate immunizations.
- Do not sort potentially infectious linen prior to washing.
- Place potentially infectious linen in a water soluble bag that can be placed straight into the washing machine.

(Wilson 1997)

- Indicate the appropriate infection control procedures in the care plan of a person with an infection.

(Truman College, 2001)

All hospitals receiving acutely ill patients must have infection control policies in place. In order to ensure the safe management of exogenous infections and to avoid exposing staff and other patients to the risk of contracting infection, the procedures must be known by all relevant staff. The movement of patients with MRSA, and other resistant bacterial infections, into the community must be taken into consideration. Increasing problems are being encountered with immunocompromised patients and those with prosthetic devices *in situ*. These patients are susceptible to endogenous infections as well as the community-acquired opportunistic infection and frequently require hospital-based management.

Infectious Disease Units

A dedicated ward with isolation and other rooms with appropriately trained staff are more effective in managing infection than a scattering of isolation rooms widely dispersed across a hospital. Individual rooms, preferably with *en suite* facilities should be available for patients with communicable disease under treatment in hospital. Patients identified as colonized with multiresistant pathogens, such as MRSA, should be managed in similar units if appropriate isolation facilities cannot be guaranteed elsewhere. A part of the Infectious Diseases Unit should be set aside to manage patients who do not need isolation once the nature of the infection is established, but who do need specialist care, for example a patient with malaria. These units have an important role in teaching doctors and nurses to diagnose and appropriately manage infection and for research in the speciality (The Scottish Office, 1998).

Treating Patients with Infectious Diseases at Home

Patients with infectious diseases might be better treated in the community rather than in hospital, according to research carried out at Coventry University. The study by hospital manager, Carl Holland, also found that a community-based approach could result in significant savings (UKCC [now known as the Nursing and Midwifery Council] *News*, 2002). The study was based upon a policy used in the United States, where patients with infectious diseases are successfully treated out of hospital, either at the patient's home or outpatient clinics. After evaluating the benefits of the scheme Carl Holland calculated that, by treating patients in the community rather than as inpatients, wards could save 2700 bed days and over £680 000 in south Warwickshire alone, reducing the strain on hospital funding. The author considered that this approach was both safe and effective and stated that patients benefited from staying at home while the hospital benefited from reduced risk of cross-infection. In a pilot community-based approach to care in south Warwickshire, nursing staff were appointed to co-ordinate and develop the service (Allerdyce, 2002). The community-based approach has the advantage of keeping infective conditions out of hospitals, where they can spread very quickly, for example, the 'winter vomiting' virus that can lead to hospital wards being closed to further admissions.

Conclusion

The emergence of the HIV in the 1980s sensitized nurses and other healthcare providers to the seriousness of infectious diseases (Murphy and McMahon, 2000). The prevalence of infectious diseases has decreased in the population, but its variety has altered with the emergence of new or antibiotic-resistant pathogens. In hospital practice and also increasingly in the community, infections occur with multiresistant bacteria, often a reflection of inappropriate or excessive use of antibiotics (The Scottish Office, 1998). Current methods may not effectively detect newly emerging infections, resurgent diseases and antibiotic-resistant pathogens or prevent the rapid importation of international outbreaks. The incubation period for many infectious diseases is considerably longer than the time taken to reach the UK from distant countries, where infectious diseases are endemic. Tuberculosis is an example of how emergence or resurgence of infection in a community can result in local outbreaks (Murphy and McMahon, 2000).

An Infectious Diseases Strategy was announced in January 2002. The Chief Medical Officer's Infectious Diseases Strategy describes the formation of the new National Infection Control and Health Protection Agency. The strategy recommends that intensified action is required to control

- Healthcare associated infection
- Tuberculosis

- Antimicrobial resistance
- Blood-borne and sexually transmitted viruses

Other recommendations include a programme of new vaccine development, a strengthened, integrated approach to infection in childhood and enhanced programmes of professional development (Department of Health, 2002). The spectrum of infectious disease is changing rapidly in conjunction with dramatic changes in our society and environment. Worldwide there is explosive population growth with expanding poverty and urban migration; international travel is increasing and technology is rapidly changing. These factors affect the risk of exposure to infectious agents, which we humans share with the environment. Despite historical predictions to the contrary, humans remain vulnerable to a wide range of new and resurgent infectious diseases (Satcher, 2001).

The education and training of healthcare staff is an important consideration in the task of preventing the spread of infectious diseases and treating those individuals who are affected. Nursing students should be exposed to core knowledge of infection control and management and regular training of nursing staff in infection control should be standard in Infectious Disease Units (The Scottish Office, 1998). In today's complex healthcare world it still remains essential to practise the most basic form of infection control, such as effective hand washing. In addition, it is prudent for all nurses to keep abreast of current literature regarding scientific studies and recommendations for ways to prevent the transmission of infection. Learning, however, is only the beginning: what has been learned must be applied in daily nursing practice.

References

Allerdyce, C. 2002, 'Cut Waiting Times by Treating Infectious People at Home'. Health-News.co.uk, http://www.druginfozone.org/news/Jan02_news176/jun02_news176.html

Bowler, I. C. J. W. and Crook, D. W. M. 2000, 'Nosocomial infections' in Ledingham, J. G. G. and Warrell, D. A. (eds), *Concise Oxford Textbook of Medicine*. 3rd edn. Oxford. Oxford University Press.

Caddow, P. 1989, 'Hospital and community acquired infection' in Caddow, P. (ed.), *Applied Microbiology*. Middlesex. Scutari Press.

Conlon, C. P. and Syndman, D. R. 2000, *Mosby's Color Atlas and Text of Infectious Diseases*. London. Mosby International Ltd.

Davey, P. G. 2000, 'Antimicrobial chemotherapy' in Ledingham, J. G. G. and Warrell, D. A. (eds), *Concise Oxford Textbook of Medicine*. 3rd edn. Oxford. Oxford University Press.

Department of Health 2002, 'CNO Bulletin – February 2002'. Crown Copyright. http://www.doh.gov.uk/cno/bulletin7.htm

Donegan, N. E. 2000, 'Management of patients with infectious diseases' in Smeltzer, S. C. and Bare, B. G. (eds), *Brunner and Suddarth's Textbook of Medical-Surgical Nursing*. 9th edn. Philadelphia. Lippincott, Williams and Wilkins.

Gormley, K. 1995, 'Adult nursing' in Basford, L. and Slevin, O. (eds), *Theory and Practice of Nursing: An Integrated Approach to Patient Care.* Edinburgh. Campion Press Limited.

Gould, D. and Brooker. C. 2000, *Applied Microbiology for Nurses.* London. Macmillan Press Ltd.

Greenwood, B. M. 1996, 'The host's response to infection' in Weatherall, D. J., Ledingham, J. G. G. and Warrell, D. A. (eds), *Oxford Textbook of Medicine.* 3rd edn. Oxford. Oxford University Press.

Greenwood, B. M. 2000, 'The host's response to infection' in Ledingham, J. G. G. and Warrell, D. A. (eds), *Concise Oxford Textbook of Medicine.* 3rd edn. Oxford. Oxford University Press.

Griffin, G. E., Sissons, J. G. P. and Chiodini, P. L. and Mitchell, D. M. 1999, 'Diseases due to infection' in Haslett, C., Chilvers, E. R., Hunter, J. A. A. and Boon, N. A. (eds), *Davidson's Principles and Practice of Medicine.* 18th edn. London. Harcourt Brace and Company.

Lambert, H. P. 1996, 'Clinical approach to the patient with suspected infection' in Weatherall, D. J., Ledingham, J. G. G. and Warrell, D. A. (eds), *Oxford Textbook of Medicine.* 3rd edn. Oxford. Oxford University Press.

Long, M. and Miller, M. D. 1995, 'Infection Control' in Potter, P. A. and Perry, A. G. (eds), *Basic Nursing Theory and Practice.* 3rd edn. London. Mosby-Year Book.

Makoni, T. 2002, 'MRSA: risk assessment and flexible management'. *Nursing Standard,* 16 (26), 39–41.

Mayon-White, R. T. 2000, 'Epidemiology and public health' in Ledingham, J. G. G. and Warrell, D. A. (eds), *Concise Oxford Textbook of Medicine.* 3rd edn. Oxford. Oxford University Press.

Murphy, D. C. and McMahon, K. 2000, 'Infectious Microbes and Diseases: General Principles'. Nursing spectrum.inc (2002). http://nsweb.nursingspectrum.com/ce/cel165.htm

Murphy, P. A. 2000, 'Physiological changes in infected patients' in Ledingham, J. G. G. and Warrell, D. A. (eds), *Concise Oxford Textbook of Medicine.* 3rd edn. Oxford. Oxford University Press.

Rice, D. and Eckstein, E. C. 1995, 'Infection' in Phipps, W. J., Cassmeyer, V. L., Sands, J. K. and Lehman, M. K. (eds), *Medical and Surgical Nursing: Concepts and Clinical Practice.* 5th edn. St. Louis, Missouri. Mosby.

Rudd, P. and Nicoll, A. 1991, *British Paediatric Association Manual on Infections and Immunizations in Children.* Oxford. British Paediatric Association.

Sansonetti, P. J. 1996, 'Biology of pathogenic microorganisms' in Weatherall, D. J., Ledingham, J. G. G. and Warrell, D. A. (eds), *Oxford Textbook of Medicine.* 3rd edn. Oxford. Oxford University Press.

Satcher, D. 2001, 'Emerging Infectious Disease Threats'. Mid-Atlantic Associates. http://www.nursingnetwork.com/threats1.htm

Scherer, J. 1991, *Introductory Medical – Surgical Nursing.* 5th edn. Philadelphia. Lippincott Company.

Stucke, V. A. 1993, *Microbiology for Nurses.* 7th edn. London. Bailliere Tindall.

Taylor, C., Lillis, C. and Le Mone, P. 1993, *Fundamentals of Nursing: The Art and Science of Nursing Care.* 2nd edn. Pennsylvania. Lippincott Company.

The Scottish Office 1998, 'Scottish Infection Manual'. Crown Copyright. http://www.scotland.gov.uk/library2/doc15/sim-07.asp

Thomlinson, D. 1989a, 'The infection process' in Caddow, P. (ed.), *Applied Microbiology.* Middlesex. Scutari Press.

Thomlinson, D. 1989b, 'Microorganisms and their properties' in Caddow, P. (ed.). *Applied Microbiology*. Middlesex. Scutari Press.

Thomlinson, D. 1989c, 'Laboratory Intervention' in Caddow, P. (ed.), *Applied Microbiology*. Middlesex. Scutari Press.

Truman College 2001, 'Infection Control'. http://faculty.ccc.edu/tr-infectioncontrol/faq.htm

UKCC-News 2002, http://www.ukcc.org.uk./cms/content/news/treat%20infections%20at%20home,%20says%20researcher.asp

Wansbrough-Jones, M. H. and Wright, S. G. 1997, 'Infectious tropical and parasitic diseases' in Souhami, R. L. and Moxham, J. (eds), *Textbook of Medicine*. London. Harcourt Brace and Company Limited.

Waugh, A. 1995, 'Science and the art of nursing' in Peattie, P. I. and Walker, S. (eds), *Understanding Nursing Care*. 4th edn. London. Pearson Professional Limited.

Wilson, J. 1997, 'Infection and disease' in Walsh, M. (ed.), *Watson's Clinical Nursing and Related Sciences*. 5th edn. London. Bailliere Tindall.

11

Tuberculosis

NORMA WHITTAKER

The World Health Organization (WHO) in 1993 took the unprecedented step of declaring tuberculosis (TB) a global emergency. Not only has tuberculosis re-emerged in developed countries, but also the world has been introduced to multidrug resistant tuberculosis (MDR-TB) strains. These are more serious because the course of treatment is longer, more costly and because the TB bacteria are unaffected by at least one of the anti-tuberculosis drugs still being used today.

Contents

Learning Objectives

By the end of the chapter you should be able to demonstrate knowledge of

- Factors associated with the epidemiology and aetiology of TB.
- The potential outcomes for individuals exposed to *Mycobacterium tuberculosis*.
- The pathophysiology of TB and the effects upon the individual.

- The potential for transmitting TB from person to person.
- How TB is diagnosed and treated.
- The role of the nurse in screening, contact tracing and encouraging adherence to treatment regimens.
- Nursing interventions that recognize the need to target high risk groups and deliver appropriate health promotion and education.
- Nursing interventions that reflect the need to support affected individuals physically and psychologically during lengthy treatment regimens.
- The role of the specialist nurse.

Definition

Tuberculosis is an infectious disease that most commonly affects the lungs but it can be transported to any number of sites around the body via the blood or lymphatic system. These include the lymph glands, kidneys, skin, bones, wounds/lesions, meninges and reproductive organs. TB is categorized as either pulmonary or non-pulmonary (Gleissberg, 1996).

Aetiology

Tuberculosis is an infectious disease caused by *Mycobacterium tuberculosis* (*M. tuberculosis*).

- *Mycobacterium tuberculosis*
- *Mycobacterium bovis*
- Atypical/opportunistic mycobacteria

More rarely TB is caused by *Mycobacterium bovis* (*M. bovis*) and opportunistic atypical mycobacteria may also cause disease in humans, especially in immuno-compromised individuals (Cook, 1996). Bovine TB rarely affects humans but affects cattle, horses and pigs and can be transmitted via the human food chain through cow's milk and beef carcasses. Infection is prevented in humans by inoculating cattle against the disease and by pasteurizing/sterilizing milk. The rare atypical bacterium causes cervical lymph node infections in children and pulmonary disease (Taylor and Littlewood, 1998).

Epidemiology

Points for consideration

- The incidence of tuberculosis is increasing
- The prevalence is high in dense inner city areas
- Certain groups of individuals have an increased risk of developing TB

Tuberculosis is the world's oldest infectious disease and remains the biggest killer in the world as a single pathogen (Rouillon, 1992). The incidence of TB is increasing to such an extent that it has been identified as a 'global emergency' by WHO, 1994. Although it is found throughout the world, TB is especially prevalent in developing countries where poverty, poor nutrition and lack of healthcare are present; there is also a higher incidence in high-density populations such as are found in inner city areas (Payling, 1997). For example, TB cases are three to four times the national average in the Leicester city area (Knott, 1999). Two hundred years ago TB caused one death in four in the UK. Since the early part of the twentieth century there has been a decline; by the 1950s there were approximately 50 000 cases annually and the introduction of effective treatment at this time led to a faster reduction until there were only 5000 cases reported in 1987 (Gleissberg, 1996). Since then there has been a gradual increase in notified cases and TB is now a recognized problem among the homeless. The extent to which homelessness and poverty contribute to the increase is uncertain, as improved reporting of cases, an ageing population, the increase in international travel and immigration of people from countries with an increasingly high incidence of TB may also influence the figures (Payling, 1997).

The number of cases of TB soared by more than one-fifth during the last decade of the twentieth century. Figures from the Public Health Laboratory Service showed an increase from 4659 cases in England and Wales in 1998 to 5658 in 1999. The indication is that the number of cases continues to rise. The rate of increase in the 1990s has been from 9.4 per 100 000 people to 10.9 per 100 000. More than half (56 per cent) of the cases are in people born outside Britain, and 40 per cent arrived in Britain in the previous five years (Bosely, 1999). There were 7300 reported cases of TB in the year 2000, with London alone accounting for 2500 cases (Hill, 2001). TB has reached its highest infection rate for 17 years in London, where two-thirds of TB cases are now found (Sadler, 2001).

Some notorious hot spots such as Leicester and Bradford actually showed a decrease of about 15 per cent between 1987 and 1993 but others such as Leeds (11 per cent), Manchester (12 per cent), inner London (25 per cent) and Liverpool (30 per cent), showed increases (Davies, 1996). Leicestershire as a whole had a higher percentage of non-pulmonary TB than the national average, which might account for the slight decrease in the incidence of TB in the county (Radwan, 1999). In 2001, however, Leicester was hit by an outbreak of what was thought to be a particularly virulent strain of TB, on a scale unheard of for many years.

Tuberculosis is 20 times more common in South Asians than in the white population and non-pulmonary tuberculosis is 100 times more common in this group in the UK. In decreasing order the sites are lymph nodes, usually cervical bone and joint (spinal disease accounts for half), abdominal abscesses, genito-urinary, meningeal and miliary (Davies, 1996).

Table 11.1 Potential outcomes of infection with *M. tuberculosis*

Level	*Classification of tuberculosis*	*Outcomes*
0	No TB exposure, not infected	No history of exposure, negative tuberculin skin test
I	TB exposure, no evidence of infection	History of exposure, negative tuberculin skin test
II	TB infection without disease	Positive tuberculin skin test, negative bacteriological studies, no evidence of TB on x-ray, no symptoms of TB
III	TB infection, with disease	Patient's current status determined by ▪ Location of the disease ▪ Bacteriological status ▪ Chemotherapy status

Billing and Stokes, 1987.

Tuberculous Infection and Tuberculosis

The process of catching TB involves two stages: first the person has to become infected; second the infection has to progress to disease. There is a difference between TB infection and TB disease (see Table 11.1). TB infection can be present with or without the disease. People may have the *M. tuberculosis* bacillus present with no clinically active disease. Such people usually demonstrate a positive reaction to a tuberculin test but are not infectious (Taylor and Littlewood, 1998). TB disease is manifest as pathological and functional symptoms indicating destructive activity of mycobacteria in host tissue (Thompson *et al.*, 1993). There are genetic variations between different strains of TB and variations between people that affect their susceptibility to the disease (HealthCentral.com, 1998).

The actual mechanisms that determine the development of the disease are poorly understood, but several risk factors are recognized.

Risk factors

- History of TB among family or friends
- Size of the infecting dose
- Place of origin having a high incidence of TB
- History of travel to an area of high incidence (Gleissberg, 1996)
- Extremes of age (particularly children under 15 years of age and young adults between 15 and 44 years of age)
- Race
- Heredity
- Alcoholism

- Drug addiction
- Pre-existing disease, for example, diabetes, chronic renal failure, silicosis, malnourishment, gastrectomy, jejunoileal bypass
- Immunocompromising factors, for example, human immunodeficiency virus (HIV), cancers, corticosteroid treatment, old age
- Smoking
- Overcrowding
- Homelessness
- Impoverishment
- Institutionalization, for example, in prisons, care facilities, psychiatric institutions
- Healthcare workers

(Smeltzer and Bare, 1996)

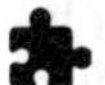 **Connection**

Chapter 1 (Social and Environmental Influences on Health and Well-being) identifies a number of issues relative to the increased incidence and prevalence of some disorders among certain groups of people.

Pathophysiology of TB

Mycobacterium tuberculosis is non-motile and rod shaped and classified as an acid-fast aerobic organism.

 **Connection**

Chapter 10 (Infectious Diseases) describes various types of microorganism.

Ziehl–Neelson or other acid-fast stains are required for staining these organisms, which have cell walls containing abundant lipids (Brunner and Suddarth, 1992). It is a Gram-positive bacillus (Cook, 1996) that is sensitive to heat and ultraviolet (UV) light (Smeltzer and Bare, 1996). The bacillus is extremely hardy, even at very low temperatures and can stay dormant for long periods. *Mycobacterium tuberculosis* has a slow rate of growth, dividing every 18–24 hours (Taylor, 1996). Infection is acquired by inhalation of droplet nuclei containing the organisms distally into the bronchial tree at the level of the respiratory bronchiole or alveolus. It is thought that droplet nuclei smaller than ten microns in diameter are capable of being deposited in the distal airways because their small size allows them to remain airborne and to pass into the small airways without being deposited on the mucous blanket of the tracheobronchial tree, which would normally remove them from the airways to be expectorated or swallowed (Gracey and Addington, 1979). Larger infected inhaled particles are removed by the mucociliary action of the respiratory airways.

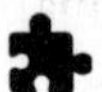

Connection

Chapter 9 (Chronic Obstructive Pulmonary Disease) for further information about the anatomy and physiology of the lungs.

Bacteria that land on furniture or other surfaces are not contagious since they cannot be inhaled and are usually killed quickly by the UV rays of sunlight or by drying. A person with active TB can spread the disease by coughing or sneezing, speaking or laughing. To become infected, a person has to come into close contact with another person who has active TB (Ames and Kneisl, 1988). Typically, a 3000-droplet nucleus results from one cough and fewer than ten are needed to cause an infection (Taylor and Littlewood, 1998). When infected droplet nuclei are inhaled into the alveoli of a susceptible person, tubercle bacilli begin to multiply slowly. The inhaled bacilli are carried to the peripheral alveoli, often in the middle to lower zones (Thompson *et al.*, 1993). Within an hour of reaching the lung, tubercle bacilli reach the draining lymph nodes at the hilum of the lung and a few escape into the bloodstream. The initial inflammatory response reaction comprises exudation and infiltration with neutrophil granulocytes. These are rapidly replaced by macrophages and blood monocytes that phagocytose the free bacilli and polymorphs that contain them. This process produces the epithelioid cells that lie around the inflammatory lesion, becoming a primary tubercle. The tubercle then becomes surrounded by lymphocytes and at around 3–8 weeks a cellular humoral response can be detected by a skin test. At this stage the classical pathology of TB can be seen. Granulomatous lesions consist of necrotic material of a cheesy nature, called caseation, surrounded by epithelioid cells and Langhans' giant cells with multiple nuclei, both cells being derived from macrophages (Dowles, 1994). *Mycobacterium*-specific lymphocytes and antibodies stimulate a fibrocystic response at the periphery of the lesion, resulting in a dense connective tissue enclosure (Thompson *et al.*, 1993). Subsequently, in most cases the caseated areas heal and may become calcified.

Connection

Chapter 10 (Infectious Diseases) explains the body's response to invasion by microorganisms.

Caseation

Blood vessels are compressed, nutrition of the tubercle is interfered with and necrosis occurs at the centre. The area becomes walled off by fibrotic tissue around the outside and the centre gradually becomes soft and cheese-like in consistency. This latter process is known as caseous necrosis. This material may become calcified or it may liquefy and is known as liquefaction necrosis. The liquefied material can be coughed up, leaving a cavity or hole in the parenchyma of the lung. The cavity or cavities are visible on x-ray and result in a diagnosis of cavitary disease (Phipps and Brucia, 1991).

Granuloma

If macrophages are unable to prevent tissue damage, the body attempts to wall off and isolate the infected site, forming a granuloma. Granulomas are formed if neutrophils and macrophages are unable to destroy microorganisms during the acute inflammatory response. Granuloma formation begins when some of the macrophages differentiate into large epithelioid cells; these cells are incapable of phagocytosis but capable of taking up debris and other small particles. Other macrophages fuse into multinucleated giant cells that are active phagocytes and can engulf larger particles than single macrophages. The granuloma itself is usually walled off by fibrous deposits of collagen and may be calcified by deposits of calcium carbonate. The TB granuloma is characterized by a wall of epithelioid cells surrounding the centre of dead and decaying tissue (caseous necrosis) and mycobacteria. Some of the cells fuse into Langhans'-type giant cells. The decay of cells within the granuloma results in the release of acids and the enzymic contents of dead phagocytes' lysozymes, resulting in liquefaction necrosis (McCance and Huether, 1994).

Primary Complex

If the initial infection is contained, the primary lesion, known as Ghon's focus, develops. Tubercle bacilli reach the draining lymph nodes at the hilum of the lung and the resulting inflammatory lesions cause their enlargement. The combination of the lesion in the lung and hilar enlargement is known as the primary complex and in most cases the primary complex heals. Healing occurs by fibrosis and the healed tuberculous lesion may calcify (Dowles, 1994). Successful encapsulation of all lesions occurs in 85–95 per cent of infected individuals. These people enter a latent stage of the disease and remain disease free for variable amounts of time; contained bacilli are, however, capable of being reactivated. For 5–15 per cent of infected persons, host responses are inadequate to contain the infection and active disease progresses in the portal of entry lesions or in all lesions in the body. Necrosis and cavitation continue in the lesions, forming caseation. The lesions may rupture, spreading necrotic residue and bacilli throughout the tissue and throughout the body.

Disseminated bacilli establish new focal lesions that progress through the stages of inflammation, non-caseating granulomas and caseating necrosis (Thompson *et al.*, 1993).

Post-primary Pulmonary TB

Progressive pulmonary TB may develop directly from a primary lesion or may occur months or years later following reactivation of an incompletely healed lesion or as a result of reinfection. Post-primary TB refers to all forms of TB that occur after the first few weeks of the primary infection when immunity to the *Mycobacterium* has developed (Dowles, 1994). The characteristic pathological feature of post-primary pulmonary TB is the tuberculous cavity, formed when the caseated and liquefied centre of a tuberculous pulmonary lesion is discharged into a bronchus. The lesions are most frequently situated in the upper lobes. The disease is often bi-lateral and occasionally the whole lobe may be consolidated in acute pneumonic TB. Extension of infection to the pleura causes tuberculous pleurisy, which may be accompanied by effusion and occasionally followed by the development of tuberculous empyema. Blood-borne dissemination to other organs is uncommon in post-primary pulmonary TB. This form of TB causes most of the morbidity and mortality from TB. Acquired-immune deficiency syndrome (AIDS) has caused an increase in the incidence of TB among young adults (Crompton *et al.*, 1999).

Progression of a tuberculous lesion can occur by

- Local progression
- Bronchogenic dissemination (dissemination of infected material into an uninfected area from an infected area via the tracheobronchial tree)
- Lymphogenous dissemination (spread to other areas via the lymphatics)
- Haematogenous dissemination (spread via the blood)

Complications of Primary Pulmonary TB

Progressive pulmonary TB

When a primary infection does not heal, particularly when it occurs during adolescence or early adult life, progressive pulmonary TB may occur. Occasionally the tuberculous node may ulcerate through the bronchial wall and discharge caseous material into the lumen, resulting in acute tuberculous lesions in the related lobe or segment. Progressive pulmonary TB may also occur as a result of reinfection or reactivation of an incompletely healed lesion months or years after the primary infection (Crompton *et al.*, 1999).

Pulmonary Collapse

A tuberculous mediastinal lymph node, especially in children, may compress a lobar segmental bronchus (rarely a main bronchus) and may produce pulmonary collapse. The collapse disappears as the primary complex heals. Persistent collapse can give rise to subsequent bronchiectasis, often in the middle lobe (Dowles, 1994).

Tuberculous Pleurisy or Pericarditis

Infection may be carried by the lymphatics from tuberculous mediastinal lymph nodes to the pleura or pericardium causing pleurisy with or without pleural effusion or pericarditis.

(Comparable complications occur when the primary lesion is in the tonsil or bowel giving rise to a 'cold' abscess, in the neck or tuberculous peritonitis.)

Erythema Nodosum

The primary infection may be accompanied by erythema nodosum. This is characterized by bluish-red, raised, tender, cutaneous lesions on the shins and sometimes the thighs and is associated in some patients with pyrexia and polyarthralgia. Erythema nodosum may be the first clinical indication of a TB infection (Crompton *et al.*, 1999).

Miliary TB

This is the result of acute diffuse dissemination of tubercle bacilli via the bloodstream. Widespread microscopic lesions are disseminated throughout the body. It can be difficult to diagnose, especially in older people, as it tends to take the form of an insidious illness, presenting in an entirely non-specific manner (Dowles, 1994).

In miliary TB multiple organs are involved. The diagnosis is most commonly suggested by the x-ray and can be confidently made when radiological examination of the chest shows the characteristic 'miliary' mottling symmetrically distributed throughout both lung fields (Crompton *et al.*, 1999). Tuberculous meningitis is relatively common (Moxham and Costello, 1997). Miliary TB may start suddenly or present in an entirely non-specific manner with the gradual onset of vague ill health, loss of weight and then fever. In children and young adults systemic disturbances rapidly become profound.

Signs and symptoms of miliary TB are

- High pyrexia with drenching sweats during sleep
- Marked tachycardia
- Weight loss
- Progressive anaemia

Liver and spleen may be enlarged and there may be choroidal tubercles in the eyes.

There may be no abnormal physical signs in the lungs, although widespread crepitations may be heard. If chemotherapy is not given, death usually occurs within days or weeks. Miliary TB has in the past occurred chiefly in children and young adults, but with the changing demography of TB miliary TB is affecting people in older age groups in whom it tends to take the form of an insidious illness that is often difficult to diagnose and not suspected during life.

The diagnosis of miliary TB

- Radiological evidence shows the characteristic 'miliary' mottling symmetrically distributed through both lung fields
- Choroidal tubercles visible on ophthalmoscopy
- Progressive clinical deterioration
- Persistent pyrexia and splenomegaly
- Bacteriological confirmation

A liver biopsy may be diagnostic in difficult cases. Although tuberculin skin test is usually positive a negative result does not exclude miliary TB, as tuberculin sensitivity is sometimes depressed in the later stages of the disease (Crompton *et al.*, 1999).

Haematogenous Lesions

If healing is incomplete, particularly in lymph nodes, viable tubercle may enter the bloodstream and in consequence tuberculous lesions may develop elsewhere. Such lesions are common in the lungs, bones, joints and kidneys and lesions may develop months or years after the primary infection.

Extra-pulmonary TB

TB can affect any organ and tissue in the body:

Gastrointestinal Tract

Mainly the ileocaecal area, but occasionally the peritoneum is affected. Diarrhoea, malabsorption and ascites can result.

Genitourinary System

Renal TB is a fairly common form of non-pulmonary TB but rarely gives rise to symptoms until the renal lesions are extensive. Haematuria and increased frequency of micturition may occur. Salpingitis and tubal abscesses and infertility in women can result. In men epididymal TB presents as a painless, craggy swelling that can subsequently form a sinus.

Central Nervous System

Tuberculous meningitis and tuberculoma.

Skeletal System

Skeletal infection is relatively common and can lead to arthritis and osteomyelitis with cold abscess formation. Vertebral collapse can occur.

Pericardium

Infection of the pericardial sac is uncommon but can give rise to pericardial effusion and tamponade. Constrictive pericarditis can be a late result of infection and is the consequence of fibrosis and calcification.

Lymph Nodes

This is a very common manifestation of tuberculous disease, especially in young adults, children and Asians. Lymph node enlargement can occur in any site but cervical node enlargement is most common. The enlargement is usually painless. Initially the nodes are firm and discrete but later they become matted and can suppurate and form sinuses.

Skin

Tuberculous infection of the skin is referred to as lupus vulgaris.

Eye

Choroiditis, iridocylitis, phlyctenular keratoconjunctivitis can result (Crompton *et al.*, 1999; Farthing *et al.*, 1994).

Clinical Manifestations

The primary stage of TB may be symptom free; a positive tuberculous skin test is the only indication of a tuberculous infection. The onset of signs and symptoms of pulmonary TB in many individuals is insidious, symptoms developing so gradually that they are not noticed until the disease is advanced. Symptoms can, however, appear in immunocompromised individuals within weeks of exposure to the bacillus (McCance and Huether, 1994). If symptoms are present they may be characterized as being vague and non-specific. A person with

TB disease may have any, all or none of the following:

- Fever (usually low grade and in the latter part of the day)
- Lassitude
- Fatigue
- Malaise
- Anorexia
- Weight loss
- Tachycardia

(Dickson, 1997)

- Night sweats and/or chills (Taylor, 1996)
- Irregular menses (Billing and Stokes, 1987)
- Swollen lymph glands (Gleissberg, 1996)

It is not unusual for individuals to attribute such symptoms to overwork or emotional distress (Billing and Stokes, 1987). (While some symptoms are common to pulmonary and non-pulmonary TB, extra-pulmonary TB symptoms will relate to the affected organs.)

As the pulmonary disease progresses and as more lung tissue becomes involved other symptoms may develop as

- Cough that may be dry and progressively becomes frequent and productive
- Chest pain (often described as being aching, dull or a tightness in the chest)
- Haemoptysis (although unusual, this may be the initial symptom prompting the individual to seek help)
- Pleuritic pain and dyspnoea (usually resulting from extensive pulmonary involvement)

(Billing and Stokes, 1987)

- The patient may look wasted but with a high colour

(Laszlo and Catterall, 1998)

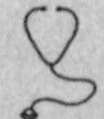

Nursing action points

- Be aware of the possibility of TB in relation to any person presenting with the following history
  - □ Weight loss
  - □ Lassitude/fatigue
  - □ A persistent cough
  - □ Haemoptysis
  - □ Spontaneous pneumothorax

(Crompton *et al.*, 1999)

Table 11.2 Diagnostic investigations

Pulmonary	*Non-pulmonary*
Sputum examination	Biopsy
Induced sputum	Fine needle aspirate
Bronchoscopy	Lumbar puncture
Gastric washing	Urine test
Chest x-ray	Radiological examination
Tuberculin skin test	Tuberculin skin test

Investigative Tests

It is important to establish a diagnosis of TB as soon as possible in order to prevent spread of the infection (refer Table 11.2).

Tests for Pulmonary TB

Sputum Examination

The most reliable way of diagnosing TB is through microscopy and culture. Diagnosis is confirmed by finding the acid-fast bacilli (AFB) in smears of sputum.

> *Nursing action points*
>
> - When sputum cannot be coughed up directly, induce sputum expectoration by the inhalation of aerosols that irritate the trachea and produce coughing.
> - Obtain an early morning specimen that has pooled overnight secretions, as this is the best specimen to examine.
> - If the patient is unable to expectorate, obtain gastric secretions containing swallowed sputum by passing a nasogastric tube (Brunner and Suddarth, 1992).
> - Ensure that the patient is fasted overnight prior to collecting swallowed sputum (Gracey and Addington, 1979).

Bronchoscopic aspirations using a fibreoptic bronchoscope or transtracheal aspiration are other options for obtaining a specimen of sputum. Children rarely produce sputum and although it is possible to obtain a specimen of sputum as described above, this may be traumatic to a child and therefore children are often treated empirically (Gleissberg, 1996).

The presence of AFB on direct microscopy indicates mycobacterial infection and will most commonly confirm a diagnosis of TB. Although there are over

40 species of mycobacteria, the others rarely infect humans in the developed world unless they are immunocompromised. Sputum is said to be 'smear positive' when AFB are seen microscopically and patients are considered to be highly infectious. It is still considered necessary for the positive specimen to be cultured in order to confirm the identity of the bacilli and to check their sensitivity to the various anti-tuberculous drugs. If AFB are not seen it is necessary to incubate the specimen for at least 8 weeks before it can be considered to be negative. Patients who are immunocompromised are more susceptible to atypical mycobacteria and it cannot always be assumed that a positive AFB smear indicates TB. It is recommended however, that patients are isolated and treated for TB until the diagnosis is confirmed by culture. If it is assumed that they have an atypical mycobacterial infection, which then turns out to be TB, treatment will have been inadequate in the initial phase of the disease. This means that the individuals concerned will have remained infectious and may have developed resistance to one or more of the drugs used to treat TB (Gleissberg, 1996).

The slow growth of *M. tuberculosis* in culture hinders the ability to make a rapid diagnosis. Radio-labelled DNA probes specific for various mycobacterial species can identify organisms in culture, providing a diagnosis within 48 hours (Dowles, 1994). Only approximately half of pulmonary TB is smear positive and bacteria can take weeks to grow. The polymerase chain reaction (PCR) is a method of DNA augmentation that can rapidly multiply the bacterial DNA potentially giving a culture result within hours of taking a specimen from the patient (Davies, 1999). The Gen-Probe Amplified Mycobacterium Tuberculosis Direct test (MTD assay) offers equivalent performance to the PCR assay for detection of *M. tuberculosis* in fresh specimens, but is faster to perform (same day). Culture is still the gold standard for detection of *M. tuberculosis*, and molecular genetic tests should be used in conjunction with culture (Leslie, 1997).

Chest X-ray

Radiological examination is of paramount importance for diagnosis in the early stages before physical signs appear and for assessment of the extent and progress of the TB (Crompton *et al.*, 1999). Findings may show

- calcification at the original site
- enlargement of the hilar lymph nodes
- parenchymal infiltrate representing extension of the original site of infection
- pleural effusion
- cavitation

(Thompson *et al.*, 1993)

The presence of cavitation in an untreated patient usually indicates active disease. When fibrosis is marked the trachea and mediastinal structures are displaced towards the side of the lesion (Crompton *et al.*, 1999).

Tuberculin Skin Test

Both the tests involve giving an intradermal injection of purified protein derivative (PPD), prepared from the heat-treated products of the *Mycobacterium*, but in different strengths (Cook, 1996). A strongly positive response indicates that an immune response to mycobacteria has been stimulated.

Heaf Test

This is the most popular method and uses a Heaf gun that makes six simultaneous shallow needle-punctures through the skin on which a small amount of tuberculin has been spread. A localized skin reaction then develops and is read after 7 days, being graded according to the size of the reaction. A minimal reaction indicates a negative result. A solid induration 5–10 millimetres (mm) wide or a wider induration sometimes with vesicles or ulceration indicates a strong positive result (Brown and Capewell, 1986).

Mantoux Test

PPD is injected intradermally into the forearm. A positive Mantoux is characterized by an area of induration greater than 5 mm in diameter over a 48–72 hour period. Induration of 0.4 mm is a negative result, while 15 mm or more is strongly positive (Brunner and Suddarth, 1992).

T-cell Responses

Differential T-cell responses to mycobacteria-secreted proteins distinguish vaccination with bacille Calmette–Guerin from infection with *M. tuberculosis*. These proteins have potential as skin test reagents for detecting infection with *M. tuberculosis* (Roche *et al.*, 1994; Arend *et al.*, 2000).

Tests for Extra-pulmonary TB

Biopsy

Needle biopsy of the pleura, liver, bone marrow and lung may establish a diagnosis of TB.

Tissue Aspirates and Body Fluids

Lymph nodes, peritoneum, joints, epididymis, pericardium and even lung may be aspirated for AFB stains and culture.

Tubercle bacilli may be cultured from ascitic fluid, pleural fluid, urine and pus that has been aspirated or drained from abscesses. Tissue such as liver, bone marrow and lymph nodes may also be cultured (Brunner and Suddarth, 1992).

Lumbar Puncture

The cerebrospinal fluid is usually clear in tuberculous meningitis. Lymphocytes predominate, protein is raised and the glucose concentration is low (Davies *et al.*, 1996).

Urine

Haematuria and increased frequency of micturition can be caused by renal TB. At least three early morning specimens should be examined (Crompton *et al.*, 1999).

Radiological Examination

Cervical or abdominal calcification may be evident and in children lesions may be evident on bones even when there is no clinical evidence of disease at that site (Davies *et al.*, 1996). Imaging, for example, computerised axial tomography (CT) and/or magnetic resonance imaging (MRI) may also be used (Gleissberg, 1996).

Treatment

Healed tuberculous lesions may still contain viable bacteria and if cellular immunity is suppressed for any reason the disease may reappear. Such people and those who have been in close contact with a patient with active TB are given chemoprophylaxis (Crompton *et al.*, 1999). The prophylactic treatment regimen involves taking isoniazid for 6–12 months. To minimize side effects, pyridoxine (vitamin B_6) is administered (Smeltzer and Bare, 1996). Chemotherapy is the mainstay of treatment although surgery for drainage of empyema, caseating lymph nodes or the prevention of spinal paraplegia is occasionally necessary. Apart from a few variations in dose and duration of treatment, the policy governing the use of antituberculosis drugs is the same for all forms of the disease (Crompton *et al.*, 1999). The two most important drugs are isoniazid and rifampicin. Isoniazid, because it kills the great bulk of bacteria, rendering the patient non-infectious within days of starting treatment, and rifampicin, because it eliminates the persisting bacteria allowing treatment to be shortened (Davies, 1999).

Second line drugs include

- Capreomycin
- Kanamycin
- Ethionamide
- Para-aminosalicylate sodium
- Amikacin

- Quinolones, for example, ofloxacin, ciprofloxacin, sparfloxacin
- Macrolides, for example, clarithromycin
- Clofazimine.

Drug Regimens

The 'short course' regimens are virtually 100 per cent effective. To avoid the emergence of drug-resistant organisms susceptibility testing is recommended for all suspected cases of TB (Phipps and Brucia, 1991). Multiple medication regimens are the recommended treatment for newly diagnosed patients.

Standard drug regimens

Total duration six months

- Pyrazinamide (plus ethambutol) together with isoniazid and rifampicin for two months.
- Isoniazid and rifampicin for four months.

Quadruple therapy should be the initial treatment if primary drug resistance is suspected. Isoniazid and rifampicin in combination with pyrazinamide during the initial two months is usually adequate for the majority of patients in the UK.

Total duration nine months

- Isoniazid plus rifampicin and ethambutol for two months
- Isoniazid plus rifampicin for seven months

(Crompton *et al.*, 1999)

Immunocompromised patients, such as HIV-positive people, are more susceptible to the development of resistant organisms. It is therefore recommended that those patients with HIV and TB be treated for a total of nine months and for at least six months after their sputum converts to negative. If drug susceptibility is not available, ethambutol or streptomycin should be considered for the entire course of therapy because of the rapid progression of TB while treatment is inadequate.

Treatment of extra-pulmonary TB is similar to that outlined, although some believe that therapy should be for nine months instead of six in cases of disseminated TB, miliary disease and TB of bones, joints and the lymph glands. Pregnant women are not treated with streptomycin because it may cause congenital deafness. Breast-feeding is possible during therapy because the concentration of drugs in breast milk is so low that drug toxicity does not occur in the infant (Phipps and Brucia, 1991).

Drug resistance

- **Primary drug resistance** is resistance to one of the first line antituberculosis drugs in a previously untreated person.
- **Secondary (acquired) drug resistance** is resistance due to one or more antituberculosis drugs in a patient undergoing therapy.
- **Multidrug resistance** is resistance to isoniazid and rifampicin, whether or not there is resistance to other drugs.

(Smeltzer and Bare, 1996)

Multidrug Resistance (MDR-TB)

The incidence of MDR-TB in the UK is between 1.5 and 3 per cent. The development of MDR-TB results from inconsistent or partial treatment. If the disease is treated with one drug or treatment regimens are inadequate, the growth of strains of *M. tuberculosis* susceptible to commonly prescribed drugs, such as isoniazid and rifampicin, is suppressed. These circumstances can lead to the multiplication of drug-resistant strains (secondary resistance). Once these strains are transmitted to others, a strain of TB that is drug resistant from the outset develops (primary resistance). Few effective drugs are available for treatment; people are therefore less likely to be cured and more likely to spread TB to other people (WHO International Union Against Tuberculosis and Lung Disease [WHO/IUATLD], 1997). The treatment of MDR-TB is specialized, complex and expensive.

Risk factors for drug-resistant TB

- Previous treatment for TB, especially if this was prolonged
- Contact with another patient known to have MDR disease
- Immigration from an area with a high incidence of MDR-TB
- HIV seropositivity
- Substance abuse
- Homelessness

If drug resistance is suspected, the patient will be prescribed at least three and preferably four drugs to which there has been no previous exposure. Isoniazid and rifampicin are usually commenced at the outset of treatment, as time will be gained if the strain is sensitive to one or both of these drugs (Davies, 1999).

TB, HIV and AIDS

The impact of HIV infection on the incidence of TB has been catastrophic from a global perspective. Although the rates for HIV-related TB in the UK are among the lowest in Europe, a rise in its incidence has been reported from the London HIV centres (Taylor and Littlewood, 1998). Approximately 10 per cent of new cases of tuberculosis infection result from existing infection with HIV (WHO/ IUATLD, 1997).

It is likely that most cases of TB in patients with HIV infection are the result of a previous tuberculous infection being reactivated (Taylor, 1996). When latent TB is reactivated by HIV, a cough could be masked by AIDS-related pneumonia (Sadler, 2001).

The role of HIV in the creation of MDR-TB is complicated (Taylor, 1996). HIV positivity does not in itself increase the chance of drug resistance, but HIV does considerably accelerate infection developing into disease. In communities where the prevalence of HIV is high the introduction of TB can swiftly result in an epidemic of the disease. If drug-resistant TB is introduced, then the epidemic will be drug resistant (Davies, 1999).

All patients with newly diagnosed TB should be encouraged to undergo HIV testing according to researchers from south London. The seroprevalence of HIV in patients with TB was found to be more than double the previous estimates with a similar distribution across ethnic groups (Bowen *et al.*, 2000).

Directly Observed Treatment (DOT)

A major cause of MDR-TB and treatment failure is patient non-adherence to prescribed treatment. The result of these can be life threatening to patients and pose other serious public health problems because they lead to prolonged infectiousness of the patient and increase the risk of transmitting TB to others.

This mode of treatment involves healthcare professionals and trained volunteers observing the patient taking medication correctly to ensure completion of the course of drugs. Patients may also be accompanied to hospital and clinic visits. This ensures attendance and the patient remains known to healthcare professionals co-ordinating treatment regimens (WHO/IUATLD, 1997). Effective use of DOT requires a setting where patients can go to receive the prescribed treatment either daily or two to three times a week according to the regimen ordered. The setting can be a TB clinic, community health centre, homeless shelter, prison, drug treatment centre or other settings that agree to serve as treatment settings. Providing transport or financial support for bus fares may prove to be an incentive and promote patient adherence to a DOT programme (Phipps and Brucia, 1991). Vagrancy, drug abuse and alcoholism can hamper management of TB (Evans, 1995).

In countries where directly observed treatment was implemented correctly, low levels of MDR-TB were observed (WHO/IUATLD, 1997). According to researchers from Leeds and Pakistan, however, direct observation of treatment in TB is not necessarily any more effective than other strategies. A randomized trial assessed the effectiveness of different packages for TB treatment under operational conditions in Pakistan. The three strategies were as follows:

- DOTS with direct observation treatment by health workers
- DOTS with direct observation treatment by family members
- Self-administered treatment

The findings were that there was little difference between the outcomes of treatment. DOTS did not give any additional improvement in cure rates (Walley *et al.*, 2001).

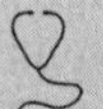

Nursing action points

- Inform patients of the potential side effects of the medication.
- Instruct patients to contact the specialist nurse or doctor as soon as possible if they experience any problems. Minor problems are as follows
  - □ discolouration of the urine
  - □ nausea and occasional vomiting
  - □ abdominal discomfort
  - □ lack of energy
  - □ mild rash.

Table 11.3 Adverse effects of antituberculosis drugs

First line drugs	*Side effects*
Rifampicin (RIF)	Hepatitis, febrile reaction, nausea, vomiting, purpura (rare), drug interactions, urine sweat and tears may turn orange/pink
Isoniazid (INH)	Peripheral neuritis, hepatitis, hypersensitivity reactions, for example, rashes, fever, lack of mental concentration
Ethambutol (EMB)	Even with relatively low doses some patients develop optic neuritis and some are left with permanent visual defect
Pyrazinamide (PZA) (particularly useful in treating tuberculous meningitis because it diffuses well into the cerebrospinal fluid)	Hepatitis, gout, hypersensitivity (rashes), arthralgias, gastrointestinal irritation
Streptomycin (SM) (rarely used except with multiple drug resistance or hypersensitivity)	Vestibular disturbance, hypersensitivity, deafness (rare)

Crompton *et al.*, 1999; Smeltzer and Bare, 1996; Phipps and Brucia, 1991.

These symptoms are not considered serious enough to stop treatment, but can be debilitating and difficult for the patient to cope with. Such patients will need a great deal of support in order to complete the treatment. Table 11.3 outlines the adverse effects of antituberculosis drugs.

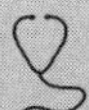 *Nursing action points*

In the event of side effects occurring

- Advise patients to change the time that medication is taken.
- Advise patients to change diet.
- Advise patients to take mild anti-emetics and antihistamines as prescribed.

When a patient experiences major side effects it is usually necessary to stop treatment and reintroduce each drug one at a time in order to identify the causative drug. This can then be removed from the regimen and an alternative can be added. This does, however, inevitably extend the treatment period.

Major side effects

- Persistent vomiting
- Hepatic toxicity
- Peripheral neuropathy
- Severe rash
- Visual impairment (if on ethambutol)
- Itching

(Gleissberg, 1996)

Nursing Interventions

Nurses have always had an important role to play in the treatment and management of TB.

Typical nursing activities

- Caring for patients in their own homes/institutions
- Contact tracing
- Administration of medication
- Working with families and communities
- Monitoring adherence to treatment regimens

- Maintaining a safe environment
- Referring patients to sources of assistance

(Taylor, 1996)

Health Promotion

Health education is a crucial part of both prevention and health promotion. Nurses must not only educate themselves but must also educate patients, their families and other colleagues. Modifying the environment with the aim of encouraging wise choices can be difficult and challenging when working with the groups of people most at risk of developing TB. Nurses must have the ability to impart information that is relevant, appropriate, accurate and current. The information, however, is only useful if the client understands it. Nurses need to ascertain the level of need and motivation as well as the existing level of understanding (Taylor, 1996). The approaches used should recognize the needs of particular groups and individuals. Community staff and outreach workers are well placed to deal with the multitude of potential and actual problems that arise as a result of TB. Those at greatest risk are people for whom access to care is not always easy and whose beliefs about health and illness differ from the general population (Taylor and Littlewood, 1998).

Connection

Chapter 1 (Social and Environmental Influences on Health and Well-being) discusses how peoples' attitudes towards health and illness can differ and how such differences can influence health and well-being.

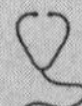

Nursing action points

- Explain the nature of the disease (be sensitive to the associated stigma of TB).
- Explain the importance of adherence to prescribed treatment (to effect a cure and to prevent MDR-TB).
- Discuss potential side effects of prescribed treatment (give relevant contact names and telephone numbers).
- Instruct the patient where to obtain further supplies of drugs.
- Emphasize the importance of attending out-patient clinics.
- Give information about the role of the specialist TB nurse
- Explain the importance and need to undertake contact tracing.

(Karim, 1995a)

Potential resources for health education

- Leaflets on childhood immunization (available from the local Health Education Authority/local health promotion department)
- Training video (produced by the Department of Health; usually available free of charge from the district immunization co-ordinator)

(Willcox, 1999)

Adherence to Treatment

Non-adherence may be influenced by

- Physical factors, for example poor eyesight, reduced strength and manual dexterity
- Social factors
- Mental factors
- Forgetfulness
- Taste, size, method of administration of medication
- Poor communication
- Unacceptable waiting times

(Taylor, 1996)

Where non-adherence to treatment is suspected it may be appropriate to implement DOT either in hospital or in the community.

Screening and Vaccination

School nurses have an important role in screening school children for TB. The presence of TB is determined by the person's response to the tuberculin skin test. A person with a positive Heaf test is referred for a chest x-ray. Bacille Calmette–Guerin (BCG) is a live vaccine administered intradermally. Department of Health guidelines recommend BCG vaccinations for all neonates in high-risk groups and all children aged 10 to 14 years that have not previously been vaccinated. Vaccination is also recommended for certain high-risk groups (Gleissberg, 1996). Pre-testing is required before the vaccine is administered; a positive test indicates past tuberculous infection or successful immunization and BCG vaccine is not required. Infants do not require pre-testing (Willcox, 1999). All healthcare staff and prison officers should be vaccinated as appropriate. However, simply relying on vaccination may not be enough. Most of the Leicester school children had been vaccinated with the BCG injection, but this does not always give complete protection (Hill, 2001).

Targeting High Risk Groups

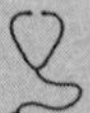

Nursing action points

- Provide care through locally organized delivery systems.
- Provide community groups with support to enable them to become active partners in primary healthcare.
- Remove financial, physical and cultural barriers to the use of primary healthcare.
- Strengthen active outreach in the community.

(Taylor and Littlewood, 1998)

Providing Care for the Infectious Patient in Hospital and at Home

Most people with TB can be successfully cared for at home. The exceptions are those who have

- Severe illness
- Adverse side effects to medication
- Poor compliance with treatment (refusal or difficulty in following instructions)

(Payling, 1997)

Patients should be informed of how the infection is spread and explanations should be given about the need to cover the mouth and nose when coughing and sneezing. Instruction should also be given in relation to the safe handling of secretions. A well-balanced diet is recommended, high in proteins, to guard against the wasting nature of TB. Intake of calcium and vitamins B, C and D must be encouraged. Misconceptions should be corrected and fears allayed. The importance of adequate ventilation should be stressed; this is essential since it reduces the number of droplet nuclei in the air. Ventilation can also be enhanced with ultraviolet radiation in the air. The question of bed rest varies with the type of disease. Many patients can be treated with little disruption to their lives and even when activity is restricted, this is usually only for a brief period (Billing and Stokes, 1987).

Hospital Care

In the initial two weeks of treatment, patients with smear-positive pulmonary TB should be segregated in a room ventilated by a mechanical extraction system, without recirculation, to a safe location (British Thoracic Society, 1994). Barrier nursing is not necessary although more rigorous measures are suggested in relation to HIV or MDR-TB patients (Taylor and Littlewood, 1998). The size of the droplet nuclei means that they can readily pass through masks, and facemasks and are therefore, of limited value. They are helpful in dealing with patients who do not comply with using tissues correctly. The mask if used must fit snugly over the mouth and nose, must filter out particles as small as one micron and be discarded immediately after use (Billing and Stokes, 1987). Copious secretions may be a problem and the nurse may assist the patient by instructing on how best to facilitate expectoration by ensuring adequate hydration (Smeltzer and Bare, 1996). Visiting should be limited to those who have had close contact with the patient. Respiratory isolation is maintained until sputum smears are negative for AFB and infection control policies should be followed in relation to any contaminated material.

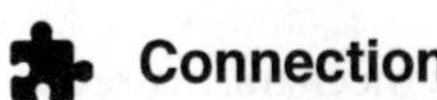

Chapter 10 (Infectious Diseases) discusses ways of preventing the transmission of infection from person to person.

Contact Tracing

Up to 10 per cent of cases are diagnosed by contact tracing and disease occurs in about 1 per cent of contacts (Taylor, 1996). Arrangements for contact tracing vary considerably in the UK. Some health authorities have contracts for a TB control programme, alternatively, contact tracing may be the responsibility of the local chest clinic or community health services and may be done by the clinical nurse specialist or non-specialist community nurse. Mackay (1993) suggests that the development of nursing standards is essential to the efficient running of a contact tracing service. The service Mackay describes included a systems approach that could be easily followed. The use of a flow chart meant that any member of the team could follow a case to its completion.

Specialist Nurses

The role of the TB specialist nurse has been well recognized as an integral part of local TB services. Specialist nurses are ideally placed to participate in the systematic collection of local data and to disseminate such information to others that may ultimately lead to more innovative ways of reversing the current upward trend in TB notifications (Karim, 1995b). There is a clear role for specialist nurses using a case management approach that involves planning and implementing the method of service provision by means of evaluating outcomes. The specialist nurse also ensures the highest possible quality of input and the assessment of clients' access to services (Taylor and Littlewood, 1998).

Sadler (2001) reports on the appointment of the UK's first TB/HIV clinical nurse specialist (CNS), with responsibility for developing a nurse-led service for people co-infected with HIV. The results of an audit and needs assessment carried out after the appointment, highlighted that the main existing problem was interdisciplinary barriers that resulted in fragmentation of care. Measures taken included improved documentation, the development of a hospital-based TB staff education programme, close co-operation with the infection control team, sustained support and encouragement during treatment, direct referrals and assessment by the nurse specialist. Also the development of a variety of TB treatment protocols, for example, empowering the CNS to manage repeat prescriptions. Sustained cross-sector, integrated health and social care is the underlying philosophy of this nurse-led seamless TB service (Sadler, 2001).

Conclusion

During the primary phase of TB the body's natural defence mechanisms resist the disease and most or all of the bacilli are walled in by a fibrous capsule. In many cases TB does not progress beyond this stage. If the immune system fails active disease occurs, sometimes after a latent period of months or years. Most forms of TB can be cured if treatment is managed correctly but this may be difficult in some cases given the necessary long treatment period and the transient and unreliable nature of some of those most at risk.

Nurses have a significant role to play in preventing the spread of TB by health education and promotion and in encouraging compliance with treatment. The British Thoracic Society (BTS) guidelines recommend one specialist nurse for every 50 notifications of the disease. A BTS survey carried out in 2000 revealed that only 14 per cent of the UK's TB hot spots have adequate staffing levels. The Leicestershire outbreak in 2001 had half the number of specialist nurses recommended in the guidelines (Akid, 2001). According to Hill (2001) there needs to be an urgent review of the shortage of TB specialists and health professionals to monitor and control the disease, otherwise more outbreaks will be inevitable. There are real concerns about the increased incidence of TB, its link with HIV and the prevalence of MDR-TB in the UK. It is therefore vital that all healthcare workers are aware of the contribution that they can make to the management and control of TB.

Tuberculosis is the leading cause of death from infectious diseases in the world, yet it has long been regarded as a problem confined to developing countries (Thompson, 1999). Until the late 1980s there was a steady decline in TB cases in the UK, however, since then there has been a steady increase; the incidence is particularly high among certain groups and the disease threatens the most vulnerable members of societies throughout the world. TB remains a significant threat to public health in the UK. Prevalence tends to reflect social and economic conditions: poor housing and overcrowding increase the risk of massive infection or reinfection (Mackay, 1993).

Socio-economic strategies to improve general health and housing have not yet adequately met the needs of the homeless, the displaced and the very poor (Willcox, 1999). Homeless people residing in shelters and hostels are at risk of developing TB and an effective interface between healthcare providers is essential to reduce its spread (Rayner, 2000).

References

Akid, M. 2001, 'TB-hit area has 50% specialist nurse shortfall'. *Nursing Times*, 97 (15), 4.

Ames, S. W. and Kneisl, C. R. 1988, *Essentials of Adult Health Nursing*. Wokingham. Addison-Wesley Publishing Ltd.

Arend, S. M., Anderson, P., van Meijgaarden, K. E., Skjot, R. L., Subronto, Y. W., van Dissel, J. T. and Ottenhoff, T. H. 2000, 'Detection of active tuberculosis infection by T cell responses to early secreted antigenic target 6-kDa protein and culture filtrate protein 10'. *Journal of Infectious Disorders*, 181 (5), 1850–4. http://www.ncbi.nlm.nih.gov/entrez/query.fcgi?cmd=Retrieve&db=PubMed&list_uids=1

Billing, D. M. and Stokes, G. L. 1987, *Medical–Surgical Nursing. Common Health Problems of Adults and Children Across the Life Span*. 2nd edn. St. Louis. The Mosby Company.

Bosely, S. 1999, 'Warning as TB cases increase'. *The Guardian*, 14 December.

Bowen, E. F., Rice, P. S., Cooke, N. T., Whitfield, R. J. and Rayner, C. F. J. 2000, 'HIV seroprevalence by anonymous testing in patients with *Mycobacterium tuberculosis* and in tuberculosis contacts'. *Lancet*, 356 (9240), 1488–9.

British Thoracic Society 1994, 'Control and prevention of tuberculosis in the United Kingdom, code of practice'. *Thorax*, 49, 1193–200.

Brown, J. and Capewell, S. 1986, 'Respiratory tuberculosis'. *Nursing*, 3 (4), 132–4.

Brunner, L. S. and Suddarth, D. S. 1992, *The Textbook of Adult Nursing*. London. Chapman and Hall.

Cook, R. 1996, 'Tuberculosis'. *Nursing Standard*, 10 (48), 49–52.

Crompton, G. K., Haslett, C., Chilvers, E. R., Hunter, J. A. A. and Boon, N. A. (eds) 1999, *Davidson's Principles and Practice of Medicine*. London. Churchill Livingstone.

Davies, P. D. O. 1996, 'Tuberculosis: no longer down and out'. Priory Lodge Education Ltd. http://www.priory.com/med/tubercul.htm

Davies, P. D. O. 1999, 'Multi-drug resistant tuberculosis'. Priory Lodge Education Ltd. http://www.priory.com/cmol/TBMultid.htm

Davies, E. G., Elliman, D. A. C., Hart, C. A., Nicoll, A. and Rudd, P., 1996, *Manual of Childhood Infections*. London. W.B. Saunders Company Ltd.

Dickson, A. 1997, 'Caring for the patient with a disorder of the respiratory system' in Walsh, M. (ed), Watson's *Clinical Nursing and Related Sciences*. 5th edn. London. Balliere Tindall.

Dowles, R. J. 1994, 'Respiratory disease' in Kumar, P. and Clark, M. (eds), *Clinical Medicine*, 3rd edn. London. Balliere Tindall.

Evans, M. R. 1995, 'Is tuberculosis taken seriously in the United Kingdom?'. *British Medical Journal*, 311, 1483–5.

Farthing, M. J. G., Jeffries, D. J. and Anderson, J. 1994, 'Infectious diseases, tropical medicine and sexually transmitted disease' in Kumar, P. and Clark, M. (eds), *Clinical Medicine*. 3rd edn. London. Balliere Tindall.

Gleissberg, G. 1996, 'A shadow of the past: tuberculosis today'. *Nursing Standard*, 11 (1), learning unit 067.

Gracey, D. R. and Addington, W. W. 1979, *Discussion in Patient management: Tuberculosis*. USA. Medical Examination Publishing Co. Inc.

HealthCentral.com 1998, 'Genes play a role in TB infection'. HealthCentral.com http://www.healthcentral.com/news/news/fulltext.cfm?id=86&StoryType=Reuters News

Hill, B. 2001, 'Global Killer'. *Nursing Standard*, 15 (37), 22.

Karim, K. 1995a, 'Beating tuberculosis'. *Journal of Community Nursing*, 9 (5), 10–14.

Karim, K. 1995b, 'Challenging beliefs about tuberculosis'. *Nursing Standard*, 9 (24), 38–41.

Knott, H. 1999, 'Rising TB rate sparks concern'. *Leicester Mercury*. 26 March, 3.

Laszlo, G. and Catterall, J. R. 1998, 'Respiratory medicine' in Jones, J.V. and Tomson, C. R. V. (eds), *Essential Medicine*. Edinburgh. Churchill Livingstone.

Leslie, D. E. (ed), 1997, 'Technical bulletin'. Mycobacterium Reference Laboratory. http://www.vidrl.org.au/mrl/mrlnews.htm

Mackay, L. 1993, 'Evaluation is the key to success'. *Professional Nurse*, 9 (3), 176–80.

McCance, K. L. and Huether, S. E. 1994, *Pathophysiology. The Biologic Basis for Disease in Adults and Children*. 2nd edn. London. Mosby-Year Book Inc.

McKinley, Health Centre Web Site 1998, 'Tuberculosis'. McKinley, Health Centre Web Site. http://www.uiuc.edu/departments/mckinley/health-info/dis-cond/tb/TB.html

Moxham, J. and Costello, J. 1997, 'Respiratory disease' in Souhami, R. L. and Moxham, J. E. (eds), *Textbook of Medicine*. 3rd edn. Edinburgh. Churchill Livingstone.

Payling, K. J. 1997, 'Tuberculosis'. *Professional Nurse*, 12 (4), 260–2.

Phipps, W. J. and Brucia, J. J. 1991, 'Management of persons with problems of the lower airway' in Phipps, W. J., Cassmeyer, V. L., Sands, J. K. and Lehman, M. K. (eds), *Medical–Surgical Nursing*. 5th edn. St. Louis. Mosby-Year Book Inc.

Radwan, K. 1999, 'Local cases of once feared killer disease on decrease'. *Leicester Mercury*. 20 February, 12.

Rayner, D. 2000, 'Reducing the spread of tuberculosis in the homeless population'. *British Journal of Nursing*, 9 (13), 871–5.

Roche, P. W., Triccas, J. A., Avery, D. T., Fifis, T., Billman-Jacobe, H. and Brittor, W. J. 1994, 'Differential cell responses to mycobacteria-secreted proteins distinguish vaccination with bacille Calmette–Guerin from infection with *Mycobacterium tuberculosis*'. *Journal of Infectious Diseases*, 170(5), 1326–30. http://www.ncbi.nlm.nih.gov/entrez/query.fcgi?cmd=Retrieve&db=PubMed&list_uids=7

Rouillon, A. 1992, 'Foreword' in Crofton, J. *et al.*, *Clinical Tuberculosis*. London. Macmillan Publishing Co. Inc.

Sadler, C. 2001, 'Breath of fresh air'. *Nursing Standard*, 15 (27), 18–19.

Smeltzer, S. C. and Bare, B. G. (eds) 1996, *Brunner and Suddarth's Textbook of Medical and Surgical Nursing*. 8th edn. Philadelphia. Lippincott-Raven Publishers.

Taylor, D. 1996, 'Tuberculosis. The role of the nurse'. *Nursing Times*, 92 (43), 5–8.

Taylor, D. and Littlewood, S. 1998, 'Tuberculosis: respiratory system: Part 2'. *Nursing Times*, 94 (11), 49–53.

Thompson, J. 1999, 'Tuberculosis: a global epidemic'. *Community Practitioner*, 72 (9), 303–4.

Thompson, J. M., McFarland G. K., Hirsch, J. E. and Tucker, S. M. 1993, *Mosby's Clinical Nursing*. St. Louis. Mosby-Year Book Inc.

Walley, J. D., Khan, M. A., Newell, J. N. and Khan, M. H. 2001, 'Effectiveness of the direct observation component of DOTS for tuberculosis: a randomised controlled trial in Pakistan'. *Lancet*, 357 (9257), 664–9.

Willcox, A. 1999, 'Defeat the world's most deadly infection'. *Practice Nurse*, 17 (5), 326–8.

World Health Organization 1994, *TB – A Global Emergency*. Geneva. WHO. World Health Organization/International Union Against Tuberculosis and Lung Disease 1997, *Global Project on Anti-tuberculosis Drug Resistance Surveillance Report*. Geneva. WHO/IUATLD. http://www.priory.com/med/tubercul.htm

Chronic Inflammatory Bowel Disease, Ulcerative Colitis, Crohn's Disease and Colorectal Cancer

12

NORMA WHITTAKER

Chronic inflammatory bowel disease is a multidimensional experience that involves a permanent alteration in a person's lifestyle. Chronic inflammatory bowel disease can have a major impact on all aspects of a person's life. Home, social, work and sex lives can be disrupted, which can lead to the impairment of emotional and psychological function, as well as physical debilitation. The consequences of inflammatory bowel disease can be costly in terms of healthcare, both in relation to primary and secondary healthcare settings and to human sufferings (Rowlinson, 1999a).

Contents

Learning Objectives

By the end of the chapter you should be able to demonstrate knowledge of

- Factors associated with the epidemiology and aetiology of ulcerative colitis and Crohn's disease.
- Differences between the pathophysiology and clinical manifestations of ulcerative colitis and Crohn's disease.
- How ulcerative colitis and Crohn's disease are diagnosed and treated.
- Nursing interventions that reflect the chronic nature of the disorders and the potential impact physically, psychologically and socially.
- The role of the specialist nurse.
- The potential complications of chronic inflammatory bowel disease, including colorectal cancer.

Definition

Inflammatory bowel disease (IBD) is an all-embracing term for the chronic inflammatory disorders of the intestine. Ulcerative colitis and Crohn's disease are idiopathic chronic inflammatory disorders of the gastrointestinal tract, characterized by periods of relapse and remission. There is some overlap in their clinical features; the major difference between them, however, is that ulcerative colitis is confined to the large bowel whereas Crohn's disease can occur in any part of the gut, from mouth to anus. Both diseases can have a major impact upon all aspects of a patient's life. There is a significant risk of carcinomatous change in patients with long standing inflammatory bowel disease.

Epidemiology

Ulcerative colitis and Crohn's disease are more prevalent in Europe and North America (Allison *et al.*, 1998). The incidence of IBD varies widely between populations: Crohn's disease appears to be rare in the underdeveloped world, yet ulcerative colitis, although still unusual, is becoming more common. In the West, the incidence of ulcerative colitis is stable at 10 per 100 000 while that of Crohn's disease is increasing and is reported to be 5–7 per 100 000 (Palmer and Penman, 1999). An exception to this trend is in Scandinavia where the incidence of ulcerative colitis has risen sharply (Allison *et al.*, 1998).

In the United Kingdom (UK) inflammatory bowel disease affects between 15 and 30 people per 10 000 of the population (Rowlinson, 1999a). Ulcerative colitis affects approximately 95 000 people in the UK, which is about 1 in 600 of the population and Crohn's disease affects approximately 55 000 people in the UK, which is about 1 in 1000 of the population. Approximately 5500 new cases of ulcerative colitis are diagnosed each year and 3000 new cases of Crohn's disease (National Association for Colitis and Crohn's Disease [NACC], 2001b). The incidence of ulcerative colitis in the UK may be as high as 26 per 100 000

Table 12.1 A comparison of the incidence of ulcerative colitis and Crohn's disease

Ulcerative colitis	*Crohn's disease*
■ Incidence stable in the West ■ Most commonly diagnosed in the 20–40 age group	■ Incidence increasing ■ Commonly presents at adolescence and in young adults. The incidence among children is rising

of the population with a prevalence of 80–120 per 100 000 of the population. The incidence of Crohn's disease is generally considered to be 5–7 per 100 000 of the population with a prevalence of 30–60 per 100 000 of the population (Table 12.1) (Allen, 1999; Long and Cooper, 1997; Clark and Kumar, 1994).

The incidence of IBD is lower in the non-white races and people of Jewish descent are more prone to IBD than non-Jewish people (Clark and Kumar, 1994). Ulcerative colitis begins most frequently in people 20–40 years of age; Crohn's disease commonly presents in puberty and young adults. Young children and the elderly, however, can be affected by both disorders (Curry, 1995). There has been a rise in the incidence of Crohn's disease among children. The first epidemiological study in children to be carried out in England and Wales showed that the incidence of Crohn's disease in South Glamorgan more than doubled in 11 years (Kmietowicz, 1997). A second incidence peak occurs in the seventh decade (Palmer and Penman, 1999). The incidence between the sexes is equal in both diseases (Finley, 1999).

Aetiology and Pre-disposing Factors

The cause or causes are unknown. Immunological and infective agents have been proposed and researched as possible causes of both conditions, but without conclusive results (Finley, 1999). It has been suggested that the pathogenesis of IBD represents an interaction between genetic and predisposing factors, exogenous and endogenous and modifying factors (Travis, 1998).

Aetiology and pre-disposing factors

- Genetics
- Immunological factors
- Microvasculature
- Infection
- Environmental factors
- Stress
- Smoking
- Dietary factors
- Geographical factors

Genetics

There is an overlap of clinical, radiological, endoscopic and histological features. In addition, shared epidemiological characteristics, such as similar distribution with respect to geography, age, gender, race, ethnicity, occupation and social class suggest the possibility that the two disorders have a common genetic basis (Jewell, 1998). While they may share some genetic predisposing factors and immunological mechanisms, the weight of evidence however, suggests that they are genetically and otherwise fundamentally distinct disease processes (Podolsky, 1991).

Familial clustering has been observed and if both parents are affected the risk to their children is very high. Also the first presentation of the disease in familial cases occurs at an earlier age compared with those without a family history (Rowlinson, 1999a). First-degree relatives of patients with IBD have a ten-fold increased risk of developing the same disease. Studies of twins confirm a strong genetic link; the risk is higher for an identical twin of an affected patient than for a non-identical twin. Among monozygotic twin pairs there is a concordance of about 25 per cent for each of the diseases. In families in which two or more relatives have one of the IBDs, the affected first-degree relatives are not always concordant with the same disease (Allison *et al.*, 1998). There appears to be a relationship in some families between ankylosing spondylitis, the HLA phenotype B27 and IBD (Walsh, 1997).

Immunological Factors

The cellular events involved in the pathogenesis of ulcerative colitis and Crohn's disease involve activation of macrophages, lymphocytes and polymorphonuclear cells with the release of inflammatory mediators (Palmer and Penman, 1999). Both food and bacterial antigens have been implicated in the disorders but there is no clear evidence for either (Long and Cooper, 1997). It has been noted that there are deficiencies and abnormalities of the intestinal mucous layer in IBD, with associated abnormality of the mucous glycoproteins. In ulcerative colitis in particular, the immune response is mounted against a specific colon-associated protein. Mucus is an essential component contributing to intestinal mucosal defence and in ulcerative colitis colonic mucus is qualitatively and quantitatively abnormal. There may also be deranged restitution of damaged mucosa in both disorders. These factors may underlie the development of IBD (Rowlinson, 1999a). It remains unclear whether immunological abnormalities are the primary or secondary event in the pathogenesis (Clark and Kumar, 1994).

Microvasculature

The study of the microvasculature of resected gut has given new insight into the pathogenesis of Crohn's disease. It suggested that vascular injury and focal arteritis were early pathological events leading to micro-infarction. It has also been shown that there is an association between ulcerative colitis and thrombotic events and histological examination of rectal biopsies have detected fibrin thrombin in the mucosa in patients with IBD. Research into the use of anticoagulants is underway (Rowlinson, 1999a).

Infection

No infectious agent has yet been shown to transmit the disease; however, infectious agents have long been considered to be a cause of Crohn's disease (Walsh, 1997). Upper respiratory tract infections, the measles virus and *Mycobacterium paratuberculosis* have all been implicated, although incontrovertible evidence of their relevance has failed to emerge (Rowlinson, 1999a).

Professor John Hermon-Taylor is convinced, however, that a human pathogen, probably the *Mycobacterium avium* subsp. *paratuberculosis* (MAP), causes 95 per cent of Crohn's disease. In Western Europe and North America, subclinical infection with *M. paratuberculosis* is widespread in domestic livestock, and infected animals shed mycobacteria in their milk. *M. paratuberculosis* causes Johne's disease in cattle and both Johne's disease and Crohn's disease are present in Scotland in almost epidemic proportions (NACC, 2001a). It is known that *M. paratuberculosis* can accumulate in the intestine and sit there for years and that it can cause chronic inflammation of the intestine in many animal species.

M. paratuberculosis has also been found in the inflamed tissue of people with Crohn's disease (Hermon-Taylor, 2000). Complete destruction of *M. paratuberculosis* by pasteurization is not assured. Studies have shown that the temperature used for pasteurization does not destroy all the mycobacteria. A study of milk bought at retail outlets, discovered that one in four bottles tested positive for *M. paratuberculosis* (NACC, 1997). *M. paratuberculosis* is quite often present in people's bodies without appearing to cause any ill effects, but Hermon-Taylor believes that drinking pasteurized milk could be a risk for people who are susceptible to Crohn's disease. *M. paratuberculosis* appears to be highly resistant to standard antituberculosis drugs but Hermon-Taylor claims that using new drugs to which MAP is more susceptible can make patients a lot better, some lastingly so. Current genetic research, funded by the Ileostomy Association, is attempting to make a therapeutic vaccine to help the immune system of people with Crohn's disease eradicate MAP themselves (Hermon-Taylor, 2000).

The role of the bacterium is not clear-cut, however, as *Mycobacterium* has not been consistently found in involved tissues of people with Crohn's. The organism has not been shown to appear, persist, or recur with the clinical course of the disease. People with Crohn's disease have been shown to improve if their immune system is suppressed. For example, people go into remission if their T-cell counts are low because of AIDS or a recent bone marrow transplant.

In these cases a *Mycobacterium* infection would worsen, but people with Crohn's improve. The heterogeneity of Crohn's may, however, allow a role for *M. paratuberculosis*, as there may be similar types of Crohn's disease, each determined by various genes. One type may involve this organism. It is also possible that the organism is one of many bacteria that may trigger the inflammatory response in Crohn's disease. It is therefore important to cast the net wider in examining the development of the disease (NACC, 2001a).

Data published by the Royal Free Hospital's Inflammatory Bowel Study Group (IBSG) suggested that measles vaccination in infancy might triple the risk of developing Crohn's disease and more than double the risk of developing ulcerative colitis (Thompson *et al.*, 1995; Wakefield *et al.*, 1993; 1998). However, other extensive research has not shown a link between measles, mumps and rubella (MMR) vaccination and bowel disease and experts from around the world, including the World Health Organization (WHO), have agreed that there is no link between MMR and bowel disease (Yarwood, 2001). Dr Andrew Wakefield, the IBSG leader, has stressed that no changes to immunization schedules should be made until the exact nature of the link has been investigated. He does, however, believe that the research conducted so far cannot simply be ignored. Studies linking prenatal exposure to measles virus and Crohn's disease have also showed conflicting results (Kmietowicz, 1997).

Research published by Scott Montgomery in 1999, found that children who had caught measles and mumps in quick succession seemed much more likely to develop IBD as adults. The statistics indicate the likelihood of developing ulcerative colitis to be seven times greater than normal and for Crohn's disease to be four times greater. The findings did not establish a link between children having measles infection on its own and the subsequent development of IBD. The study looked at viruses caught naturally and not weakened viruses contained in the MMR vaccination and it was not therefore possible to make any conclusion about MMR on the basis of this study. As with any new research, this finding will need to be tested in other groups of people and by other researchers before it can be accepted as a certain cause of IBD (NACC, 1999).

Data collected by Health Promotion England show that when parents turn to health professionals for advice they want clear, consistent information based on facts.

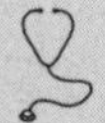

Nursing action points

- Advise clients that
  - extensive research has failed to show a link between MMR and IBD.
  - measles kills and disables children. In nearly 30 years, more than 500 million doses of MMR have been given in over 90 countries.

(Yarwood, 2001)

The increase in IBD over the past 50 years parallels the increasing use of antibiotics in human and veterinary medicine. Antibiotics can promote the proliferation of toxic bacteria and make them more invasive. It has also been suggested that Crohn's disease is an infectious disease caused by a mutated form of an organism of the normal bacterial flora, which becomes a super germ under constant selection pressure from antibiotics (Hoffman, 1997).

Environmental Factors

Evidence suggests that the cause is environmental. When a population migrates from areas of low to high incidence, the incidence in that population subsequently rises (Long and Cooper, 1997). A seasonal variation of relapses, with the highest relapse rate occurring from September to February has been suggested. This may indicate that microbiological factors are involved in the exacerbation of symptoms as some infectious agents occur with seasonality, peaking in late summer and autumn. Also patients may be less inclined to seek help during holiday periods or have less access to medical help (Rowlinson, 1999a).

Stress

Emotional factors and stress have not been shown to cause IBD, despite the demonstrated link between stress and bowel disorders. Although life stressors have not implicitly been shown to influence the clinical course of ulcerative colitis, the regulatory effects of stress on the neurogenic system and the inflammatory response cannot be discounted (Walsh, 1997).

Smoking

Ulcerative colitis is commoner in non-smokers and ex-smokers and there also appears to be a rebound effect in smokers that quit (Rowlinson, 1999b). Studies have suggested that smokers were more likely to develop Crohn's disease; heavy smokers had a higher risk of relapse and smokers with small bowel involvement had more frequent bowel movements, suffered more pain, were admitted to hospital more frequently and had an increased risk of surgical intervention. There may also be a tendency to arterial thrombosis in patients with IBD who smoke and multifocal gastrointestinal infarction has been demonstrated in Crohn's disease and proposed as a possible pathogenic mechanism (Rowlinson, 1999a).

Dietary Factors

Dietary factors are thought to play a role. Swedish researchers have found that people who eat at fast food restaurants regularly and who eat too much sugar may increase their risk of developing Crohn's disease. New unnatural substances have been introduced into the diet of people in the West, including fluoridated and chlorinated water, the residue of dental fillings and many common antacids containing aluminium and other hazardous materials. Toothpaste, food additives and synthetic food ingredients are possible dietary elements requiring further research. Infant feeding patterns may be related to the incidence of IBD according to some studies that have found a correlation between lack of breast-feeding and susceptibility to IBD. Also, the premature introduction of allergenic food such as cow's milk, soy and difficult to digest fruit juices may accelerate the development of IBD in children (Hoffman, 1997).

Geographical Factors

The incidence of Crohn's disease is higher in urban than in rural areas but no such geographical relationship has been shown in ulcerative colitis. Migrant studies have shown that environmental factors play a role in the development of these disorders. Crohn's disease is rare in Hong Kong Chinese yet is more common among Chinese migrants in Vancouver. People who migrate from the West Indies to Europe may increase their risk of developing Crohn's. Although there is a low prevalence of ulcerative colitis among Bangladeshi immigrants to the UK, the incidence of the disease among Sikhs and Hindus from Asia living in the UK is higher than among those remaining in Asia (Allison *et al.*, 1998).

Anatomy and Physiology of the Intestinal Tract

The Small Intestine

The small intestine is a convoluted tube extending from the pyloric sphincter in the epigastric region to the ileocaecal valve in the right iliac region where it joins the large intestine. It is the longest part of the alimentary canal, but its diameter is only about two and a half centimetres (Marieb, 2001) (Figure 12.1).

The small intestine is subdivided into three parts:

- The duodenum
- The jejunum
- The ileum

The duodenum is about 25 centimetres long. It is the first part of the small intestine; it is a short curved portion, roughly C-shaped and curves around the head of the pancreas (Jackson and Bennett, 1988). At its mid point there is an

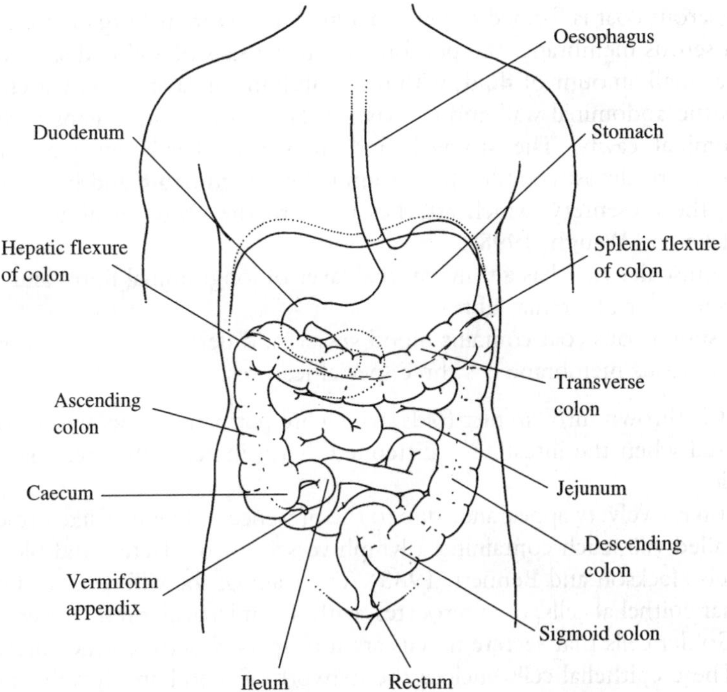

Figure 12.1 Digestive tract in body outline

opening, to the pancreatic duct and the bile duct, guarded by the hepatopancreatic sphincter.

The jejunum is the middle part of the small intestine and is about two metres long.

The ileum or terminal part is about three metres long and ends at the ileo-caecal valve, which controls the flow of material from the ileum to the caecum and prevents regurgitation (Wilson and Waugh, 1998).

Structure of the Small Intestine

The wall of the small intestine has the same four coats as the rest of the alimentary canal.

Coats of the small intestine:

- Serous coat
- Muscular coat
- Sub-mucous coat
- Mucous membrane lining

- The serous coat is formed of peritoneum. The abdominal organs are covered by a serous membrane, the peritoneum. It consists of a closed sac, containing a small amount of fluid, within the abdominal cavity. The parietal layer lines the abdominal wall and the visceral layer covers the organs within the abdominal cavity. The stomach and intestines, deeply invaginated from behind, are almost completely surrounded by peritoneum and have a double fold, the mesentery, which attaches them to the posterior abdominal wall (Wilson and Waugh, 1998).
- The muscular coat has a thin external layer of longitudinal fibres and a thick internal layer of circular fibres.
- The submucous coat contains blood vessels and nerves.
- The mucous membrane has three special features:

  1. It is thrown into circular folds, which are permanent and are not obliterated when the intestine is distended. They increase the area for absorption.
  2. It has a velvety appearance due to the presence of fine hair-like projections called villi, each containing a lymph vessel called a lacteal and blood vessels (Jackson and Bennett, 1988). The walls of the villi consist of columnar epithelial cells, or enterocytes, with tiny microvilli on their free border. Goblet cells that secrete mucus are interspersed between the enterocytes. These epithelial cells enclose the network of blood and lymph capillaries (Wilson and Waugh, 1998). Digested foodstuffs are absorbed through the epithelial cells into both the capillary blood and the lacteal. Between the villi, the mucosa is studded with pits or openings that lead into tubular intestinal glands called intestinal crypts or crypts of Lieberkuhn. The epithelial cells that line these crypts secrete intestinal juice (Marieb, 2001).
  3. It is supplied with simple tubular type glands that secrete intestinal juice (Jackson and Bennett, 1988).

The small intestine contains considerable amounts of lymphoid tissue that deals with bacteria that may be absorbed through the intestinal wall. The lymph nodes are numerous in the mucosa at irregular intervals throughout the length of the small intestine. The smaller ones are known as solitary lymphatic follicles and larger nodes, situated towards the distal end of the ileum are called aggregated lymphatic follicles or Peyer's patches (Wilson and Waugh, 1998). The Peyer's patches increase in abundance towards the end of the small intestine, reflecting the fact that the large intestine contains huge numbers of bacteria that must be prevented from entering the bloodstream (Marieb, 2001).

Functions of the small intestine:

- Onward movement of its contents, which is brought about by peristalsis, segmental and pendular movements.

- Completion of chemical digestion of carbohydrates, protein and fats in the enterocytes of the villi
- Protection against infection by microorganisms that have survived the antimicrobial acid in the stomach, by the solitary and aggregated lymph follicles
- Secretion of the hormones cholecystokinin and secretin. These hormones are produced by cells in the walls of the duodenum and stimulate the secretion of pancreatic juice. The presence in the duodenum of acid material from the stomach stimulates the production of these hormones
- Absorption of nutrient material

(Wilson and Waugh, 1998)

The Large Intestine

The large intestine is about one and a half metres long. It begins at the caecum in the right iliac fossa and terminates at the rectum and anal canal, deep in the pelvis (see Figure 12.1). Its diameter is greater than that of the small intestine but it is less than half as long. It forms an arch round the coiled up small intestine. Its major function is to absorb water from indigestible foodstuffs and eliminate them from the body as semisolid faeces. Over most of its length the large intestine exhibits features not seen elsewhere. Except for its terminal end, the longitudinal muscle layer of its muscularis is reduced to three bands of smooth muscle called teniae coli. Their tone causes the wall of the large intestine to pucker into pocket like sacs called haustra. A unique feature of the large intestine is its epiploic appendages. These are small, fat filled pouches of visceral peritoneum that hang from the surface. Their significance is not known (Marieb, 2001).

Parts of the Large Intestine

The large intestine is divided into seven parts.

- The caecum
- The ascending colon
- The transverse colon
- The descending colon
- The sigmoid colon
- The rectum
- The anal canal

- The caecum lies in the right iliac fossa. It is a dilated portion, which has a blind end inferiorly and is continuous with the ascending colon superiorly. Just below the junction of the two the ileocaecal valve opens from the ileum (Wilson and Waugh, 1998). Attached to its posteromedial surface is the blind, wormlike vermiform appendix, which contains masses of lymphoid tissue (Marieb, 2001).
- The ascending colon passes upwards from the caecum to the level of the liver where it bends acutely to the left at the hepatic flexure to become the transverse colon.
- The transverse colon is a loop of colon, that extends across the abdominal cavity in front of the duodenum and stomach to the area of the spleen where it forms the splenic flexure by bending acutely downwards to become the descending colon.
- The descending colon passes down the left side of the abdominal cavity then curves towards the midline. After it enters the true pelvis it is known as the sigmoid colon.
- The sigmoid describes an S-shaped curve in the pelvis then continues downwards as the rectum.
- The rectum is a slightly dilated part of the colon that is about 13 centimetres long. It leads from the sigmoid colon to the anal canal.
- The anal canal is a short canal and leads to the exterior. There are two sphincter muscles that control the anus. The internal sphincter consists of smooth muscle and is under the control of the autonomic nervous system and the external sphincter, formed by striated muscle is under voluntary nerve control (Wilson and Waugh, 1998).

The Structure of the Large Intestine

- Outer serous coat of peritoneum
- Muscular coat
- Sub-mucous coat
- Mucous membrane lining

The arrangement of the longitudinal muscle fibres is modified in the colon. They do not form a smooth continuous layer of tissue but are collected into three bands, called teniae coli, situated at regular intervals round the colon. They stop at the junction of the sigmoid colon and the rectum. As these bands are slightly shorter than the total length of the colon they give a sacculated or puckered appearance to the large intestine. The sacculations are called haustrations or haustra (Wilson and Waugh, 1998). The longitudinal muscle fibres spread out and completely surround the rectum and anal canal. Thickening of the circular muscle layer forms the anal sphincters. In the submucous coat there is more lymphoid tissue than in any other part of the alimentary tract, providing non-specific defence against invasion by resident and other microorganisms. In the mucosa that lines the colon and upper part of the rectum there are large numbers of goblet cells forming simple tubular glands, which secrete mucus. They are not present beyond the junction between the rectum and the anus. The lining membrane of the anus consists of squamous epithelium, which is continuous with the mucous membrane lining of the rectum above and merges with the skin beyond the external sphincter (Wilson and Waugh, 1998).

Functions of the Large Intestine

- Absorption of water and salts
- Defecation
- Microbial activity

Absorption. Absorption of water continues in the large intestine along with mineral salts, vitamins and some drugs.

Defecation. The large intestine does not exhibit peristaltic movement as seen elsewhere in the digestive tract. Only at fairly long intervals does a wave of strong peristalsis sweep along the transverse colon forcing its contents into the descending and sigmoid colon. This is known as mass movement and when this forces faeces into the rectum, nerves endings in its wall are stimulated. Defecation is a reflex action but the brain can inhibit the reflex until it is convenient to defecate. If defecation is delayed the sensation of fullness in the rectum passes and more water is absorbed (Jackson and Bennett, 1988).

Contents of faeces

- Water makes up 60–70 per cent of the weight
- Fibre
- Dead and live microorganisms
- Epithelial cells from the walls of the tract
- Fatty acids
- Mucus, which helps to lubricate the faeces

Microbial Activity. Although most bacteria entering the caecum from the small intestine are dead some are alive. Together with bacteria that enter via the anus, these constitute the bacterial flora of the large intestine. These bacteria colonize the colon and ferment some of the indigestible carbohydrates, releasing irritating acids and a mixture of gases. About 500 millilitres of gases are produced each day, much more when certain carbohydrate-rich foods are eaten. The bacterial floras also synthesize B complex vitamins and most of the vitamin K the liver requires to synthesize some of the clotting proteins (Marieb, 2001). These bacteria are commensals in humans; they include *Escherichia coli*, *Enterobacter aerogenes*, *Streptococcus faecalis* and *Clostridium perfringens*. They may become pathogenic if transferred to another part of the body (Wilson and Waugh, 1998).

Pathophysiology

In both diseases the intestinal wall is infiltrated with acute and chronic inflammatory cells, however, there are differences in the distribution of disease and in histological features (Palmer and Penman, 1999) (see Table 12.2).

Ulcerative colitis is predominantly a mucosal disease of the colon. The rectum is almost always involved; proximal extension occurs in about half of patients who present initially with disease confined to the rectosigmoid region. In some cases the whole colon may be affected (pancolitis). There is usually an abrupt cut off between affected and unaffected colon. A variety of appearances may be encountered depending upon the activity and duration of the disease. In acute-onset severe disease (toxic megacolon) most of the bowel is distended and plum-coloured and the walls are paper thin and friable. More usually, the disease is confined to the mucosa, with only mild reactive changes in the submucosa. In contrast to Crohn's disease, the bowel wall is not thickened and fibrous, and the outer surface of the bowel may appear normal (Allison *et al.*, 1998). Initially there is reddening and oedema of the mucosa with bleeding points. This is followed by ulceration, which is usually superficial. In long standing pancolitis the bowel becomes shortened and narrowed with lack of haustrations (Miller *et al.*, 1994). The mucosal surface is characterized initially by hyperaemia and capillary fragility. With advancing disease these changes lead to irregular ulceration, which may become confluent, with undermining of the adjacent mucosa. Residual mucosal bridges then disappear and areas of the mucosal surface become denuded. This means that most of the mucosa has been lost leaving only small islands of congested mucosa, overlying a smooth and inflamed submucosal base (Allison *et al.*, 1998). Inflammation at the base of the crypts of Lieberkuhn damages the epithelial cells in the crypts and forms abscesses. The mucosa surrounding the ulcerations may appear 'heaped up', because the muscularis

Table 12.2 A comparison of ulcerative colitis and Crohn's disease

Ulcerative colitis	*Crohn's disease*
▪ Mucosal involvement	▪ Transmural involvement
▪ Inflammation is confluent	▪ Skip lesions
▪ Granulomas absent	▪ Granulomas present
▪ Crypt abscesses common	▪ Crypt abscess uncommon
▪ Reduced number of goblet cells	▪ Normal number of goblet cells
▪ Colon affected	▪ Any part of the gastrointestinal tract affected
▪ Strictures uncommon compared with Crohn's disease	▪ Strictures (narrowing of the lumen of the bowel)
▪ Anal lesions such as fissures and fistulas are less severe and less common	▪ Fistulas and fissures are features
▪ Curative surgery	▪ No cure

mucosa tends to contract. These are known as pseudopolyps and are a diagnostic finding (Doughty and Jackson, 1993). Acute and chronic inflammatory cells infiltrate the lamina propria and the crypts. Goblet cells lose their mucus and may become distorted in long-standing cases Inflammation is confluent and is more severe distally (Palmer and Penman, 1999).

In Crohn's disease any part of the gastrointestinal tract from mouth to anus can be affected but the commonest site is the terminal ileum. In some cases the whole of the colon and/or the small intestine can be involved (Clark and Kumar, 1994). The inflammatory changes affect isolated segments of all layers of the intestinal wall, which becomes oedematous and thickened. Crohn's disease can involve one small area or multiple areas with relatively normal bowel in between (skip lesions). The change from the affected area is abrupt. The mesenteric lymph nodes are enlarged and the mesentery thickened (Palmer and Penman, 1999). Aphthous ulcers are probably the earliest pathological finding. These begin as microabscesses in lymphoid follicles and develop into superficial ulcers surrounded by normal or mildly oedematous mucosa. As the disease process continues, the ulcers become more invasive forming fissures that may extend into the submucosal layer (rake ulcers). The rake ulcers run longitudinally and transversely and tend to coalesce, creating a 'cobblestone' appearance of the bowel wall. With advanced disease, fissures can penetrate the bowel wall to create fistulas or abscesses. Narrowing (strictures) of the lumen of the bowel wall also occurs as the disease advances (Doughty and Jackson, 1993). Fistulas can develop between adjacent loops of bowel or between affected segments of bowel and the bladder, uterus or vagina and may appear in the perineum (Palmer and Penman, 1999). There are focal aggregates of epithelioid histocytes, which may be surrounded by lymphocytes and contain giant cells. These are non-caseating granulomas and are a hallmark of Crohn's (Clark and Kumar, 1994). This feature is seen in about 50 per cent of cases (Allison *et al.*, 1998).

Clinical Manifestations

Ulcerative Colitis

The first attack is usually the most severe and in most cases will be followed by relapses and remissions of the disease. Emotional stress, infection, gastroenteritis, antibiotics or non-steroid anti-inflammatory drugs may provoke a relapse (Palmer and Penman, 1999). The usual presenting symptom is the passage of frequent loose, small volume, brown motions with fresh blood and mucus either on the surface of the stools or intermixed with them. Patients with mild attacks open their bowels up to five times a day, with moderate attacks up to ten times a day and with severe attacks over ten times a day (Long and Cooper, 1997). In an acute attack, 20 liquid stools a day may be passed and diarrhoea occurs at night, with urgency and incontinence that is severely disabling for the patient. Occasionally blood and mucus alone are passed (Clark and Kumar, 1994). The pain is usually located in the lower left quadrant and is colicky in nature. After defaecation, pain may subside. In very severe cases tenderness in the left lower quadrant, guarding and abdominal distension may occur (Walsh, 1997).

The clinical features depend upon the site and activity of the disease:

Proctitis

Proctitis causes rectal bleeding and mucus discharge accompanied by tenesmus. Some patients pass frequent, small volume liquid stools but some may experience constipation and pass small pellet stools. No constitutional symptoms occur.

Proctosigmoiditis

Proctosigmoiditis causes bloody diarrhoea with mucus. Most patients are well, having no constitutional symptoms. Small minorities of patients, who have very active, limited disease, develop fever, lethargy and abdominal discomfort.

Extensive Colitis

Extensive colitis causes bloody diarrhoea with mucus. In severe cases anorexia, malaise, weight loss and abdominal pain occur. The patient is toxic with fever, tachycardia and signs of peritoneal inflammation. Fever and tachycardia, usually indicate severe widespread and active disease rather than infection. Anaemia is usually hypochromic and microcytic and due to blood loss (Palmer and Penman, 1999).

Toxic Megacolon

This is a rare, very serious complication resulting from a spread of the mucosal inflammation to the submucosal, muscular and possibly the serosal layers of the colon; the smooth muscle is paralysed allowing the colon to passively dilate and the barrier functions of the epithelium appears to be lost, permitting the uptake of bacterial toxins and antigens. Clinical manifestations include:

- Severe abdominal distention
- Abdominal pain and tenderness
- Chills
- Fever
- Anorexia
- Nausea and vomiting
- Bloody diarrhoea
- Leucocytosis

The goal of treatment is to prevent perforation and peritonitis, which carries a high mortality rate (Doughty and Jackson, 1993).

Crohn's Disease

The patient with Crohn's disease may have occasional acute episodes of illness but more often has mild intermittent symptoms. The commonest initial presentation is with terminal ileum disease, often with coexistent oral and anal involvement. Less common initial presentations are acute right iliac fossa pain simulating acute appendicitis and acute colitis identical to ulcerative colitis. General symptoms include the following:

- Fever
- Malaise
- Weight loss (may be due to malabsorption or avoidance of food, since eating provokes pain. Some patients present with features of fat, protein or vitamin deficiency)
- Amenorrhoea
- In children: failure to thrive, growth retardation, delayed puberty
- In pre-pubertal and pubertal children there may be no history of diarrhoea or abdominal pain (Long and Cooper, 1997)

Gastrointestinal Symptoms

As a result of stricture formation many patients with ileal disease complain of colicky abdominal pain, usually in the right iliac fossa. Diarrhoea is usually moderate and may contain excess fat. Flatulence, nausea, borborygmus and increased peristalsis may be present (Walsh, 1997). Urinary frequency and dysuria may result from inflamed bowel adjacent to the urinary tract. Air in the urine and faeces via the urethra or vagina indicate a fistula from bowel to genitourinary tract (Long and Cooper, 1997).

The gastrointestinal symptoms depend primarily upon the site of disease.

Ileal Disease

Ileal disease causes colicky, abdominal pain, principally due to subacute obstruction, although an inflammatory mass, intra-abdominal abscess or acute obstruction may be responsible (Palmer and Penman, 1999). Pain is often associated with diarrhoea that is soft or semi-liquid and does not contain blood or mucus. If steatorrhoea is present the stools will be foul smelling and fatty. When the terminal ileum is involved, the pain is in the periumbilical region. Initially the ileal pain is peristaltic and intermittent; later it becomes more constant and may be noticed in the lower right quadrant. Cramps of regional enteritis are not closely associated with defaecation, and unlike cramps with colonic disease are not relieved by passing stool or flatus. A constant aching soreness or tenderness usually indicates advanced disease (Walsh, 1997).

Crohn's Colitis

Crohn's colitis presents in an identical way to ulcerative colitis with bloody diarrhoea, passage of mucus and constitutional symptoms including lethargy, malaise, anorexia and weight loss. Rectal sparing and the presence of perianal disease favour a diagnosis of Crohn's disease rather than ulcerative colitis. Many patients present with symptoms of both small and large bowel disease. A few have isolated perianal disease, vomiting from jejunal strictures or severe oral ulceration.

Physical examination often reveals evidence of weight loss, anaemia with glossitis and angular stomatitis. Abdominal tenderness, most marked over the inflamed area is present. An abdominal mass due to matted loops of thickened bowel or an intra-abdominal abscess may occur. Perianal skin tags, fissures or fistulae are found in at least 50 per cent of patients (Palmer and Penman, 1999).

Acute arthritis, portal pyaemia, liver abscess, and dermatological, ocular and vascular complications tend to occur during acute relapse of bowel disease. IBD can be considered as a systemic illness and in some patients extraintestinal complications are a dominant clinical feature. Some occur during a relapse of intestinal disease; others appear unrelated to intestinal disease (see Table 12.3) (Palmer and Penman, 1999).

Table 12.3 Complications of inflammatory bowel disease

Intestinal	*Extraintestinal*
Inflammation ▪ Severe, life-threatening inflammation of the colon (occurs in ulcerative colitis and Crohn's disease) **Perforation** ▪ Perforation of the small intestine or colon (can occur without the development of toxic megacolon) **Haemorrhage** ▪ Life-threatening acute haemorrhage (due to erosion of a major blood vessel) **Fistula and perianal disease** ▪ Fistula and perianal disease (specific complications of Crohn's disease and not ulcerative colitis)	**Seronegative arthritis** ▪ Acute arthritis affecting medium sized joints ▪ Ankylosing spondylitis ▪ Sacroilitis **Dermatological** ▪ Erythema nodosum ▪ Pyoderma gangrenosum ▪ Oral aphthous ulcers **Ocular** ▪ Conjunctivitis ▪ Iritis ▪ Episcleritis **Hepatic and biliary** ▪ Primary sclerosing cholangitis (ulcerative colitis only) ▪ Gallstones ▪ Autoimmune hepatitis ▪ Fatty liver ▪ Portal pyaemia and liver abscesses ▪ Amyloidosis ▪ Cholangiocarcinoma

Table 12.3 (Contd.)

Intestinal	*Extraintestinal*
Cancer ■ Cancer (patients with extensive colitis of more than eight years duration are at increased risk of colon cancer). The cumulative risk for patients with ulcerative colitis may be as high as 20 percent after 30 years but is probably less for Crohn's colitis	**Renal** ■ Oxalate calculi (small bowel Crohn's) ■ Amyloidosis ■ Ureteric obstruction (Crohn's)
	Vascular ■ Deep vein thrombosis ■ Portal or mesenteric vein thrombosis

Investigative Tests

History

After taking a history the doctor will assess each individual to decide the type and extent of investigations required (Table 12.4).

Medical and Surgical Treatment

Medical Management

Aims are to bring about remission and maintain this for as long as possible. This may involve correcting fluid and electrolyte balance, malnutrition and anaemia.

Table 12.4 Investigative tests

Tests	*Investigations*
General examination	■ Recent weight change ■ Appetite ■ Bowel frequency ■ Pain ■ Energy levels/altered lifestyle
Abdominal observation and palpation	Observable abdominal distention or visible peristalsis. Palpable mass or areas of tenderness.
Ano-rectal examination	
Visual inspection	Inspection of perianal skin, noting any skin tags, anal fissure, anal fistula, skin discolouration.
Protoscopy	Visual examination of the rectal mucosa.
Sigmoidoscopy	Direct examination of the anal canal rectum and sigmoid colon, using a rigid or flexible instrument.

Table 12.4 (Contd.)

Tests	*Investigations*
	Rectal sparing, perianal disease and discrete ulcers suggest Crohn's disease rather than ulcerative colitis.
Rectal biopsy	Taken during sigmoidoscopy to determine disease extent, as this is underestimated in endoscopic appearance alone and to seek dysplasia in patients with long-term disease.
Colonic examination	
Plain abdominal x-rays	In severe colitis to observe for any colonic dilatation and assess the extent of the disease, which can be judged by the distribution of air in the colon.
Barium enema	Less sensitive than colonoscopy for the investigation of colitis. In long standing ulcerative colitis the bowel becomes shortened and loses haustra to become tubular and pseudopolyps are visible. In Crohn's disease the appearance may be similar to ulcerative colitis but skip lesions, strictures and deep ulcers are characteristic Contrast studies of the small bowel are normal in ulcerative colitis. Barium enema is contraindicated in acute disease.
Colonoscopy	The whole bowel can be viewed with a fibreoptic scope. May show active inflammation with pseudopolyps or a complicating carcinoma. In ulcerative colitis the macroscopic and histological abnormalities are confluent and most severe in the distal colon and rectum. In Crohn's colitis the endoscopic abnormalities are patchy with normal mucosa between the areas of abnormality and 'cobblestoning' of the mucosa. Aphthoid or deep ulcers are common.
Radionucleide scans	Radio-labelled white cell scans can show areas of active inflammation. This test is less sensitive than conventional tests but is useful in severely ill patients in whom invasive tests are to be avoided.
Ultrasound and CT scanning	Helpful in delineating abscesses, masses, thickened mesentery or other extraluminal problems in Crohn's disease.
Small bowel examination	
Barium enema and follow through	To identify disease in the upper gastrointestinal tract.
Specimens	
Stool analysis and culture	
Observation	To observe consistency and presence of blood, mucus, pus or steatorrhoea.
Microbiological examination	To rule out infective agents.
Stool weight	Measure stool weight per 24 hours.
Blood analysis	
Full blood count (FBC)	For noting any anaemia, raised white cell count or raised platelets.
Erythrocyte Sedimentation Rate (ESR) or C Reactive Protein (CPR)	ESR or CPR may be raised in active disease.
Liver Function Test (LFT)	Particularly noting albumin level as a nutritional indicator.
Urea and electrolytes (U & E)	To indicate fluid balance deficiencies and general state of health.

Palmer and Penman, 1999; Curry, 1995; Clark and Kumar, 1994.

The principles of drug treatment are similar for ulcerative colitis and Crohn's disease.

Drug therapy

- Corticosteroids
- Aminosalicylates
- Immunosuppressants
- Antibiotics
- Nicotine

Corticosteroid Therapy

Corticosteroids are first line treatment and are prescribed for their anti-inflammatory and immunosupressant actions. Steroid foam or liquid retention enemas, from which systemic corticosteroid absorption is insignificant, are used to treat active proctosigmoiditis. In severe proctosigmoiditis, where patient is unable to retain enemas or patient has active, extensive colitis, oral corticosteroids are given. Severe active colitis can be treated with intravenous methylprednisolone. Once improvement occurs, a reducing regimen of oral prednisolone is commenced.

Systemic Steroid Side Effects: Mood changes, acne, weight gain and dyspepsia are common but resolve as soon as the dosage is reduced. More rarely, hypertension and hyperglycaemia may result. Long term, high dose therapy is avoided because of the risks of metabolic bone disease and infection (Palmer and Penman, 1999).

Aminosalicylate Therapy

Sulphasalazine, mesalazine, balsalazineside or olsalazine are given during an attack of ulcerative colitis and for long-term use to keep the disease in remission to prevent inflammation from developing. These are also given for Crohn's colitis. For small intestine Crohn's disease, a slow release mesalazine preparation is used. These drugs may be given as tablets, enemas or suppositories.

Side Effects. Headaches, nausea, skin rashes, diarrhoea, anorexia, oligospermia, renal toxicity, blood dyscrasias.

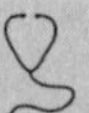

Nursing action points

- Be aware that side effects such as headaches, nausea and anorexia are dose related.
- Inform young male patients of the potential side effect of oligospermia, with sulphasalazine therapy, though this is reversible once the drug is withdrawn.
- Be aware that the newer range of drugs are as effective as sulphasalazine but have significantly lower side effects.

(Rowlinson, 1999b)

Immunosuppressant Therapy

Immunosuppressant therapy with drugs such as azathioprine, methotrexate or cyclosporine is valuable in refractory inflammatory bowel disease in helping to achieve and maintain clinical remission, reducing steroid use and avoiding surgery. These drugs work by blocking the immune reaction that contributes to inflammation.

Side Effects. Nausea, vomiting, diarrhoea and a lowered resistance to infection (Rowlinson, 1999b).

Antibiotic Therapy

A fistula complicated by infection or a stagnant area or loop of intestine in which there is an overgrowth of bacteria may be treated with antibiotics such as, metronidazole, ampicillin, cephalosporin, tetracycline or sulphonamide (Walsh, 1997). The use of antibiotics may be to eradicate atypical mycobacteria. Rifambutin and clarithromycin have been used to treat people with Crohn's disease and analysis of the outcomes showed significant improvement in disease severity and a reduction in inflammatory markers. However, not all people respond to the treatment, possibly due to existing drug resistance (Hermon-Taylor, 2000).

Nicotine

In various clinical trials both nicotine gum and transdermal patches have been found to be clinically effective in the treatment of ulcerative colitis, although there was a high incidence of side effects, especially among those patients that had never smoked (Rowlinson, 1999b).

Infliximab, the first treatment approved specifically for the treatment of Crohn's disease is an anti-tumour necrosis factor (anti-TNF) substance. TNF is a protein produced by the immune system that may cause the inflammation associated with Crohn's disease. Anti-TNF removes TNF from the bloodstream before it reaches the intestines. It has been used to treat moderate to severe cases that do not respond to standard therapies.

Nutrition

There is no specific therapeutic diet for patients with IBD. Many patients find that certain foods aggravate their symptoms and these are therefore best avoided. Such foods vary widely from patient to patient but include fatty foods, dairy products, caffeine or raw, high fibre foods that are difficult to digest.

Sometimes IBD is treated with an elemental diet, which is a liquid consisting of all the nutrients in a pre-digested form, ready for absorption through the wall of the small intestine. Usually nothing but the diet and water are allowed for weeks or months at a time. The diet can be rather unpalatable and should be taken in sips to avoid increasing the diarrhoea. In some cases it may be given via a nasogastric tube.

Medical intervention may be necessary in order to restore nutritional and electrolyte balance during active disease. Nutritional deficiencies are common due to

- Decreased nutritional intake
- Increased nutritional requirements due to inflammation, infection and fever
- Increased nutritional losses due to malabsorption, diarrhoea, bleeding
- Nutritional interference by drugs, for example, steroids

(Curry, 1995)

In fulminating disease, enteral nutrition may not be possible and total parenteral nutrition (TPN) will be required. If enteral nutrition is possible, an elemental residue free diet may be necessary for a short while until a low residue diet can be introduced. As the inflammation settles dietary restrictions can be reduced. During periods of remission a normal well-balanced diet is recommended. It should contain sufficient kilocalories to restore and maintain weight, as well as being high in protein and carbohydrates and low in fat. Supplements of vitamins, iron, folic acid, zinc and potassium may be required (Miller *et al.*, 1994).

Fish oil preparations have been shown to have anti-inflammatory properties and have been recommended for use in a number of chronic inflammatory diseases and it is claimed that they may have some positive benefits in prolonging periods of remission in patients with Crohn's disease (Medicinenet.com, 1999).

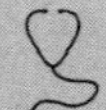

Nursing action points

- Identify what type of diet the patient normally has.
- Advise the patient to note food or drinks that aggravate their symptoms so that they can be avoided in future.
- Note how much of a normal diet is eaten and tolerated.
- Record prescribed supplements on the appropriate chart.
- Be aware that nutritional supplements may be recommended, especially for children whose growth has been slowed. Special high-calorie liquid formulas may be used for this purpose.

Surgical Management

Surgery may be appropriate in the following situations:

- Loss of occupation or education.
- Disruption of family life.
- Disease complications such as arthritis and pyoderma gangrenosum that are unresponsive to medical treatment (Palmer and Penman, 1999).
- Imminent risk of perforation.
- A long history of moderately active disease with few or no periods of remission.
- Failure to respond to medical treatment.
- Intestinal obstruction and abdominal or perianal fistulae.
- Pre-cancerous change or cancer (Curry, 1995).

The type of surgery will depend upon the specific diagnosis. Up to 60 per cent of patients with extensive ulcerative colitis eventually require surgery, involving removal of the entire colon and rectum, which cures the patient. The choice of procedure is either panproctocolectomy with ileostomy or proctocolectomy with ileo-anal pouch anastomosis.

The indications for surgery in Crohn's disease are similar to those for ulcerative colitis. Operations are often necessary for dealing with fistulae, abscesses or perianal disease and may be necessary to relieve small or large bowel obstruction. Up to 80 per cent of patients eventually require some form of surgery, but unlike ulcerative colitis surgery does not cure the patient. Surgical intervention should therefore be conservative in order to conserve as much viable intestine as possible and to avoid a short bowel syndrome.

Surgical procedures

- Localized segments of Crohn's colitis may be managed by segmental resection.
- Extensive colitis may require total colectomy (ileo-anal pouch is to be avoided because of the high risk of disease recurrence in the pouch and subsequent fistula, abscess formation and pouch failure).
- Perianal disease is managed as conservatively as possible by drainage of the abscess and avoidance of resection or reconstructive procedures.
- Obstructing or fistulating small bowel disease may require resection of affected tissue.
- Multiple or recurrent strictures may require strictureplasty in which the stricture is not resected but incised in its longitudinal axis and sutured transversely (Palmer and Penman, 1999).

Nursing Interventions

Nursing care will inevitably be determined by the presenting symptoms.

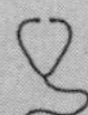 *Nursing action points*

Symptoms	Nursing interventions
Diarrhoea The need to defecate is often associated with a degree of urgency and tenesmus. The stool may also have an offensive smell.	■ Position the patient close to a lavatory. ■ If the patient is unable to reach a lavatory due to weakness or urgency, provide a bedside commode. ■ Monitor faecal loss on a stool chart, recording consistency, presence of blood, mucus and pus. ■ Provide soft tissues and wipes. ■ Provide a pleasant air freshener; this may alleviate embarrassment. ■ Maintain privacy and dignity. Patient may monitor his or her own stool output if appropriate.
Faecal incontinence This may be a problem. Incontinence associated with frequent bowel movements can lead to excoriated perianal skin.	■ Assist the patient to maintain personal hygiene. ■ Provide disposable pants and pads. ■ Help the patient to wash perianal skin and apply barrier cream if excoriation or soreness is a problem.
Weakness and general malaise due to a combination of inflammatory disease, frequent bowel movements and weight loss. Interrupted sleep adds to the tiredness.	■ Give assistance with maintaining the activities of living; ensure that the patient has adequate rest. ■ Provide a quiet environment.
Loss of appetite The disease process may suppress appetite	■ Offer small appetizing meals that are light and easy to digest.

and patients may be reluctant to eat as they have a misconception that eating will increase bowel frequency. Nausea and vomiting may also be experienced.

- In between snacks may be required.
- Be aware that dietary supplements may be prescribed to maintain nutritional intake.
- Administer prescribed anti-emetics as appropriate.
- Monitor body weight.

Abdominal pain

Persistent, colicky abdominal pain is characteristic of Crohn's disease. The pain of ulcerative colitis is severe prior to defecation and is usually relieved by defecation.

- Monitor the patient's pain and report any changes.
- Encourage the patient to report any aggravating factors.
- Ensure the patent's comfort by providing extra pillows.

Anxieties

These may be related to lack of understanding of the disease, fears of having to have a stoma or fears of being unable to cope with work or taking care of the family. Altered body image due to weight loss may be a problem. The increasing incidence of Crohn's disease among young children can lead to problems at adolescence. This can be a very difficult time as changes in nutritional state may lead to a pallid and sickly appearance that the adolescent perceives as decreasing body image (Pullen, 1999).

- Give full explanations of planned treatment and investigations.
- Correct any misconceptions.
- Give time for patient to express any anxieties and discuss the effects that the disease has upon the individual and significant others.
- Identify specific psychological problems and provide the relevant support, for example, counselling.
- Liaise with stoma therapist if a stoma is indicated.
- Liaise with a medical social worker.
- If appropriate and desired arrange a meeting with another person who has had similar experiences of the disease and treatment. Contact NACC for further patient information (Curry, 1995).

A professional and caring approach will help the nurse to establish a trusting partnership in care. This is essential for those practitioners involved in the long-term care of patients, as compliance with maintenance drug therapy and other relevant advice will determine the potential course of the disease. A prime aim will be to reduce stress, as there is growing evidence that both chronic and everyday stress can cause psychophysiological reactions such as colonic hyperactivity. Patient participation in care gives back an element of control over his or her life. While not all patients will want to be fully informed or involved in decision-making they should be given the choice. The role of the nurse is to support those individuals who wish to be fully involved, while relieving those for whom this responsibility is perceived to be too overwhelming. The effects upon the family should also be taken into account. It is not uncommon for family members, in caring for the individual with IBD to overlook their own needs. This can result in family tensions, fatigue, feelings of resentment and decreased ability to cope (Walsh, 1997).

 **Connection**

Chapter 2 (Family-Centred Care) discusses how the health of relatives can be compromised by the burden of care and explores ways in which nurses can support such family members.

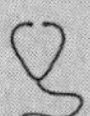 *Nursing action points*

- Encourage patients to take control of their own lives where appropriate.
- Discuss stress management techniques.
- Assess how relatives are coping with the impact of caring.

The Impact of IBD

Some individuals may feel it necessary to hide their illness from employers for fear of discrimination or due to the socially unaccepted nature of the disease and the associated embarrassment. Despite poor attendance, affected children show a normal educational outcome in terms of leaving age and the uptake of further education (Mayberry *et al.*, 1992). The fear of diarrhoea and incontinence may inhibit social life. It is common for individuals to locate the nearest lavatory in any new situation. Personal relationships can be affected. Fear of faecal incontinence, abdominal pain, dyspareunia and perianal disease can have a major impact upon sexuality. Fertility in male patients has not been shown to be different from the normal population and women with IBD have the ability to conceive. Fewer children are born to such women, possibly through choice or medical advice (Rowlinson, 1999c).

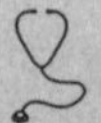

Nursing action points

- Be aware of the potential embarrassment that this condition may cause patients.
- Be aware that patients may find it difficult to initiate discussion relative to sexual dysfunction.

The Role of the Clinical Nurse Specialist

In adapting to a chronic illness or significantly altered body function, feeling understood and supported is of prime importance. This is difficult to achieve if patients see different staff at each clinic attended. Many patients only ever attend an outpatient clinic or their GP's surgery and even then may not see the same doctor. The need for continuity and the benefits of being seen by a familiar person have been recognized and nurse specialist posts are being developed in many gastroenterology departments. These posts will enable patients to obtain specialist advice and pastoral care. They will enable patients to make informed choices on future treatment and complementary therapies. Nurse specialists will be able to make referrals to other specialists, ward and community nurses and to disseminate their expertise to an array of practitioners (Finley, 1999).

A nurse whose role is totally devoted to patients with IBD can be invaluable in providing educational, emotional and psychological support. Such nurses do not replace doctors or 'general' nurses but provide a complementary service. Drawing upon research, and their own experience and intuition, they are in a unique position to influence the quality of care offered to patients. By combining both medical and nursing functions to provide a service that is acceptable to patients, the specialist nurse can assist patients to attain a higher quality of life through purposeful interventions designed to minimize symptoms, reduce the frequency and intensity of exacerbations and enhance psychosocial well-being (Rowlinson, 1999c).

Conclusion

There are marked differences in the manifestations and severity of the disease and in the ways that individuals adapt and cope with symptoms. The fact that only the worst exacerbations require serious medical intervention may lead to both patients and healthcare professionals underestimating the physical and psychological impact that the chronic disease has upon the individual and his or her family. It may be true that individuals do not often feel very ill but they may not often feel entirely well, such is the nature of IBD.

Colorectal Cancer and IBD

Individuals with chronic ulcerative colitis are at increased risk of developing colorectal carcinoma, particularly if there is long-standing or extensive colitis. It is generally accepted that the risk of colorectal cancer does not begin until eight to ten years after ulcerative colitis is diagnosed. Thereafter the risk increases by approximately 0.5–1.0 per cent, per year. The risk is smaller and less well defined (Solomon and Schnitzler, 1998). The relative risk of colorectal cancer is increased in both ulcerative colitis and Crohn's disease in those patients whose colitis started before the age of 25 years. Whether the absolute risk is greater in the younger age group or merely reflects the fact that the expected number of carcinomas increases with age is uncertain. The number of patients with Crohn's disease who actually develop cancer is small because many patients with extensive colitis undergo colectomy early in the course of the disease to relieve persistent symptoms that do not respond to medical treatment (Gillen *et al.*, 1994).

Aetiology

Epithelial cells lining the colon are normally subject to rapid turnover. They form and mature and are then lost by a process of sloughing within a period of two to three days. This rapid turnover prevents the accumulation of damaged or defective cells. In some cases the renewal cycle breaks down and abnormal tissue structures begin to appear. This can range from hyperplasia (excessive production of normal cells) to dysplasia (clumps of abnormal cells) to polyps, comprised of dysplastic cells (Campbell, 1999). The increased cell proliferation that occurs in ulcerative colitis may predispose the mucosa to mutational events, thereby increasing the risk of cancer (Noffsinger *et al.*, 1996). Histopathological grading of tumour tissue gives a measure of its aggressiveness and may relate to prognosis and treatment.

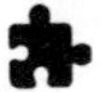

Connection

Chapter 14 (Cancer – an Overview) addresses the aetiology and pathophysiology of malignant changes in body cells.

Screening

The signs and symptoms of IBD may mask any symptoms of malignancy and monitoring any changes in the pattern of disease is important. The most significant predictor of the risk of malignancy is the presence of dysplasia in colonic biopsies; there is however, controversy over the efficacy of colonoscopy and the role of prophylactic surgery. Research is underway to identify genetic and biochemical markers that may prove useful for predicting cancer risk (Solomon and Schnitzler, 1998).

Treatment

Recent research into colorectal cancers has resulted in the increased use of combination therapies, which incorporate local treatments (surgery and radiotherapy) and systemic therapy (cytotoxic chemotherapy), either to cure or offer palliation for the disease. The choice will depend upon the stage of the disease and the prognosis at the time of presentation. The primary treatment for potentially curable cancer is resection of the tumour, the surrounding tissue and the draining lymph nodes, followed by restoration of intestinal continuity. The location of the tumour determines the surgical approach. If the tumour is extensive, palliative resection of the affected portion of the bowel can relieve obstruction, alleviate the local effects of the tumour and prevent perforation and haemorrhage.

Radiotherapy may be given pre-operatively to downstage a tumour or make it smaller. Post-operative radiotherapy is given less frequently and is reserved for patients considered to be at high risk of residual disease, for example when histology demonstrates the presence of malignant cells at the margins of the resected tissue. Palliative radiotherapy provides relief from symptoms of colorectal cancer and for the treatment of distant metastases.

Chemotherapy may be commenced prior to surgery to reduce the tumour size and offers early systemic treatment for undetectable micro-metastases if given at a time when malignant cells are likely to be more responsive to treatment. Adjuvant chemotherapy attempts to treat occult metastases following surgery or radiotherapy with curative intent. Palliative chemotherapy aims to improve the duration of survival and the quality of life in advanced disease when a high incidence of toxicity and patient distress is clearly inappropriate (Lunn *et al.*, 1999).

The Role of the Nurse

Health Promotion

Nurses have a role to play in making patients and family aware of the potential significance of changes in the pattern of symptoms and the importance of colonoscopic surveillance.

Surgical Intervention

The patient will require physical and psychological support during the pre- and post-operative periods. A greater degree of spiritual well-being may help to mitigate the demands of illness imposed by colorectal cancer according to a study by Fernsler *et al.* (1999). They also point out that younger patients with colorectal cancer may experience more intense illness-related problems than older patients. It is important for nurses to be aware of this and to plan appropriate assessment and interventions accordingly.

Side Effects of Treatments

Patients having radiotherapy or chemotherapy are likely to experience one or more of a range of common physiological toxicities and a range of psychological reactions. In addition to the patient's response to the disease itself, nursing assessment, within a structured theoretical framework, enables monitoring and recording of toxicity. This enables prompt nursing interventions to resolve problems and alleviate patient distress. Information and support are key elements of the nursing role, enabling the patient to prepare for the experience of toxicity, to take preventative measures and to develop coping strategies (Campbell and Lunn, 1999).

Colorectal Cancer Nurse Specialist

In many cases the colorectal cancer nurse specialist takes a technical role and is involved in screening and follow up endoscopy. Other key functions involve health education and the provision of information prior to screening and following diagnosis (Campbell and Borwell, 1999).

Conclusion

Patients with IBD have an increased risk of developing colorectal cancer. If the disease is detected at an early stage it is easily treated and potentially curable. People with colorectal cancer have specific needs at each stage of the disease and as patients will be nursed in a variety of settings. It is important that all nurses who come into contact with them have a clear understanding of the nature of the disease, its treatment and impact upon the patient and his or her family. The specialist nurse has an important role to play in providing expertise and continuity of care for the patient and family. This allows for sensitive issues around sexuality and continence to be discussed (Campbell and Borwell, 1999). A holistic and individualized approach to care will take account of the potential impact that a diagnosis of colorectal cancer may have upon a person who has already experienced perhaps many years of IBD.

References

Allen, S. 1998, 'Ileostomy'. *Professional Nurse*, 14 (2), 107–9.

Allison, M. C., Dhillon, A. P., Lewis, W. and Pounder, R. E. 1998, *Inflammatory Bowel Disease*. London. Mosby International Limited.

Bonner, G. 1999, 'Current medical therapy for inflammatory bowel disease'. http://www.sma.org/smj/96jun2.htm

Campbell, T. 1999, 'Colorectal cancer Part 1: epidemiology, aetiology, screening and diagnosis'. *Professional Nurse*, 14 (12), 869–74.

Campbell, T. and Borwell, B. 1999, 'Colorectal cancer Part 4: specialist nurse roles'. *Professional Nurse*, 15 (3), 197–200.

Campbell, T. and Lunn, D. 1999, 'Colorectal cancer Part 3: patient care'. *Professional Nurse*, 15 (2), 117–21.

Clark, M. L. and Kumar, P. J. 1994, 'Gastroenterology' in Kumar, P. and Clark, M. (eds), *Clinical Medicine. A Textbook for Medical Students and Doctors*. 3rd edn. London. Bailliere Tindall.

Curry, A. 1995, *Caring for Patients with Ulcerative Colitis and Crohn's Disease. A Guide for Nurses*. St. Albans. The National Association for Colitis and Crohn's Disease.

Doughty, D. B. and Jackson, D. B. 1993, *Gastrointestinal Disorders*. St. Louis. Missouri. Mosby-Year Book, Inc.

Fernsler, J. L., Klemm, P. and Miller, M. A. 1999, 'Spiritual well being and demands of illness in people with colorectal cancer'. *Cancer Nursing*, 22 (2), 134–40.

Finley, T. 1999, 'Inflammatory bowel diseases'. *Nursing Times*, 95 (8), 51–3.

Gillen, C. D., Walmsley, R. S., Prior P., Andrews, H. A. and Allan, R. N. 1994, 'Ulcerative colitis and Crohn's disease: a comparison of the colorectal cancer risk in ulcerative colitis'. *Gut*, 35, 1590–2. PubMed QUERY http://www.ncbi.nlm.nih.gov/htbin-post/Entrez/query old?db=m_d

Hermon-Taylor, J. 2000, 'We know what is causing Crohn's disease'. *ia Journal*. 168, 29–35.

Hoffman, R. 1997, 'Inflammatory bowel disease update'. http://www.consciouschoice.com/holisticmd/hmd101.html

Jackson, S. M. and Bennett, P. J. 1988, *Physiology with Anatomy for Nurses*. London. Bailliere Tindall.

Jewell, D. 1998, 'Crohn's disease'. *Medicine*, 26(9), 87–92.

Kmietowicz, Z. 1997, 'Are you prepared for the measles vaccine debate?'. *Nurse Prescriber/Community Nurse*, 3 (7), 31–4.

Long, R. G. and Cooper, B. T. 1997, 'Gastrointestinal disease' in Souhami, R. L. and Moxham, J. (eds), *Textbook of Medicine*. 3rd edn. Edinburgh. Churchill Livingstone.

Lunn, D., Hurrell, C. and Campbell, T. 1999, 'Colorectal cancer Part 2: treatment'. *Professional Nurse*, 15 (1), 53–7.

Marieb, E. N. 2001, *Human Anatomy & Physiology*. 5th edn. London. Benjamin Cummings, an imprint of Wesley Longman Inc.

Mayberry, M. K., Probert, C., Srivastava, E. *et al.*, 1992, 'Perceived discrimination in education and employment by people with Crohn's disease'. *Gut*, 33, 312–14.

Medicinenet.com 1999, 'Which watch?' http://www.medicinenet.com/Script/Main/Art.asp?li=MN1&ag+Y&ArticleKey=583.

Miller, R., Howie, E. and Murchje, M. 1994, 'The gastrointestinal system, liver and biliary tract' in Alexander, M. F., Fawcett, J. N. and Runciman, P. J. (eds), *Nursing Practice. Hospital and Home. The Adult*. Edinburgh. Churchill Livingstone.

National Association for Crohn's and Colitis. 1997, 'Mycobacterium paratuberculosis and Crohn's disease'. http://www.nacc.org.uk/serv_info_milk.asp

National Association for Crohn's and Colitis. 1999, 'Debate about MMR and IBD continues'. http://www.nacc.org.uk/research_debate.asp

National Association for Crohn's and Colitis. 2001a, 'US Debate on mycobacterium para TB'. http://www.org.uk/research_usdebate.asp

National Association for Crohn's and Colitis. 2001b, 'Fact sheet on inflammatory bowel disease'. http://www.nacc.org.uk/about_ccfact.asp

Noffsinger, A. E., Miller, M. A., Cusi, M. V. and Fenoglio-Preiser, C. M. 1996, 'The patterns of cell proliferation in neoplastic and nonneoplastic lesions in ulcerative colitis'. *Cancer*, 78 (11), 2307–12. American Cancer Association. http://www3.interscience.wiley.com/cgi-bin//abstract/59219/START

Palmer, K. R. and Penman, I. D. 1999, 'Diseases of the alimentary tract and pancreas' in Haslett, C., Chilvers, E. R., Hunter, J. A. A. and Boon, N. A. (eds), *Davidson's Principles and Practice of Medicine*. 18th edn. Edinburgh. Churchill Livingstone.

Podolsky, D. K. 1991, 'Inflammatory bowel disease: the surgical pathology of Crohn's disease and ulcerative colitis'. *Human Pathology*, 6, 7–29.

Pullen, M. 1999, 'Nutrition in Crohn's disease'. *Nursing Standard*, 13 (27), 48–52.

Rowlinson, A. 1999a, 'Inflammatory bowel disease: aetiology and pathogenesis'. *British Journal of Nursing*, 8 (13), 858–62.

Rowlinson, A. 1999b, 'Inflammatory bowel disease 2: medical and surgical treatment'. *British Journal of Nursing*, 8 (14), 926–30.

Rowlinson, A. 1999c, 'Inflammatory bowel disease 3: importance of partnership in care'. *British Journal of Nursing*, 8 (15), 1013–18.

Solomon, M. J. and Schnitzler, M. 1998, 'Cancer and inflammatory bowel disease: bias, epidemiology surveillance and treatment'. *World Journal of Surgery*, 22(4), 352–8. PubMed QUERY http://www.ncbi.nlm.nih.gov/htbin-post/Entrez/query_old?db=m_d

The National Digestive Diseases Information Clearinghouse 1998, 'Introduction to Crohn's disease'. http://members.aol.com/bospol/homepage/crohnsl/crohnsinfo.htm

Thompson, N. P., Montgomery, S. M., Pounder, R. E. and Wakefield, A. J. 1995, 'Is measles vaccination a risk factor for inflammatory bowel disease?'. *Lancet*, 345, (8957), 1071–4.

Travis, S. 1998, 'Ulcerative colitis'. *Medicine*. 26 (9), 81–6.

Wakefield, A. J., Pittilo, R. M. and Sim, R. 1993, 'Evidence of persistent measles virus infection in Crohn's disease'. *Journal of Medical Virology*, 39 (4), 345–53.

Wakefield, A. J., Murch, S. H., Anthony, A., Linnell, J., Casson, D. M., Malik, M., Berelowitz, M., Dhillon, A. P., Thompson, M. A., Harvey, P., Valentine, A., Davies, S. E., Walker-Smith, J. A. 1998, 'Ileal-lymphoid nodular hyperplasia, non-specific colitis and pervasive developmental disorder in children'. *Lancet*, 351 (9103), 637–41.

Walsh, M. (ed.) 1997, *Watson's Clinical Nursing and Related Sciences*. 5th edn. London. Bailliere Tindall.

Wilson, K. J. W. and Waugh, A. 1998, *Ross and Wilson Anatomy and Physiology in Health and Illness*. London. Harcourt Brace and Company Limited.

Yarwood, J. 2001, 'Take my advice'. *Nursing Standard*, 15 (32), 20.

13

Diabetes Mellitus

PHILIPPE MARIE AND NORMA WHITTAKER

Diabetes mellitus (diabetes) is a serious disease accounting for about 9 per cent of hospital costs although the total cost is much greater. Less than a hundred years ago diabetes was invariably fatal and while enormous strides have been made in terms of increasing knowledge about the disorder and the most effective ways to improve the quality of the lives of those affected, there is still no cure for diabetes. It can have a major impact on the physical, psychological and material well-being of individuals and their families. Life expectancy is reduced, on average, by more than 20 years in people with type 1 diabetes and by up to ten years in people with type 2 diabetes. Mortality rates from coronary heart disease are up to five times higher for people with diabetes and the risk from stroke is up to three times higher. Prompt diagnosis, regular checks to identify serious complications at an early stage and treatment to control blood glucose and hypertension can reduce the risk of serious complications and increase life expectancy (Department of Health [DOH], 2001).

Much of the burden of care falls upon individuals who have to manage the disease themselves on a day-to-day basis. Support and education are crucial in order for individuals to manage this complex disorder effectively. Not all patients receive the best care, according to a study of diabetes services (Audit Commission, 2000). The National Service Framework for Diabetes sets out a number of standards to ensure that people receive high-quality care at the right time and the right place. The document clearly sets out the partnerships that must be at the centre of modern diabetes services: partnerships between people with diabetes and professionals; between primary care and specialist services and between doctors, nurses and allied health professionals (DOH, 2001).

Contents

Learning Objectives

By the end of this chapter you should be able to demonstrate knowledge of

- The different types of diabetes.
- The impact diabetes has on the individual.
- The potential complications of diabetes.
- The overall management of diabetes, including nursing contributions.

Definition

Diabetes mellitus is a disorder of carbohydrate, protein and fat metabolism resulting from an imbalance between insulin availability and insulin need. It can represent an absolute insulin deficiency, impaired release of insulin by the pancreatic beta cells, inadequate or defective insulin receptors or the production of inactive insulin or insulin that is destroyed before it can carry out its action. Although diabetes is clearly a disorder associated with insulin, it is probably not a single disease (Guven and Kuenzi, 1998). It has been referred to as a syndrome with metabolic, vascular and neuropathic components that are interrelated (Davidson, 1998).

Epidemiology

The number of people developing diabetes is increasing around the world. Diabetes is a very common disorder that currently affects 1.4 million people in the United Kingdom (UK) which is about three in every 100 people. In England alone, currently there are more than a million people affected by diabetes. This number continues to grow and is expected to double by 2010 (Diabetes UK, 2000a). There are an estimated one million people in the UK who are unaware that they have diabetes. Whilst the risk of developing diabetes increases with age, anyone can develop it. Diabetes is found disproportionately in people from minority ethnic groups and socially excluded groups. Type 2 diabetes is up to six times more common in people of South Asian descent and up to three times more common amongst those of African and African–Caribbean origin. It is also more common in Chinese and other non-white groups. Morbidity from diabetes complications is three and a half times higher amongst the poorest people than the richest (DOH, 2001).

 **Connection**

Chapter 1 (Social and Environmental Influences on Health and Well-being) and Chapter 3 (Health Issues Related to Ethnic Minority Groups) highlight differences in the prevalence of some disorders among certain groups within the general population.

The incidence of type 1 diabetes is increasing in children, particularly in the under-five age group. Diabetes type 2 is increasing across all groups, including children and young people and particularly among black and ethnic minority groups (DOH, 2001). Over three-quarters of people with diabetes have type 2 (Diabetes UK, 2000a). A population of 100 000 would be expected to include between 2000 and 3000 people with diabetes and approximately 25–30 will be children. These numbers will be significantly higher in areas with a high proportion of black and ethnic minority groups. The incidence of diabetes in England is higher in men than women; however, women are at a relatively greater risk of dying. This may be because gender compounds other aspects of inequality (DOH, 2001).

Aetiology

Classification of Diabetes

The reclassification of diabetes in 1997 moved from the previous classification system, which had focused on the pharmacological treatment used in the management of diabetes, to one based on the disease aetiology (see Table 13.1).

Table 13.1 Types of diabetes based on disease aetiology

Types of diabetes	*Disease aetiology*
I. Type 1 (previously known as insulin-dependent diabetes (IDDM) and juvenile-onset diabetes)	Beta cell destruction leading to absolute insulin deficiency • Immune mediated (autoimmune destruction of beta-cells) • Idiopathic (cause unknown)
II. Type 2 (previously known as non-insulin dependent diabetes (NIDDM) and mature-onset diabetes)	May range from predominantly insulin resistance with relative insulin deficiency to a predominantly secretory defect with insulin resistance
III. Other specific types	A. Genetic defects of beta-cell function B. Genetic defects in insulin action C. Diseases of the exocrine pancreas D. Endocrinopathies E. Drug or chemical induced F. Infections G. Uncommon forms of immune-mediated diabetes H. Other genetic syndromes associated with diabetes
IV. Gestational diabetes	Any degree of glucose intolerance with onset or first recognition during pregnancy

Guven and Kuenzi, 1998; Solares *et al.*, 2002.

Type 1 Diabetes

Type 1 diabetes is characterized by autoimmune destruction of pancreatic beta cells. Type 1 can be subdivided into 1A, immune-mediated diabetes and 1B, idiopathic diabetes. Circulating antibodies to islets cells, to endogenous insulin and/or to other antigen components at the time of diagnosis would suggest an autoimmune cause (Guven and Kuenzi, 1998). Viral infections may be involved in the destruction of beta cells. In some instances, there may be a hereditary tendency to beta-cell destruction even in the absence of viral infection or autoimmune disorders (Guyton and Hall, 2000). Only a few people with diabetes fall into the 1B category and they are mostly of African or Asian descent. Type 1B diabetes is strongly inherited (Guven and Kuenzi, 1998).

Type 1 diabetes occurs more commonly in young people but can occur at any age. Although less common than type 2 diabetes, it is more immediately evident. It is a catabolic disorder characterized by an absolute lack of insulin, an elevation in blood glucose and a breakdown of body fats and proteins. In the absence of insulin, ketosis develops when fatty acids are released from fat cells and converted to ketones in the liver. The absolute lack of insulin means that people with this type of diabetes are particularly prone to develop ketoacidosis. All persons with type 1 diabetes require exogenous insulin replacement

(Guven and Kuenzi, 1998). Diagnosis has a seasonal distribution, with more cases reported during autumn and winter in the Northern hemisphere. Diagnosis is rare during the first nine months of life and peaks at age 12 years (Ludwig-Beymer *et al.*, 1994).

Characteristics of type 1 diabetes

- Age of onset usually before 30 years
- Autoimmune response evident by antibodies to insulin and islet cell proteins (Mera, 1997)
- Weight loss/not obese
- Effects are usually apparent immediately
- Absolute lack of insulin
- Ketosis is common
- Exogenous insulin replacement required

Type 2 Diabetes

Type 2 diabetes comprises a group of disorders characterized by relative insulin deficiency, high hepatic glucose output and insulin resistance. People with type 2 diabetes are usually over the age of 40 at the time of diagnosis, have a family history of type 2 diabetes and are overweight or obese (Solares *et al.*, 2002). This type of diabetes is disproportionately high in ethnic minority groups and often appears before the age of 40 (Diabetes UK, 2000b). It has a much more insidious onset than type 1, but it is sometimes not diagnosed until irreversible complications have occurred (Mera, 1997). Genetic factors, environment and lifestyle factors play a role in the development of this type of diabetes. Although type 2 diabetes is familial, a specific genetic marker has not yet been identified. Exogenous insulin replacement is not usually required but some people may require insulin or hypoglycaemic medication to control blood glucose levels (Solares *et al.*, 2002). The increased insulin resistance found in obese people has been attributed to increased visceral (intraabdominal) fat detected on CT scan. In addition to increased insulin resistance, insulin release from beta cells in response to glucose is impaired (Guven and Kuenzi, 1998).

Characteristics of type 2 diabetes:

- Impaired insulin secretion
- Insulin resistance
- Increased glucose production from the liver (Seely and Olefsky, 1993)

- No evidence of autoantibodies
- Diagnosis usually occurs around the age of 40 years
- Insidious onset
- Tends to run in the family
- People with this type of diabetes are often overweight
- The person can secrete insulin; Beta cells may need to be stimulated
- Insulin injections are not usually needed

Other Specific Types

This category was formally known as secondary diabetes and describes diabetes that is associated with other conditions and syndromes.

Gestational Diabetes

This refers to glucose intolerance of various degrees that occurs during pregnancy. It most frequently affects women with

- A family history of diabetes
- Glycosuria
- A history of stillbirth, spontaneous abortion, fetal abnormalities in a previous pregnancy, or a previous large or heavy-for-date baby
- Obesity
- Advanced maternal age
- Five or more pregnancies

Risk Factors Associated with Diabetes

- Family history
- Obesity
- Sedentary lifestyle
- Ethnicity
- Ageing

Family History

Family history is a significant but non-modifiable risk factor. Studies of identical twins have established an underlying contribution of inherited genetic factors. In type 1 diabetes there has been shown to be a 25–35 per cent concordance rate in twins. In type 2 diabetes, a 95–100 per cent concordance rate in twins has been found (Solares *et al.*, 2002). Concordance in non-identical twins is less than 20 per cent (Mera, 1997).

Obesity

Obesity is an important modifiable risk factor in type 2 diabetes. Approximately one in five adults in England is now obese and two in five are overweight (DOH, 2001). The presence of obesity and the type of obesity are important considerations in the development of type 2 diabetes. People with upper-body obesity, particularly fat stored around the waist, have a greater risk of developing type 2 diabetes than persons with lower-body obesity. Diabetes type 2 can also happen in non-obese individuals or even thin individuals, as is often the case in elderly people. Over time, insulin resistance may decrease with weight loss to the point that the condition can be managed with a weight reduction and exercise programme (Guven and Kuenzi, 1998). The United Kingdom Prospective Diabetes study (1998), showed that the greater the weight loss, the greater the reduction of fasting hyperglycaemia. Several studies have also demonstrated that weight loss reduces insulin resistance and increases peripheral glucose uptake. Even a minimal weight loss can be beneficial in this respect (Henry *et al.*, 1986).

Sedentary Lifestyle and Exercise

Obesity, sedentary lifestyle and fat distribution are very much interrelated. Many people with sedentary lifestyle tend to be fat around the waist. Diabetics with adiposity develop resistance to insulin and oral diabetic medications. Many diabetes patients are sedentary because of their obesity. Exercise is therefore an essential component of the management of diabetes unless contraindicated in certain individuals. Regular exercise has numerous potential benefits.

Connection

Chapter 4 (Hypertension) discusses nursing intervention with regard to the potential risks of obesity and sedentary lifestyle.

Benefits of regular exercise

- Improved glucose tolerance
- Weight control
- Better response to medication
- Improvement in quality of life and a sense of well-being

Ethnicity and Socially Excluded Communities

As previously identified there is a higher than average risk of diabetes, particularly type 2, among certain races. Socially excluded communities, including prisoners, refugees and asylum seekers and people with learning disabilities or mental health problems, may receive poorer quality care. Risk may accumulate if an individual belongs to one of these groups (DOH, 2001).

Ageing

The prevalence of diabetes rises steeply with age. One in 20 people over the age of 65 in the UK has diabetes and in people over the age of 85 this rises to one in five. The diagnosis of diabetes may be delayed in the elderly with symptoms being wrongly attributed to age. Discrimination may also occur with regard to the active management offered to older people in comparison with younger people. Standard 1 of the National Service Framework for Older People sets out a programme to eliminate any such discrimination (DOH, 2001).

Anatomy and Physiology

The pancreas is a complex organ composed of both endocrine and exocrine tissue that performs several functions (Figure 13.1) (Seeley *et al.*, 1992). It is a flattened organ that measures about 12.5–15 centimetres in length. It is located posterior, and slightly inferior, to the stomach and consists of a head, a body and a tail. Roughly 99 per cent of the pancreatic cells are arranged in clusters called acini; these cells produce digestive enzymes that enter the digestive tract through a series of ducts. Scattered among the exocrine acini are one to two

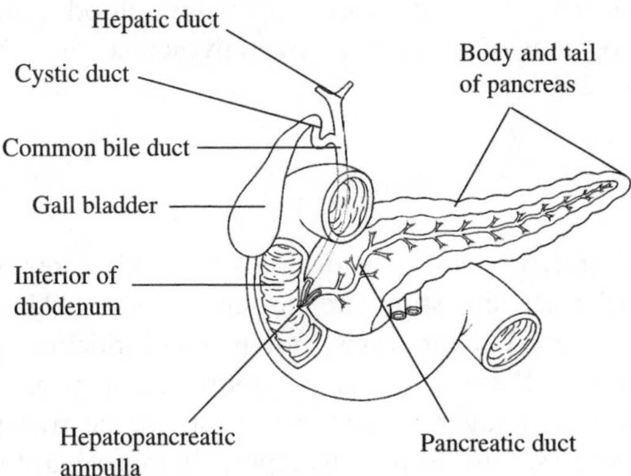

Figure 13.1 The pancreas

million tiny clusters of endocrine tissue known as pancreatic islets or the islets of Langerhans. Both the exocrine and endocrine portions of the pancreas have an abundant supply of capillaries (Tortora and Grabowski, 2000).

The islets contain two major populations of hormone-producing cells, the glucagon-synthesizing alpha cells and the more numerous insulin-producing beta cells. These cells act as tiny fuel sensors, secreting glucagons and insulin appropriately during the fasting and fed state. Insulin and glucagon are closely but independently involved in the regulation of blood glucose levels. Insulin is a hypoglycaemic hormone, whereas glucagon is a hyperglycaemic hormone (Marieb, 2001). Some islets also synthesize other peptides in small amounts. These include stomatostatin and pancreatic polypeptide. Stomatostatin inhibits insulin and glucagon release from neighbouring beta and alpha cells and it is also thought to slow absorption of nutrients from the gastrointestinal tract. Pancreatic polypeptide inhibits stomatostatin secretion, gall bladder contraction and the secretion of digestive enzymes by the pancreas (Tortora and Grabowski, 2000).

Glucagon

One molecule of this hormone can cause the release of 100 million molecules of glucose into the blood. Glucagon targets the liver, where it promotes

- The breakdown of glycogen to glucose.
- The synthesis of glucose from lactic acid and from non-carbohydrate molecules, such as the glycerol portion of fats and amino acids (gluconeogenesis).
- The release of glucose to the blood by the liver cells, which causes blood sugar levels to rise.

Secretion of glucagon by the alpha cells is prompted by falling blood sugar levels. High levels of amino acids, for example following a high protein meal can also stimulate the secretion of glucagon, which then promotes rapid conversion of the amino acids to glucose, thus making even more glucose available to the tissues. Glucagon release is suppressed by rising blood glucose levels and somatostatin. People with persistent hypoglycaemia may be deficient in glucagon (Marieb, 2001).

Insulin

Soon after a meal, glucose, amino acids and fatty acids enter the bloodstream from the intestinal tract and stimulate insulin secretion. The main effect of insulin is to lower blood sugar levels, but it also influences protein and fat metabolism. Insulin's effects are most obvious after a meal. The circulating insulin lowers the blood sugar by enhancing membrane transport of glucose and other simple sugars, into body cells, especially muscle and fat cells. It does not accelerate glucose entry into the liver, kidney and brain tissue, all of which have easy access to glucose regardless of insulin levels. Insulin inhibits the breakdown of glycogen to glucose and the conversion of amino acids or fats to glucose. Insulin therefore, counters any metabolic activity that would increase plasma levels of glucose. After glucose enters the target cells, insulin binding triggers enzymic activities that

- Catalyse the oxidation of glucose for adenosine triphosphate (ATP) production.
- Join glucose together to form glycogen.
- Convert glucose to fat, particularly in adipose tissue.

Usually energy needs are met first and then glycogen deposit occurs. If excess glucose is still available, fat deposit occurs. Insulin also stimulates amino acid uptake and protein synthesis in muscle tissue. Beta cells are stimulated to secrete insulin chiefly by elevated blood sugar levels, but also by rising plasma levels of amino acids and fatty acids. In this instance glucagon and insulin responses are not opposite. As body cells take up sugar and other nutrients, insulin secretion is suppressed (Marieb, 2001).

Insulin secretion is under chemical, neural and hormonal control. Since parasympathetic stimulation is associated with food, its stimulation is associated with increased insulin secretion. Sympathetic innervation inhibits insulin secretion and helps to prevent a rapid fall in blood glucose. Other hormones that directly or indirectly influence the release of insulin include adrenaline, thyroxine and growth hormone (Seeley *et al.*, 1992). In essence, insulin removes glucose from the blood, causing it to be used for energy or converted to other forms (glycogen or fats) and promotes protein synthesis and fat storage (Marieb, 2001).

Pathophysiology

Initially the liver produces glucose through the breakdown of glycogen (glycogenolysis). After 8–12 hours without food, the liver forms glucose from the breakdown of non-carbohydrate substances, including amino acids (Smeltzer and Bare, 2000).

Most of the pathological conditions in diabetes mellitus can be attributed to one of the following three major effects of insulin lack:

1. Decreased utilization of glucose by body cells, with a resultant increase in blood glucose concentration.
2. Markedly increased mobilization of fats from the fat storage areas, causing abnormal metabolism of fat as well as deposition of lipids in the vascular walls, resulting in atherosclerosis.
3. Depletion of protein in the body tissues.

(Guyton and Hall, 2000)

Connection

Chapter 5 (Coronary Heart Disease) explains the pathogenesis of atherosclerosis.

When insulin is absent or deficient, blood sugar levels remain high after a meal because glucose is unable to enter most tissue cells. Ordinarily when blood sugar levels rise, hyperglycaemic hormones are not released, but when hyperglycaemia becomes excessive the person begins to feel nauseous, which precipitates the 'fight-or-flight response', which results in all the reactions that normally occur to make glucose available, including glycogenolysis, lipolysis and gluconeogenesis. The already high blood sugar levels increase even further and excess glucose begins to be excreted in the urine (Marieb, 2001).

To meet the rising need for energy, which cannot be obtained from glucose, fats and proteins are metabolized. Normally when fat is metabolized, ketones are formed in the liver and transported to muscle and other tissue, where they serve as a source of energy. Ketones are chemical intermediate products in the metabolism of fat, such as beta-hydroxybutyric acid, acetoacetic acid and acetone. All three are toxic and if they accumulate in the body, they give rise to a condition called ketoacidosis (Timby *et al.*, 1999).

Clinical Manifestations

The initial manifestations of type 1 diabetes are generally acute and the individual often has the classic symptoms of polyuria, polydipsia and polyphagia (Ludwig-Beymer *et al.*, 1994). The onset of type 2 diabetes is more insidious and may be detected at a routine medical check (see Table 13.2).

Table 13.2 Symptoms/related pathophysiology

Symptom	*Related pathophysiology*
Polyuria	Some glucose in the blood is excreted by the kidneys. When the quantity of glucose entering the kidney tubules in the glomerular filtrate exceeds the renal threshold, usually 9.9–11.1 millimoles per litre, a significant proportion of glucose enters the urine (Smeltzer and Bare, 2000). The loss of glucose in the urine causes diuresis, because the osmotic effect of glucose in the tubules inhibits water reabsorption. The overall effect is dehydration of the extracellular space, which then causes dehydration of the intracellular spaces as well. The person experiences

Table 13.2 (Contd.)

Symptom	*Related pathophysiology*
	urinary frequency and large amounts of urine are passed each time (Guyton and Hall, 2000). The frequency of nocturia is a relatively good guide to the severity of hyperglycaemia (Tattersall and Gale, 1990).
Polydipsia	Dehydration stimulates the hypothalamic thirst centres, causing polydipsia, or excessive thirst. This then causes the patient to drink excessively.
Abdominal pain and vomiting	The loss of water due to polyuria is accompanied by a loss of electrolytes. Serious loss of electrolytes can occur as the body rids itself of excess ketones, which are negatively charged and carry positive ions out with them. As a result, sodium and potassium ions are also lost from the body. This may lead to abdominal pain and vomiting and the stress reaction increases (Marieb, 2001).
Polyphagia and weight loss	While the glucose is unable to be utilized, the body's requirements for energy continues, and the body starts to utilize fat and protein stores for energy. The person feels hungry and eats more (polyphagia), but hunger and weakness increase and weight is lost.
Tiredness	The abnormal metabolic changes mean that food products are not being used, resulting in lethargy and tiredness (Ludwig-Beymer *et al.*, 1994).
Pruritis vulvae/balanitis	This is a common presenting symptom and is caused by the irritating effect of the urine with its high sugar content.
Candida infections	The external genitalia are especially prone to fungal infection, which flourish on the mucous membranes contaminated with glucose. Frequent candida infections are common among women (Patel, 2002).
Visual blurring	The changes in blood glucose concentrations cause changes to occur in the lens of the eye. The first sign of this is the fluctuation between normal and blurred vision that some people experience when blood glucose is too high or too low. Large variations in glucose concentration cause the lens to take up or expel water, altering its curvature, which is experienced as blurred vision (Mera, 1997). Visual blurring usually clears as the diabetes is brought under control (Tattersall and Gale, 1990).
Ketoacidosis	If ketones are produced faster than they can be oxidized in tissues, they accumulate in tissues and body fluids. An increase in ketones in the blood causes a decrease in alkali (base) reserve. If treatment is not initiated, circulatory collapse, renal shutdown and death will occur. This complex is known as diabetic coma, although severe acidosis can be present without coma (Timby *et el.*, 1999). If the pH of the body falls below approximately 7.0 the person with diabetes will lapse into a coma Dehydration is thought to exacerbate the coma (Guyton and Hall, 2000). (See acute complications for further details.)

Chronic Complications of Diabetes

Macrovascular Disease

Diabetes is a risk factor for the development of atherosclerosis. Stroke, coronary heart disease and peripheral vascular disease are two to five times more common in people with diabetes than in the general population.

Peripheral Vascular Disease. This is very often a contributory factor in 'diabetic foot', a condition characterized by pain, gangrene and infection (Mera, 1997).

Microvascular Disease

Microvascular lesions do not occur in non-diabetics. Tissue damage in organs is caused by a combination of atherosclerotic changes in large vessels and defects in the microcirculation. The retina, kidney and nerves are particularly damaged (Blevins and Cassmeyer, 1995).

Retinopathy. Destruction in the macular retina results in loss of central vision. Diabetes is the leading cause of blindness in people between the ages of 20 and 65 years of age. In addition, cataract formation is more common, probably due to prolonged hyperglycaemia that results in swelling of the lens and opacity formation (Blevins and Cassmeyer, 1995). Laser treatment of damaged blood vessels has been known to reduce severe vision loss by as much as 60 per cent (Nathan, 1993).

Nephropathy. One of the major results of microvascular changes is alteration in renal structure and function. Nephropathy affects up to 30 per cent of people with type 1 diabetes. Although it does not affect such a high proportion of people with type 2 diabetes the numbers are greater because type 2 is more common. It is a major cause of kidney failure and death. The onset is typically within 10–20 years of the initial diagnosis. One of the manifestations is the presence of protein in the urine (Mera, 1997).

Neuropathy. Diabetes may affect peripheral sensory and motor nerves, the autonomic nervous system or the central nervous system. Multiple and varied symptoms may result, depending on the neurones involved. The most common type of diabetic neuropathy is symmetric peripheral polyneuropathy (Blevins and Cassmeyer, 1995). Impotence affects up to 30 per cent of men with diabetes, usually in combination with other features of neuropathy or peripheral vascular disease. Urinary retention caused by bladder paralysis reflects the loss of the normal ability of the nerves to respond to pressure as the bladder fills (Mera, 1997).

Acute Complications of Diabetes

Diabetic Ketoacidosis (DKA)

Diabetic ketoacidosis usually develops over a period of 12–24 hours, during which the symptoms of hyperglycaemia develop, followed by the onset of vomiting and acidotic breathing. Previously undiagnosed people with type 1 diabetes may present with DKA and it may be precipitated by intercurrent illness (Page and Hall, 1999). Sporadic changes in metabolic rates of the cells, such as might occur during bouts of fever, can precipitate dehydration and acidosis. If diabetes is not controlled satisfactorily, severe dehydration may result, even when the person is receiving treatment (Timby *et al.*, 1999). In children DKA can develop within a few hours and symptoms of DKA in the elderly may be less obvious than in younger people. In pregnancy the development of DKA is associated with fetal mortality of up to 50 per cent. The clinical features include

- Polyuria, nocturia
- Polydipsia
- Cramps in the legs
- Dyspnoea
- Nausea and vomiting
- Abdominal pain

In severe DKA the typical patient is drowsy, flushed and dehydrated with fast, deep, laboured breathing (Kussmaul respirations). Acetone, which is volatile can be detected on the breath by its characteristic odour (pear-drops). The ability to smell acetone on the breath is idiosyncratic and should not be relied upon as a substitute for measuring urine or plasma ketones. Tachycardia, peripheral cyanosis and cool peripheries are further signs (Page and Hall, 1999).

Hyperosmolar Non-ketotic Diabetic Coma (HONK)

This is less common than DKA and almost exclusively seen in patients over 60. Elderly patients are more at risk because of potential impaired perception of thirst, resulting in progressive dehydration as a result of osmotic diuresis. Osmotic diuresis is central to the pathogenesis, but it develops slowly. The condition may progressively worsen with increasing confusion over two to three weeks. HONK is characterized by marked hyperglycaemia and loss of water, up to 25 per cent of body weight in severe cases (Page and Hall, 1999). Treatment is similar to the treatment for DKA, but smaller doses of insulin are generally required (Blevins and Cassmeyer, 1995).

Nursing action points

- Assess for signs of DKA.
- Assess for signs of HONK.
- Administer insulin as prescribed.
- Administer fluid and electrolyte replacement as prescribed.
- Monitor fluid balance and record it.
- Monitor vital signs.
- Assess the precipitating factors to prevent recurrence.

(Valentine, 1996)

Hypoglycaemia

In hypoglycaemia blood sugar levels are too low. If allowed to continue the brain is starved of glucose, resulting in coma and possibly death. The initial symptoms are hunger and light-headedness, which should prompt the person to take some glucose. As blood sugar levels drop even further adrenaline is released in an attempt to mobilize glucose reserves. This gives rise to sweating, palpitations and tremor. As the condition worsens blurred vision and speech, headache, tiredness and unsteady gait occur. In severe hypoglycaemia the brain suffers from severe deprivation of glucose and the patient becomes incapacitated and disoriented and may start to have seizures and lose consciousness. The condition may arise because insulin doses are too high, or in type 2 diabetes due to use of sulphonylurea drugs (Mera, 1997).

Most diabetic patients will experience hypoglycaemia and more than half of the cases occur during the night (nocturnal hypoglycaemia) (Peragallo-Dittko, 1993). More particularly it tends to affect those who take intermediate acting insulin at evening mealtime. This is because the effect of the insulin peaks during the night as the body's need for insulin decreases. There is also a problem with adjustment not being made for certain important factors such as alcohol intake, delayed meal consumption, prolonged exercise and medication for other ailments. Hypoglycaemia is sometimes induced in patients to give them an idea of the symptoms so that they can recognize these and take appropriate actions.

A quick acting carbohydrate source such as one cup of milk, or 200 millilitres of orange juice to quickly reverse the hypoglycaemia is given orally if the person is alert enough to swallow and repeated within 10–15 minutes if there is no improvement. If the person is comatose subcutaneous injection of glucagon, or intravenous glucose may be prescribed.

Investigative Tests

History

Diabetes is normally diagnosed on the basis of the patient's clinical symptoms in combination with hyperglycaemia.

Urinalysis

Normally urine contains no detectable glucose or ketones; both may be present in the urine of someone with diabetes. A simple test using a sensitive glucose-specific reagent strip can reveal the presence of glucose and ketones in the urine. Because glucose in the urine is not always an indication of diabetes and not all people with diabetes excrete glucose in urine, other tests are necessary to establish a diagnosis.

Random Blood Glucose

Random is defined as any time of day without regard to time since the last meal. Diagnosis is based upon the presence of symptoms and a random plasma glucose concentration greater than or equal to 11.1 millimoles per litre. In a post-prandial glucose test, a blood sample is taken two hours after a high carbohydrate meal.

Fasting Blood Glucose

A blood specimen is obtained eight hours after fasting. A positive plasma glucose test indicates a fasting plasma concentration greater than or equal to 7.0 millimoles per litre (Smeltzer and Bare, 2000). Normal fasting plasma glucose is between 3.3 and 5.9 millimoles per litre.

Oral Glucose Tolerance Test

This method is used if the patient can eat and does not have any gastrointestinal malabsorption problems. The patient should also be in a normal nutritional state and not bedridden, as inactivity can interfere with glucose tolerance (Kee, 1995). A diet high in carbohydrate is eaten for three days. The person then fasts for eight hours. A baseline specimen of blood is taken and a urine sample is collected. An oral glucose solution (containing the equivalent of 75 grams of anhydrous glucose dissolved in water), is given and the time of ingestion recorded. Blood is taken at 30 minutes and at one, two and three hours after the ingestion of the glucose solution. Urine is collected simultaneously. The individual shows a positive glucose tolerance test when baseline blood glucose is greater than 6.7 millimoles per litre and increases to 11.1 millimoles per litre two hours after ingesting the glucose. This test is not recommended for routine clinical use (Smeltzer and Bare, 2000; Timby *et al.*, 1999). Feelings of weakness, dizziness and sweating may be experienced during the two to three hours of the test. These are usually transitory, but should be recorded. Activity during the test should be restricted as it could affect the results.

Intravenous Glucose Tolerance Test

The person is fasted for eight hours before the test. An infusion of 50 per cent glucose is administered over three to four minutes. Blood and urine samples are collected after five minutes and after one and two hours (Kee, 1995).

Monitoring Blood Glucose Levels

Blood glucose levels can be monitored by using a drop of capillary blood, obtained by pricking the finger with a special needle or lancet. Small trigger devices make use of the lancet virtually painless. The drop of blood is placed on or absorbed by a reagent strip and glucose levels determined electronically using a glucose meter or visually using a colour chart. This has provided a quick and relatively economical means for monitoring blood glucose and has given people with diabetes a way of maintaining near-normal blood glucose levels through self-monitoring (Guven and Kuenzi, 1998).

Glycosylated Haemoglobin Test

This test is a means of measuring how well blood glucose is controlled over a period of time. Glycosylated haemoglobin accumulates during the lifespan of red blood cells and reflects the average glucose level over several weeks (Blevins and Cassmeyer, 1995).

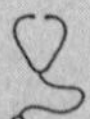

Nursing action points

Prior to testing

- Explain the procedure for the test.
- Explain what fasting involves, for example when to stop taking food or fluids other than water, and when smoking is restricted during a test.
- Give clear instructions with regard to, if and when a meal is to be taken and what it should consist of.
- Inform the patient what time to attend for the test if he or she is to come to the hospital/clinic for the test.
- If appropriate, warn the patient that feelings of faintness may be experienced during the test, which are usually transitory but should be reported to the nurse.
- If appropriate, warn the patient to minimize activities during the test.

(Kee, 1995)

Treatment

Aims of Treatment

1. To maintain blood glucose levels as near to normal as possible by balancing food intake with insulin, either endogenous or exogenous, or oral glucose lowering medications and activity levels.
2. To achieve optimum serum lipid levels.
3. To ensure that calorie intake is adequate for maintaining or attaining a reasonable weight for adults, normal growth and development for children

and adolescents, increased metabolic demands during pregnancy and lactation or recovery from illness.
4. To prevent and treat the acute and chronic complications of diabetes.
5. To improve the overall health through optimal nutrition (Valentine, 1996).

Treatment

- Dietary management
- Exercise
- Oral medication
- Insulin
- Pancreas transplantation

Dietary Management

Diet and weight control constitute the foundation of diabetes management. Diet therapy is usually prescribed to meet the specific needs of the individual concerned. Goals and principles will differ between type 1 and type 2 diabetes, as well as for lean and obese persons. A coordinated team effort is required to individualize the nutrition plan (Guven and Kuenzi, 1998). Formulation of a diabetic diet depends on the individual's sex, age, height and weight, activity level, occupation, state of health, former dietary habits and cultural background. When dietary allowances, calories, percentages of carbohydrates, fats and proteins are prescribed, the individual is given a formal diet to follow and a list of substitutions to vary the diet. Some people with mild diabetes, where there is some insulin being produced, can control their blood glucose levels by diet alone. Overweight people will need to be placed on a weight reduction diet (Timby *et al.*, 1999).

Exercise

Exercise helps to metabolize carbohydrates, thus decreasing insulin requirements. It improves circulation, which is compromised in people with diabetes and also lowers cholesterol and triglyceride levels. The exercise programme should be tailored to the individual and specify the type of exercise and the length of time the exercise should be carried out (Timby *et al.*, 1999).

Oral Medication

Oral medication is a supplement to treatment not a substitute, and it will not be successful without diet and exercise.

Sulphonylureas

Sulphonylureas are used to treat type 2 diabetes when diet alone has failed. They can be used alone or in combination with metformin or insulin (Patel, 2002). They work by increasing the sensitivity of the pancreatic beta cells to glucose, so that more insulin is released. This is accompanied by an increase in tissue sensitivity to insulin. The main difference between the different sulphonylureas is their duration of action. Examples include tolbutamide, glibenclamide and gliclazide.

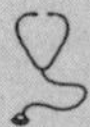

Nursing action points

When sulphonylureas are prescribed to the patient in hospital or clinic:

- Observe the patient for side effects, such as nausea, vomiting and skin rash.
- Ensure that the patient understands the potential side effects, particularly the symptoms of hypoglycaemia, which is a potentially serious side effect.
- Monitor the patient for weight gain, which may render the drug inactive, particularly if the person is already obese.

(Mera, 1997)

Metformin

Metformin is used when diet has failed and is particularly useful in obese persons. It has been found to have a beneficial effect on overall mortality in obese patients (Mooradian and Chehade, 2000). Metformin is a biguanide which increases insulin sensitivity and is only effective in the presence of insulin, enhancing the effect of insulin at the post-receptor level in peripheral tissue such as muscles, where it increases insulin-mediated glucose uptake. Biguanides also inhibit gluconeogenesis occurring in the liver (Patel, 2002). The drug is effective in obese and non-obese people. It is contraindicated in pregnancy and any degree of renal impairment (Mera, 1997). Lactic acidosis is a potential serious complication of biguanide therapy and the patient must be monitored carefully when treatment is initiated or when drug dosage is changed (Smeltzer and Bare, 2000).

Acarbose

Acarbose is used in combination with other antidiabetic drugs for the reduction of post-prandial hyperglycaemia. It is a reversible competitive inhibitor of alpha-glucosidase enzymes which are located in the small intestines. Acarbose reduces the absorption of glucose from the diet by blocking the action of enzymes in the small intestines responsible for cleaving polysaccharides and disaccharides into glucose prior to absorption (Patel, 2002).

New Developments

Amylin Analogues

Amylin is a hormone that modulates the action of insulin.

Glucagon-like Peptide

This has been shown to reduce hyperglycaemia in type 2 diabetes after intravenous or subcutaneous administration. It does not cause hypoglycaemia as it requires glucose to be present in order to stimulate insulin release from pancreatic beta cells.

Miglitol

Like acarbose, it inhibits alpha-glucosidase enzymes but unlike acarbose it is completely absorbed (Patel, 2002).

Insulin Therapy

Exogenous insulin is given as replacement to compensate for the absolute lack of endogenous insulin in type 1 diabetes and the relative lack of endogenous insulin, due to insulin resistance or a defect in the insulin release mechanism, in type 2 diabetes. The disadvantage of insulin therapy is that it must be administered subcutaneously by injection, although research is being carried out on a peptide delivery system, oral or intra-nasal route (Patel, 2002).

There are different types of insulin preparation available including beef and pork derivatives. Human insulin is now available for clinical use and is becoming the predominant form used. Human insulin is very useful for patients of certain religious beliefs which may prohibit the use of insulin derived from animals. The normally acting pancreas continuously secretes small amounts of insulin during the day and night. In addition, whenever blood glucose rises after ingestion of food, there is a rapid burst of insulin secretion in proportion to the glucose-raising effect of the food. The goal of all but the simplest of injection regimens is to mimic the normal pattern of insulin secretion as closely as possible in response to food intake and activity patterns (Smeltzer and Bare, 2000).

Insulin action can be short, intermediate or long and may be used in combination. Insulin regimens vary from one to four injections per day. There may be a combination of short acting insulin and longer acting insulin. In the latter case, once the total dose is calculated it is normally given as two-thirds intermediate or long acting insulin before breakfast and one-third short acting before the evening meal. Once the regimens have been established they may be adjusted according to the person's glycaemic profile, the aim being to obtain the best glycaemic control within reasonable limits. The alternative approach is a multiple injection regimen, where short acting insulin is administered before each meal and intermediate acting or long acting insulin at bedtime (Patel, 2002). Using a more intensive regimen is likely to achieve better control of blood glucose levels and allows more flexibility to change insulin doses from day to day in accordance with eating and activity patterns and as needed for variations in the prevailing glucose level (Smeltzer and Bare, 2000). Blood glucose levels should be assessed prior to insulin administration. The initial dose in type 1 diabetes can range from 0.5 to 0.8 units per kilogram per day, but can be higher depending on the person's health (Patel, 2002).

Complications of Insulin Therapy

- Local allergic reaction to the protein components of the insulin preparation.
- Systemic allergic reaction (rare).
- Insulin lipodystrophy – loss of subcutaneous fat or the development of fibro fatty masses. The use of human insulin has almost eliminated this condition. If insulin is injected into scarred areas, absorption may be delayed. Hypertrophied sites should be avoided and the injection sites should be rotated.
- Insulin resistance – most patients have some degree of insulin resistance at one time or another. The commonest cause is obesity. Immune antibodies develop in most people taking insulin and these antibodies bind to the insulin, decreasing the amount of insulin available for use. Very few develop high levels of antibodies.
- Morning hyperglycaemia.

(Smeltzer and Bare, 2000)

Pancreas Transplantation

Pancreas transplants, when successful, can restore carbohydrate metabolism to normal. Pancreas transplantation is not a life-saving procedure, but it does have the potential to significantly improve the quality of life for the patient. The most serious problems are the requirement for immunosuppression and the need to diagnose and treat rejection. A more recent development is the potential to transplant islet cells (Guven and Kuenzi, 1998).

Nursing Interventions

Health Promotion and Maintenance of Health

The role of the nurse in health promotion and maintenance relates to the identification, monitoring and education of the people at risk of developing diabetes and support in the self-management of the disease for those already diagnosed. Whenever possible education programmes should involve family members, particularly if the family member is likely to assume some or all of the responsibility for the treatment regimen.

Connection

Chapter 2 (Family-centred Care) discusses the implications of treatment regimens for other family members.

School nurses, community nurses and hospital-based nurses have opportunities for raising awareness about obesity, healthy food and exercise.

Many people who have diabetes are undiagnosed and many more are only diagnosed after they have had the disorder for many years by which time they would have developed complications. Practice nurses are well placed to initiate screening programmes, particularly focussing on clients considered to be in a high risk group.

Diet

Patients may not only have to follow new constraints with regard to what they can and cannot include in their diet but also have to take a much reduced calorie intake. Nurses should take account of the potential impact that this has on the psychological well-being of the patient. Reasonable weight should be viewed as weight that the individual and nurse acknowledge as achievable and maintainable in both the short and long term. This may not conform to what is usually defined as desirable or ideal body weight. A weight loss of five to ten kilograms has been shown to improve glucose control, even if desirable weight is not achieved (Valentine, 1996). Since many patients may find a weight reduction diet difficult, especially at the beginning, it is important that the nurse emphasizes the benefits and importance of sticking to the regimen. The dietary regimen demands patience and perseverance and a lot of encouragement and support for the patient may be needed. Cultural preferences and dietary constraints should also be taken into account when developing dietary regimens.

Exercise

The nurse should explain that it is most important that the exercise should be taken consistently each day. Sporadic periods of exercise are discouraged because wide fluctuations in blood glucose levels can occur. Food and insulin levels should be regulated during times of increased activities (Timby *et al.*, 1999).

Habitually sedentary adults should be advised to increase activity gradually and work up to 30 minutes of brisk walking, swimming or low impact aerobic activities. Elderly and/or physically disabled patients can be encouraged to do a range of motion and leg raising exercises (Blevins and Cassmeyer, 1995).

Health Education to Prevent the Complications of Diabetes

Maintaining blood glucose levels as close to normal as possible prevents or slows down the progression of long-term diabetic complications (Smeltzer and Bare, 2000). Peripheral vascular changes are one of the more common complications of diabetes. Because of the diminished blood supply the extremities are often pale and cool and gangrene can develop. Foot care is therefore very important. Eye problems are also a complication and any visual changes should be reported, and an appointment with an ophthalmologist made.

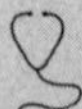

Nursing action points

- Teach the patient how to self-administer insulin.
- Teach the patient how to monitor blood or urine for glucose levels.
- Explain to the patient the importance of adhering to the prescribed treatment.
- Explain the importance of rotating the injection sites.
- Advise the patient not to inject into a hypertrophied area.
- Advise the patient to report any changes over insulin injection sites, for example skin breaks that are slow to heal or any signs of infection.
- Explain when to take oral medication.
- Ensure that the patient knows the symptoms of hyper- and hypoglycaemia.
- Explain other potential side effects of prescribed medication.
- Advise the patient to do the following: wear well-fitting shoes, inspect the feet daily, wash and dry the feet thoroughly, cut toe nails carefully and cut straight across, not attempt to remove corns or calluses, visit a podiatrist regularly, cover any injuries with a sterile dressing and seek advice, report any blister or abrasion (Timby *et al.*, 1999).
- Advise the patient to pay attention to general personal hygiene.

Psychological Issues

Self-esteem disturbance related to lifestyle changes imposed by diabetes and its treatment, the stigma of having a chronic illness and frustration at the progression of the disease despite careful management, can be manifested by negative feelings about self, resistance to make lifestyle changes and refusal to accept the diagnosis. Sexual concerns should be acknowledged and referral to an appropriate counsellor made.

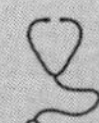

Nursing action points

- Encourage the patient to discuss the diagnosis and its implications.
- Refer to a counsellor if considered appropriate and acceptable to the patient.
- Assure the patient of continued value and self-worth.

Acute Intervention

The nurse is involved with the diabetic patient in many acute situations, such as when DKA and hypoglycaemia occur. Other areas of intervention relate to management during potentially stressful times, such as during an acute illness and surgery. Both emotional and physical stress can increase the blood glucose level and result in hyperglycaemia. Diabetic patients who smoke have been shown to exhibit more depressive symptoms than those who do not smoke. In addition the number of cigarettes smoked increased as the severity of depression increased. Assessing the number of cigarettes smoked may assist the nurse in assessing the patient's anxiety state or level of depression. The mood-altering effects of nicotine may encourage smoking among patients trying to deal with complicated self-management tasks and lifestyle changes (Valentine, 1996).

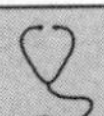

Nursing action points

- Review the effect of stress on glycaemic control so that the patient is aware that stress increases the glucose level.
- Discuss with the patient ways of managing glucose control during an illness.
- Discuss the symptoms of DKA with the patient.
- Discuss different coping strategies with the patient.

(Valentine, 1996)

The Role of the Specialist Nurse

The role of the nurse as an educator in the effective management of diabetes cannot be underestimated. Central to the teaching and counselling of the newly diagnosed patient, is the diabetic specialist nurse. Many NHS Trusts have appointed diabetic specialist nurses for children as well as adults. They are well placed to teach patients and their carers and to support and advise generic nurses in developing a better understanding of diabetes and its management. Imparting knowledge effectively empowers the individual concerned. Among the factors that must be considered in educating the patient are the patient's health beliefs and the readiness of the patient to accept change and to achieve self-efficacy. Such an approach to patient education can be beneficial with regard to improving weight loss and glycaemic control and reducing healthcare costs.

Conclusion

Estimates of the precise cost of diabetes vary but are considerable. Costs fall broadly into three categories. These include costs linked directly to the diagnosis itself, for example, the cost of inpatient and outpatient care and the cost of medication. There are costs related to the complications of diabetes, and costs related to the inability of those with diabetes to work and their poor quality of life (Diabetes UK, 2000c). People with diabetes are admitted to hospital twice as often and stay twice as long as those without diabetes. They occupy one in ten acute hospital beds. They also frequently describe poor experiences of inpatient care, particularly in relation to inadequate knowledge of diabetes among hospital staff, inappropriate amounts and timing of food and inappropriate timing of medication, lack of information provided and delay in discharge resulting from their diabetes, especially when the admission was unrelated to the diabetes. Timely liaison with a diabetes team can both prevent the need for a diabetic related admission and where admission is necessary avoid complications and delayed discharge. The diabetic specialist nurse should oversee the management of people with diabetes during their hospital admission. This can reduce the length of stay and release bed space. The National Service Framework for Diabetes sets out 12 new standards and the key interventions necessary to raise the standards of diabetes care. By improving blood glucose and blood pressure control in people with diabetes, the complications of diabetes can be reduced. The associated number of myocardial infarctions and strokes, blindness and renal failure might be reduced by as much as a third. Targeted foot care for people at risk could save hundreds of amputations a year (DOH, 2001). Nurses have a crucial role to play in achieving the standards set out in the framework.

Since there are so many cases of diabetes that remain undiagnosed and come to light only when complications have already set in, management costs are a lot greater and more importantly, the quality of life of such patients could be seriously affected. Screening the high-risk groups could lead to early detection and prevent complications. While there can be no doubt about the big threat to health that diabetes poses, there can be little doubt either that it is a condition that can be effectively managed by the individual if the appropriate support and expertise are available to them (Davidson, 1998). Empowering patients to take control over the day-to-day management of the condition in a way that enables them to experience the best possible quality of life is a key role for nurses.

References

Audit Commission 2000, *Testing Times: A Review of Diabetes Services in England and Wales.* London. Audit Commission.

Blevins, D. and Cassmeyer, V. L. 1995, 'The patient with diabetes mellitus' in Long, B. C., Phipps, J. W. and Cassmeyer, V. L. (eds) *Adult Nursing. A Nursing Process Approach.* London. Times Mirror International Publishers Ltd.

Davidson, M. B. 1998, *Diabetes Mellitus: Diagnosis and Treatment.* 4th edn. London. W. B. Saunders Co.

Department of Health (DOH) 2001, *National Service Framework for Older People.* London. DOH.

Department of Health (DOH) 2001, *National Service Framework for Diabetes: Standards.* London. DOH.

Diabetes UK 2000a, 'Who gets diabetes and what causes it?' http://www.diabetes.org.uk/diabetes/get.htm

Diabetes UK 2000b, 'Understanding diabetes'. http://www.diabetes.org.uk/diabetes/under.htm

Diabetes UK 2000c, 'Diabetes: costs and complications'. http://www.diabetes.org.uk/diabetes/infocentre/fact/fact3.htm

Guven, S. and Kuenzi, J. 1998, 'Diabetes mellitus' in Porth, C. M. (ed.), *Pathophysiology. Concepts of Altered Health States.* 5th edn. Philadelphia. Lippincott-Raven Publishers.

Guyton, A. C. and Hall, J. E. 2000, *Textbook of Medical Physiology.* 10th edn. London. W. B. Saunders Co.

Henry, R. R., Wallace, P. and Olefsky, J. M. 1986, 'Effects of weight loss on mechanisms of hyperglycaemia in obese non-insulin-dependent diabetes mellitus'. *Diabetes*, 35, 990–8.

Kee, J. L. 1995, *Laboratory and Diagnostic Tests with Nursing Implications.* 4th edn. Connecticut. Appleton & Lange.

Ludwig-Beymer, P., Heuther, S. E. and Gray, D. P. 1994, 'Alterations of hormonal regulation' in McCance, K. L. and Heuther, S. E. (eds) *Pathophysiology. The Biological Basis for Disease in Adults and Children.* 2nd edn. London. Mosby-Year Book Inc.

Marieb, N. E. 2001, *Human Anatomy and Physiology.* 5th edn. London. Pearson Education Inc. publishing as Benjamin Cummings.

Mera, S. L. 1997, *Understanding Disease.* London. Stanley Thornes (Publishers) Ltd.

Mooradian, A. D. and Chehade, J. 2000, 'Implications of the UK Prospective Diabetes Study; questions answered and issues remaining'. *Drugs and Aging*, 16 (3), 159–64.

Nathan, D. 1993, 'Long term complications of diabetes mellitus'. *New England Journal of Medicine*, 328 (23), 1676.

Page, S. R. and Hall, G. M. 1999, *Diabetes – Emergency and Hospital Management.* London. BMJ Books.

Patel, M. 2002, 'Diabetes'. http://members.aol.com/m4ynk/introl.html

Peragallo-Dittko, V. 1993, *A Core Curriculum for Diabetes Education.* Chicago. American Association of Diabetes Educators.

Seeley, R. R., Stephens, T. D. and Tate, P. 1992, *Anatomy and Physiology.* London. Mosby-Year Book Inc.

Seely, B. L. and Olefsky, J. M. 1993, 'Potential cellular and genetic mechanisms for insulin resistance in common disorders of obesity and diabetes' in Moller, D. (ed.) *Insulin Resistance and its Clinical Disorders.* London. John Wiley & Sons.

Smeltzer, S. C. and Bare, B. G. 2000, *Bruner & Suddarth's Textbook of Medical–Surgical Nursing.* 9th edn. Philadelphia. Lippincott, Williams and Wilkins.

Solares, M., Agana-Defensor, R., Song-Mayeda, C. and Canada, L. D. 2002, 'Endocrine-metabolic system' in Thompson, J. M., McFarland, G. K., Hirsch, J. E. and Tucker, S. M. *Mosby's Clinical Nursing.* 5th edn. London. Mosby Inc.

Tattersall, R. and Gale, E. 1990, 'The new patient: assessment and investigation' in Tattersall, R. and Gale, E. (eds) *Diabetes Clinical Management*. London. Churchill Livingstone.

Timby, B. K., Scherer, J. C. and Smith, N. E. 1999, *Introductory Medical–Surgical Nursing*. 7th edn. Philadelphia. Lippincott, Williams and Wilkins.

Tortora, G. J. and Grabowski, S. R. 2000, *Principles of Anatomy and Physiology*. 9th edn. London. John Wiley and Sons Inc.

Tortora, G. J. and Grabowski, S. R. 2001, *Introduction to Human Physiology*. 5th edn. London. John Wiley and Sons.

United Kingdom Prospective Study (UKPDS) Group 1998, 'Effects of intensive blood glucose control with metformin on complications in overnight patients with type 2 diabetes (UKPDS 34)'. *Lancet*, 352, 854–65.

Valentine, V. 1996, 'Nursing role in management of patients' in Lewis, S. M., Collier, I. C. and Heitkemper, M. M. (eds), *Medical–Surgical Nursing*. 4th edn. London. Mosby-Year Book Inc.

Cancer – an Overview

14

Sandra Johnson

Cancer is a disease that is universally known and its progressive nature has been recorded and investigated for thousands of years. David (1995) indicates that signs of cancer have been discovered in ancient skeletal remains and that the disease was named and classified by the Greeks as long ago as the sixth century BC.

Contents

- Definition of cancer
- Epidemiology
- Aetiology of cancer
- Physiology and pathophysiology
- Investigative tests
- Nursing interventions

Learning Objectives

By the end of the chapter you should be able to demonstrate knowledge of

- The cell cycle and how carcinogens affect its normal growth pattern.
- How cancers are classified, staged and graded.
- A variety of investigations used to detect cancer.
- The nurse's role in health promotion and risk reduction for cancer development.

Many myths and misunderstandings have persisted over the centuries and this chapter aims to enlighten the reader regarding the epidemiology and pathophysiology of the disease in order to reduce some of the common misconceptions still held today. Additionally, some of the more general investigations that can assist with the diagnostic process will be explained together with an examination of the role of the nurse in health promotion and cancer prevention measures. Volumes have been written about cancer and caring for the patient who has developed the disease, therefore the reader must view this text as an introduction to cancer in order to encourage further reading and advancement of personal knowledge and thus be better equipped to educate others, encourage the uptake of available screening and holistically care for those who have developed the disease.

Although globally cancer kills roughly six million people annually according to the Imperial Cancer Research Fund [ICRF] – now known as Cancer Research UK – 1998, some cancer deaths have decreased significantly during the 1990s, for example, Burkitt's lymphoma, Hodgkin's disease, testicular cancer, some bone and muscle cancers and a variety of paediatric cancers.

The mystery of how cancer develops is no longer the enigma that it once was. During the most recent two decades researchers have made impressive progress in determining the cancerous process at the molecular level, that in turn has led to revolutionary and exciting new treatments. These necessarily take time to be translated into wide practice, since the development of understanding and safe application of these innovations is complex and expensive.

Definition of Cancer

Cancer is the word most often used by the general public to describe a neoplasm or new growth, which consists of a mass of cells that have proliferated without normal organization or normal control and have an altered function. These cells are then able to migrate from their original site and invade nearby tissues and to form masses at distant sites in the body. This abnormal proliferation continues even when the original stimulus to the growth ceases. In addition, cancer cells become increasingly aggressive and disruptive on the tissues needed for survival and thus have a lethal potential.

Cancer refers to over 200 forms of malignancy with almost every tissue in the body having the capacity to develop the disease process, some even able to produce several types. Whilst each cancer has inimitable characteristics, the fundamental processes that produce malignant disease appear to be comparable. For that reason, most authors talk of cancer in general terms, highlighting one or other type to demonstrate what appear to be universal conditions.

Epidemiology

Although no race, culture, age group or gender is exempt from the development of cancer, these features play a role in the incidence of certain types of cancer, their frequency and severity. Cancer morbidity and mortality increases with age with well over 50 per cent of deaths from cancer occurring in those aged over 65 years and the cancer rate for people in the 65–69 years age range being almost double that for people in the 55–59 years age group (McCaffrey *et al.*, 1993). The disease varies in site frequency between males and females (ICRF, 1998) and although women are more likely to develop cancer than men, the mortality rate in men is greater. There are also variations in incidence between cultures; the incidence of melanoma (a skin cancer) is 9.2 per 100 000 in white Americans, but only 0.8 per 100 000 in black Americans (Otto, 1994). Some of these cancer variations can be linked to cultural differences of behaviour, for example diet, smoking and occupational hazards (Doll and Peto, 1986). Otto (1994) estimates that about 50 per cent of all cancers in men and women are diet related. It would appear that dietary fat is carcinogenic since foods with a high fat content have been associated with rising incidences of prostate, breast and large bowel cancers, although hormonal influences may also be interlinked.

Analysis of the data from the Office of Population Censuses and Surveys (OPCS) (the body responsible for collating annual figures for all causes of death) indicate that approximately one in three people will develop malignant disease at some stage during life and that it is known to be the cause of 20 per cent of all deaths (Richardson, 1995).

Perspectives of cancer have been known and documented for thousands of years, with much of the early recording attributed to the ancient Greeks. The use of the word cancer, which originates from 'carcinos', meaning crab, implies a comparison between the action of crabs and cancer and the concept of the hidden nature, unpredictable spread and infiltration of the disease. Probably because of this unpredictability, together with the fact that cancer is a common disease frequently associated with pain, distress and death, a conspiracy of silence often surrounds the disease which may heighten the distress and turmoil being experienced by a sufferer at a time when guidance and practical and emotional assistance are prime needs.

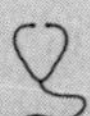

Nursing action points

Have a good factual knowledge of

- The manifestations of the disease itself.
- The types of investigations that may be instigated to achieve an accurate diagnosis.
- Methods, effects and side effects of treatments prescribed.
- The available human, practical and financial resources that can provide support for the cancer patient.

Despite recent advances in knowledge and treatment outcomes, many people view cancer as a sentence rather than a word with fear being evoked in terms of the effects of the treatment and the disease process. Much of the uncertainty surrounding the progress of the disease and its response to treatment is rooted in the fact that many members of the general public and indeed numerous professionals within the Health Service hold largely uninformed attitudes and outdated beliefs regarding the development and progression of cancerous disease (Richardson, 1995).

Cancer is a common disease but Speechley and Rosenfield (1992) have attempted to dispel some of the frequently associated misconceptions, for example people can 'catch' cancer from being in contact with a person who has the disease, but there is no evidence of such a link.

While the knowledge and understanding of cancer, its progress and treatment have advanced considerably over the last decade, their effects take time to filter through to the general public's perceptions. Yet the reaction of fear, distress, loss of control and ultimately, death, are the instant responses of most people following a diagnosis of cancer, either of themselves or their loved-ones (Richardson, 1995).

Many of these negative responses are due to the fact that malignant disease follows no regular pattern among people living in similar areas, neither among family members nor within ethnic situations. Such are the disparities, that the only certainty that a person will not die from a cancerous disease is that death will occur earlier from a different cause (Richardson, 1995).

ICRF (1998) stated that: 'One in three people in Britain will have a cancer diagnosed at some time in their life' and that the proportion of the population who will eventually die from cancer has increased from one in five to one in four. This is not because cancer survival rates are getting worse, but because fewer people are dying from other illnesses.

The ICRF (1998) fact sheet publicized the most recent five year survival statistics for all cancers in England and Wales, as diagnosed in 1981, but stated categorically that, due to advanced treatments, the expectation is that the survival rates for many cancers, having improved, will continue to do so, adding that 90 per cent of men with testicular cancer are now cured.

However, lifestyle habits continue to influence the development and progression of cancer, for example, in the 1950s early reports of a link between lung cancer and cigarette smoking (Doll and Hill, 1950; Wynden and Goldsmith, 1950), began to emerge; these links were further supported by Doll and Peto, (1976). Cigarette smoking continues at a relatively high level and the most common environmental carcinogen now is tobacco smoke, despite repeated attempts to educate the public about the dangers of this habit (Campbell, 1999).

Aetiology of Cancer

Cancers develop from a disorganization of the process that reproduces new cells from an identical original cell. Normal cells are known as differentiated and have specific structural and functional properties.

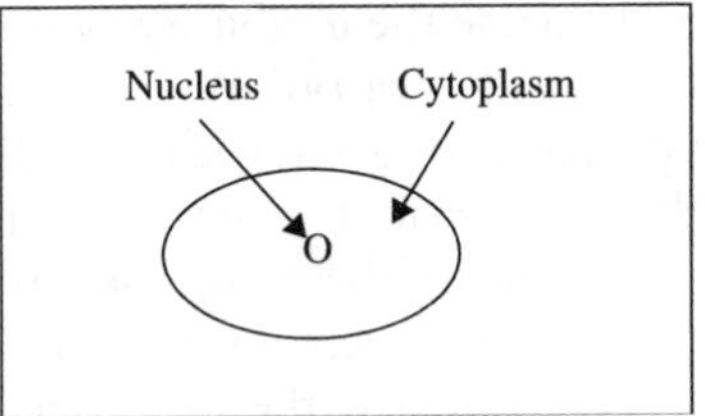

Figure 14.1 The basic cell

All cells in the body have the same basic structure. This comprises a nucleus that contains: deoxyribonucleic acid (DNA), which stores the information for cell activity and ensures that the cell behaves in the designated manner; ribonucleic acid (RNA), which is a messenger that ensures transference of the stored information to the cytoplasm surrounding the nucleus. Cytoplasm forms the bulk of the cell (Figure 14.1).

Many cells in the body have a specific life span and eventually have to be replaced. Replacement by new cells is generally co-ordinated with the loss of dying cells, thus there is a 1 : 1 'new for old' system that ensures viability of tissues. There are over 100 different types of cells in the human body, each having its own function and specific life span, reproducing at different rates, some rapidly, for example, skin and gastro-intestinal tract, some very slowly, for example, bone and others that do not reproduce at all, for example, neurones and heart muscle.

The normal metabolic activity of cells is controlled largely by enzymes, but the trigger factor to the differentiation process and growth from immaturity to maturity remains obscure. Normally, cells of the same specific tissue recognize each other and stay within the tissue boundary, they do not move into the boundaries of other tissues. This property is known as contact inhibition. It ensures that each organ composed of different tissues continues to function in the way that it should and does not interfere with the physiological processes of adjacent organs.

Physiology and Pathophysiology

The Cell Cycle

The cell renewal process is carefully regulated and consists of a sequence of activities that result in the formation of two 'daughter' cells having identical DNA and chromosome contents as the original cell. These daughter cells are exact replicas both structurally and functionally, a process known as differentiation. The cell nucleus normally integrates stimulatory and inhibitory messages;

if the stimulatory messages override the inhibitory factors, the cell will continue through its cycle of growth and division. Progression through the cycle is stimulated by a group of proteins known as cyclins. Cells having fully matured, proceed to undertake their designated activity for days, weeks or months depending upon the demands made of them; this is known as the G0 (Growth 0) stage or resting stage. When cell replacement is needed the cell enters the cell cycle at Growth stage 1 (G1) which is the preparation stage where the cell increases in size and prepares to move to the next stage of synthesis (S). The synthesis stage enables the cell to reproduce precisely its chromosome complement. It is followed by a second growth stage (G2) when the cell gathers more nutrients and prepares for the final stage of mitosis (M) and divides into two identical daughter cells. Cells that are not needed for division, to replace damaged or worn out cells of the same tissues, remain out of the cell cycle (in G0) and continue their normal activity within the tissue.

A well-differentiated cell is one that matches its parent cell well and therefore undertakes well the designated function of the cell. Poorly differentiated cells are those that, at the end of the cell cycle, for some reason, do not contain identical genetic material and therefore do not undertake the function for which they were designed. The cell that fails to follow the normal cell cycle (for whatever reason) is the cell that is potentially carcinogenic. Potential cancer cells appear to devise several means by which the destruction of a damaged cell, which would normally die and be disposed of by the normal phagocytic process of leucocytes, can be bypassed.

A protein known as P53, the actions and interactions of which are complex, is known to help induce death of these carcinogenic cells and malignant tumours are therefore evaded. However, potential carcinogenic cells appear to be able to produce excessive amounts of a counteractive protein Bcl-2 which antagonizes P53 and allows continued cell cycling in a disorganized fashion (Strachan and Read, 1996).

A second defence mechanism to stop cell reproduction is also built into the cell physiology. Normally, those cells that are able to reproduce do so for a limited number of times (between 50 and 60) – a fact that has been learned from laboratory cell culture studies (Grieder and Blackburn, 1996). After the predictable number of cell divisions a situation of senescence occurs and cell growth and reproduction ceases, provided that there is intact and balanced Bcl-2 and P53 activity.

Grieder and Blackburn (1996) found that an enzyme known as telomerase is present in almost all cancer cells and is responsible for the removal of the reproductive monitoring of cells and therefore allows endless cell replication. An imbalance between Bcl-2 and P53, coupled with the presence of telomerase, allows time for precancerous or already cancerous cells to accumulate additional mutations that might increase the size of the cell mass (tumour) and its ability to replicate and invade the surrounding tissues and organs. This knowledge has encouraged scientists to attempt to develop drugs that will inhibit the action of telomerase that will stop cells endlessly replicating. There may be cells, however, that sustain through their genetic make-up, the ability to inactivate Bcl-2 or P53 that will then allow continued cell division after senescence, but even then, surviving cells will enter a critical stage when mortification of these rogue cells occurs. The occasional cell will, however, slip through the mortification net and continue to multiply, almost becoming immortal.

Because it usually takes many years for potentially malignant cells to collect all of the properties required to mutate into cancers, the disease most frequently occurs in middle to old age. However, carcinogenesis can be accelerated with malignancies developing in early life and in many such cases this can be explained by an inherited mutant carcinogenic gene (Strachan and Read, 1996). During division of the fertilized ovum following conception, the complement of genes produced by the pairing of the sperm and ovum is copied and distributed to all cells in the body. If a genetic mutation has already occurred, this aberration can therefore be found in all body cells, resulting in a more rapid accumulation of factors that can produce a cancerous tumour, because this predisposition is already present. Consequently, a malignant condition that might otherwise have taken 30 or 40 years to present itself could become evident in the first one or two decades of life. The nature of inheritance of mutant genetic material means that several members of a family could be at risk of developing cancer at a much younger age than would have been expected.

Oncogenes

An oncogene is a gene that drives an otherwise normal cell to become cancerous, by interacting with the growth-controlling mechanism of the cell cycle (Taylor, 1992).

Proto-oncogenes

These are genes whose mutation can cause malignant change in cells and about 30 of these had been identified by 1986 (Prescott and Flexer, 1986).

Anti-oncogenes

These are growth-controlling genes and, together with tumour-suppressor genes, regulate normal cell function. Disruption or loss of these genes can result in disablement of the normal cell cycle and can lead to bizarre growth and reproduction of cells that culminates in a cancerous tumour.

Some known inheritable carcinogenic factors

Carcinogenic agent	Cancer development site
Genes	
(a) P53 located on chromosome 17	Breast, bowel, kidney, lung
(b) *RBI*	Retina, kidney
(c) *C-erb B2*	Breast
(d) *BRCA1* located on chromosome 17q	Breast (in females) ovary
(e) *BRCA2* located on chromosome 13q	Breast (male and female)
(f) Adenomatous polyposis coli located on chromosome 5q	Colon
(g) *K-ras*	Colon and rectum
Chromosomes	
(a) Philadelphia involves chromosomes 9a and 22a	Bone marrow (chronic myeloid leukaemia)

Further situations to be considered when addressing carcinogenesis

- Initiation or 'trigger' factors
- Promotional factors
- Factors that ensure tumour progression

Initiation/Trigger Factors

Once a cell is exposed to a carcinogen its nuclear material is changed, leading to a positive programming of the oncogenes or a negative programming of the tumour-suppressor and anti-oncogenes. This programmed cell then divides and daughter cells are produced that will either stay in G0 phase and not undergo any further cell cycles, or will continue growing but in a slower than normal way. In some people no further development happens and a cancerous tumour does not occur.

Promotional Factors

Promotion can occur in two ways

(a) Further genetic alteration develops over a period of time which encourages tumour formation.
(b) The slightly altered daughter cells interact with other environmental carcinogens promoting cancerous growth.

It is thought that in some instances both of these processes are working in harmony with the promotional factors, increasing the likelihood of cancer development by changing the rate at which normal cell cycling proceeds. This subsequently increases the chance of genetic errors and further disruption to normal cell division.

Progression

At the stage when the cell has cancerous characteristics, for example, a more rapid cell cycle process and disorganized function, it is then able to invade adjacent organs and tissues and also spread and metastasize in different and distant body parts.

There are numerous carcinogens and other factors involved in the development of malignant tumours, including environmental, physical and genetic contributors, all of which have been identified as having a probable part to play in the three stages of cancerous tumour development (Doll and Peto, 1986). It is thought that at least 80 per cent of malignant tumour growth is attributable to environmental carcinogens. Very early associations between the inhalation of snuff and nasal cancers were recognized by Hill (1761). Also, the association of the incidence of scrotal cancer and skin contact with coal soot experienced by chimney sweeps who would climb naked inside chimneys in order to clear soot from nooks and crannies in the chimney stacks (Pott, 1775). Kennaway and Hieger (1930) identified the specific chemical carcinogens in coal products, thus indicating the difficulty in processing and linking data within a time span where personal, local, national and international measures can coincide with efforts to prevent or reduce cancer-promoting agents or behaviours.

The last hundred years has led to an improved understanding of how cancer develops together with the main factors involved, such as environmental carcinogens, chemical agents, viruses and hereditary influences, or more usually, combinations of these (see Table 14.1) (Knudson, 1986). Despite this, nurses and other healthcare professionals continue to have a large problem in convincing the general public to engage in healthy lifestyles by which a number of potentially carcinogenic risk factors can be generally avoided. These risk factors include tobacco smoking, high-saturated fat diets, multiple sexual partners, especially when these are frequently advertised in the media as highly desirable, ego boosting and satiable.

Health professionals themselves, of course, may find it very difficult to disengage from the aforementioned, thus reducing their credibility when attempting to help patients to move towards healthy living. Nurses and members of the multidisciplinary team do need to be role models and lead by example. A twenty-stone nurse, breathless having extracted herself from her car in the hospital car park, arriving blue in the face for the late shift with her breath smelling of stale lager and a half-used packet of cigarettes tucked into her ill-fitting uniform belt is hardly likely to inspire confidence in any patient that she is attempting to instruct about issues of 'being healthy'.

Table 14.1 Some known dietary, environmental and viral carcinogens and associated tumour sites

Site of tumour	*Carcinogenic agent*
Lung	■ Tobacco smoke ■ Tar products ■ Diesel exhaust fumes ■ Pesticide chemicals
Skin	■ Sunlight radiation ■ Mineral oils ■ Tar products
Digestive Tract	■ Tobacco smoke (pancreas) ■ Sodium chloride – dietary salt (stomach) ■ Saturated animal fat (colon and rectum) ■ Alcohol (mouth and digestive tract)
Bladder	■ Tobacco smoke
Respiratory tract	■ Alcohol ■ Sodium chloride (naso-pharynx)
Scrotum	■ Tar products
Bone marrow (leukaemia)	■ Benzene
Prostate gland	■ Saturated animal fat
Various sites	■ Ionizing radiation
Viruses	
Epstein-Barr virus	■ Lymphoid tissue
Herpes virus	■ Cervix uteri
Human T-cell lymphotrophic virus (1)	■ Bone marrow (T-cell leukaemia)
Human immuno-virus	■ Various

Scientific American, 1997; Wyke, 1991.

The Development of Metastases

Metastasis

Metastasis is the spread of the malignancy to sites other than the original (primary) tumour site occurrence, for example, a stomach cancer may spread (metastasize) to the liver; prostatic cancer may spread to femoral or pelvic bones; lung cancer may spread to the brain. It is this propensity for cancerous cells to spread to other sites, distant from the primary organ in which it has developed, which makes cancer so difficult to gauge and treat. Removal of many primary tumours is a relatively easy surgical procedure, but since metastases can spread widely throughout the body, curative surgery can become impossible. It is the ability of the malignant tumour to metastasize that makes it so different from the benign tumour where other similarities might exist (Table 14.2).

Table 14.2 Comparisons and contrasts between benign and malignant tumours

Benign tumours	*Malignant tumours*
Growth rate	
Usually slow	Slow, moderate or rapid
Differentiation	
Very similar to original tissue	Dissimilar to original tissue often bizarrely so
Progression	
Progresses slowly and may stop or even regress	Progresses usually to fatality unless treated
Not usually fatal unless tumour is inaccessible	Infiltrates and metastasizes commonly causing necrosis and ulceration
Grows by expansion and is encapsulated. Rarely recurs	Recurrence is common

Metastases develop from cells that have detached themselves from the original tumour mass and travel through a blood or lymphatic vessel to a distant site, where they come to rest and re-establish growth. In so doing, these cells evade many of the mechanisms that maintain normal cellular stability.

In normal tissues there is a base membrane to which cells are attached; cells also adhere to each other, with any spaces between them being filled by a protein, extracellular matrix. Cell-to-cell adhesion molecules that normally keep all of these cells in place appear, in cancer, to have stopped or altered their normal roles. If a cell detaches itself from the base membrane or from its adjacent cell, it usually stops growing because one of the nuclear proteins that control growth closes down. This ensures stability of tissues and organs with any stray cell virtually 'committing suicide'. Cancer metastasizing cells appear to be able to maintain the activity of the nuclear proteins that would normally cause death of a membrane-detached cell. How these cells bypass the 'cell suicide' process is not fully understood, but it is believed that oncogenes falsely inform the cell nucleus that the cell is adequately adhered, when in fact it is not, thus evading the arrest of self-growth.

Following the breach of the base membrane by a cell, it rapidly meets other base membranes, all having good blood supplies. The cancer cell then penetrates the wall of a local blood vessel gaining access to the bloodstream and is then transported to other body organs. However, even when these rogue cells enter the bloodstream there are more difficulties for them to encounter; each rogue cell needs to adhere to the endothelial lining of the blood vessel, move through it and then invade the adjacent tissues and commence multiplication. All of these barriers cause distress to the marauding cancer cell that may cause its ultimate collapse, and Ruoslahti (1997) estimates that less than one in 10 000 of these rogue cells that reach the circulatory system manage to set up a new colony of cancer cells at a locality distant from the primary site.

Understanding of the circulatory system, arterial supply and venous drainage, and of the lymphatic system can help to explain the spread of metastases from a particular site of origin to a favoured second or subsequent areas. Cancer cells that break away from the primary tumour frequently become entangled in the first network of capillaries that they encounter in the venous drainage system. Commonly this is the lungs, but the portal venous drainage system of the gastrointestinal tract (from the lower one-third of the oesophagus to the anus) diverts the blood to the liver so that nutrients absorbed through the gut wall can be metabolized and synthesized in the liver. These factors account for the lungs being the most common metastatic site, followed by the liver, although bone metastases are not uncommon.

It would appear that the surface of the cancer cells lose some of the adhesion fibronectin which encourages initial disconnection from the primary tumour (Belcher, 1992), but later are able to produce chemicals that stimulate thrombocytes (platelets) to migrate towards them and become attached. This action increases the size of the already large cancer cell and also its adhesive ability; in addition, the thrombocytes manufacture growth compounds that may further increase the size of the circulating mass. Some tissues appear to possess a propensity to attract these adhesive circulating cellular collections, which may further help to explain their colonization of distant organs.

The movement of metastases via the lymphatic drainage system is likely to manifest in a similar manner to venous spread, but secondary tumours arise in lymph nodes, which filter foreign material from the circulating lymphatic fluid. Seeding is a third means by which metastases may develop. Clumps of tumour cells detach from the primary site and float across serous membranes such as the peritoneum, until they collect sufficient extraneous material, such as platelets, to achieve adhesiveness. They settle, become fixed to a basement membrane and recommence growth.

During surgery a further possibility for metastatic spread arises. Surgical instruments to which they adhere may disturb tumour cells. The instruments are then used to operate in an adjacent body area and cells are detached and deposited in the new site. Surgeons' handling of organs during operative procedures may act similarly, thus a process of metastatic transplantation is effected.

As yet, the mechanisms that convert a primary malignant tumour into a fatal metastatic disease, at molecular level, are poorly understood. However, some of the genetic influences that contribute towards malignant cells becoming immune to growth control and escape cell suicide are of obvious significance, since they allow cells to survive in the free-floating (unattached to basement membranes) manner described. Genetic studies have uncovered oncogenes, proto-oncogenes and tumour-suppressor genes which are implicated in the development of primary malignant tumours and it is possible that further research will indicate genetic involvement in the development of the ultimately fatal secondary or metastatic depositions of the disease.

Cancerous tumours appear to develop as a result of the influences of two independent events, which must coincide in order for a normal cell to transform into a malignant unit. This coincidence may be simultaneous or, more frequently, separated by months or years according to Knudson's 'two hit' theory (Knudson, 1986). Epidemiologists must be aware of this phenomenon otherwise these links may be overlooked.

Doll and Peto (1986) however, hypothesize that there are three predispositions to the development of malignant disease; 'nature, nurture and luck'. Nature relates to the genetic influences (defective or mutated inherited genes); nurture is associated with environmental elements to which all living organisms are exposed, for example, sunlight, air pollution, food additives; and luck reflects the risk factor that a cell that has been influenced by one potential carcinogen may well be exposed to another.

Malignant tumours are frequently classified according to the tissue of origin, as identified by microscopic examination in the laboratory from biopsied tissue (Table 14.3) (Belcher, 1992).

The importance of identifying the original tissue is emphasized since the tissues respond differently to available therapies.

Connections

Chapter 15 (Women's Cancers) and Chapter 16 (Men's Cancers) discuss a number of available therapies.

Staging of cancerous tumours is essential, as cure versus palliation may need to be considered at some stage of a patient's total care (Table 14.4). The TNM system is used internationally to indicate the tumour's invasive situation, the nodular (lymph node) involvement and the metastatic (or distant) deposits that can be identified.

Modifications may be made to these tables to indicate variables such as 'a' or 'b'. For example, N1a = nodes not suspected or, N1b = nodes suspected or proven, and some clinicians add further to the stages shown in order to improve clarity of diagnosis.

Table 14.3 Classification of tumours, benign and malignant

Tissue of origin	*Benign*	*Malignant*
Adipose (fatty)	Lipoma	Liposarcoma
Bone	Osteoma	Osteosarcoma
Bone marrow	–	Multiple myeloma
Cartilage	Chondroma	Chondrosarcoma
Fibrous	Fibroma	Fibrosarcoma
Glandular	Polyp/adenoma	Adenocarcinoma
Muscle (smooth)	Leiomyoma	Leiomyosarcoma
Muscle (striated)	Rhabdomyoma	Rhabdomyosarcoma
Nerve	Neuroma	Neurosarcoma
Pigmented skin	Naevus	Melanoma
Skin and mucous membrane	Papilloma	Squamous cell carcinoma

Table 14.4 The TNM staging system

Tumour (T) staging is measured from 0–4

T0	No evidence of a primary neoplasm
T1	Tumour localized to organ of origin with no evidence of invasion of adjacent structures
T2	Tumour has invaded adjacent structures and tissues but is still fairly localized
T3	A more advanced tumour that has progressively increased in size and has become regional rather than local. It is often characterized by becoming attached to a fixed structure such as bone, muscle or cartilage, thus the tumour has become immobile
T4	An advanced tumour which has extended into several surrounding structures and has invaded blood vessels, nerves and possibly bone. It is a very large, fixed mass at this stage
Tx	A tumour that cannot be assessed

Node (N) Staging is measured from 0–3

N0	Invasion of regional lymph nodes is not demonstrable
N1	Palpable and mobile lymph nodes are evident, but close to the site of the original tumour. These nodes are between 1–3 cm, mobile, firm but not hard or irregular in shape
N2	Nodes that are 3–5 cm in size, unilateral or bilateral, very firm to hard and possibly adhered together in a mass
N3	Large nodes of more than 6 cm in size, fixed to underlying and surrounding structures. These may no longer be confined to the site of the primary tumour, but found in various parts of the body
Nx	Regional lymph nodes cannot be clinically assessed

Metastatic (M) staging ranges from 0–3

M0	No metastases evident
M1	A single metastatic deposit identified at one site
M2	Several metastatic sites identified but the affected organs continue to function normally
M3	Many organs have been invaded by metastatic deposits which have caused moderate to severe functional impairment

Before treatment commences staging is carried out along with grading. Grading indicates the level of differentiation of the tumour; the better the differentiation of the tumour, the better the behaviour of the cell is understood therefore appropriate therapeutic interventions can be prescribed with greater ease, accuracy and confidence, generally offering a good prognosis (Eriksson, 1990).

Investigative Tests

A wide range of investigations is available to assist in the diagnosis of cancer, the nature and extent of which may vary according to the suspected site of tumour origin. Non-invasive investigations include taking a history, noting any changes from the normal pattern of life. Changes such as unexplained loss of appetite and weight, altered sleep pattern or bowel habit, lethargy, oedema, persistent cough, headaches and palpitations are symptoms that might be associated with malignant disease, but may also be due to other, less serious health problems. However, further physical examination is probably advisable, followed by medical investigations as deemed necessary. Generally, visual inspection and organ palpation will lead to the request for appropriate tests depending upon the site of the suspected malignant disease.

Types of investigations

- X-ray
- Body fluids
- Endoscopies
- Biopsies

X-ray

Various x-ray techniques are employed to detect tissue density changes, contour irregularities, surface erosions and changes in shape, neoplasia and the presence of fluid in cavities that are normally fluid-free.

Plain X-rays

These are the simplest and probably most commonly employed type of radiation imagery which clearly shows skeletal tissue and areas of calcification in the body, for example renal calculi (kidney stones) and can also indicate the need for further investigation, by revealing abnormal fluid-filled spaces, such as abdominal ascites. Although relatively safe, radiation from x-rays can accumulate and offer a potential health hazard, and in pregnant women should be employed with extreme caution.

Contrast X-rays

Techniques used to identify soft tissue that would be otherwise undetectable by plain x-ray, for example, intravenous pyelography (IVP). An x-ray opaque dye is intravenously injected which circulates around in the bloodstream, and, as it reaches the kidneys, is filtered out as it is detected as a foreign body. The dye is concentrated in the renal tissue and when exposed to x-ray clearly outlines renal structures. Lymphangiography and barium studies are similarly employed to illustrate otherwise x-ray transparent structures.

Computerized Axial Tomography (CT)

Produces sectional views of soft tissue by passing a number of x- rays through the body at different angles, this can also be undertaken using a contrast medium or in combination with ultrasonography.

Mammography

This also employs radiation and provides images of breast tissue and aids the diagnosis of breast cancer, cysts, fibrous changes and benign tumours, within the breast.

Magnetic Resonance Imaging (MRI)

Similar to computerized axial tomography, except ionizing radiation is not involved. An electromagnet is used to measure the vibrations of particular atoms in the body and produces computerized cross-sectional views in any body plane.

Ultrasonography

Ultrasonography is a non-invasive investigation that uses direct contact, high-frequency sound wave scanning of a body organ to produce cross-sectional images without ionizing radiation. It poses less risk to the patient and technician than the use of traditional x-rays.

Bone Scan

A radioactive substance is intravenously injected and concentrates in bone tissue. The scanner is passed over the body and identifies areas of increased uptake of the substance that may be indicative of a tumour or metastatic deposit.

Body Fluid Investigations

Blood Tests

A variety of blood tests may identify abnormalities that, in some cases can diagnose, for example, leukaemia, or in others will indicate the need for further investigations, for example, abnormal results from liver function blood tests.

Lumbar Puncture

Cerebrospinal fluid (CSF) withdrawn from the subarachnoid space via a spinal tap can show increased pressure within the subarachnoid space, increased or decreased levels of the normal constituents of the fluid, or the presence of white blood cells (leucocytes) or shed malignant cells, all of which suggest the need for further investigation.

Paracentesis Abdominis

This is a collection of fluid (ascites) from the abdominal cavity. Any pooling of abdominal fluid is abnormal and requires microscopic examination; fluid is withdrawn using a strictly aseptic procedure and the sample is visualized microscopically in the laboratory. The presence of abnormal cells may confirm the diagnosis of malignant disease. A similar procedure, thoracocentesis or pleural tap may be employed to withdraw a sample of an abnormal collection of fluid (pleural effusion) from the pleural cavity.

Cytology

Secretions containing shed cells from organ surfaces are collected and viewed microscopically for potential or actual changes in cell structure. The most common of these investigations is the cervical smear or Papanicolou test. Cells contained within the secretions from the cervix uteri are collected via a wooden or plastic spatula or a tiny brush-edged instrument; the secretions are then chemically fixed to a glass slide and microscopically examined for the presence of suspicious, altered or frankly malignant cells. Similarly, secretions from the gastrointestinal and urinary tracts and other parts of the reproductive tracts can be collected for laboratory investigation.

Endoscopies

A series of endoscopic investigations can be undertaken to view internal organs and sample suspect tissue without the need for major surgical intervention and general anaesthesia. The lungs, abdominal cavity, pelvic cavity and gastrointestinal tract can all be accessed via endoscopic instrumentation.

Biopsy

Small sections/samples or slices of tissue or cells can be removed from an organ by the use of a blade to incise a solid lesion, a small brush or spatula to gather cells from the surface of a mass, or a syringe and needle to aspirate fluid from cavities or to take minute samples of tissue for examination under the microscope.

Nursing Interventions

The nurse's role in health promotion

- Primary
- Secondary
- Teritary

The United Kingdom (UK) government has recognized the need to reduce the incidence of cancer and, in 1993, published 'The Health of the Nation' document (Department of Health [DOH], 1993), in which the role of nurses in promoting health was highlighted. Concepts were outlined that aimed to lower the occurrence of skin, lung, cervical and breast malignancies. In 1998 the sequel, 'Our Healthier Nation' (DOH, 1998) saw the government set a target to try to reduce the cancer mortality rate for people under 65 years by at least one-fifth by 2010, and again recognized the essential contribution that nurses could make in achieving this objective.

Primary

Wilby (1998) identified that over 60 per cent of all cancers are linked to lifestyle factors, for example, tobacco smoking, dietary intake and social behaviours. Nurses have an important part to play in educating the public about known predisposing carcinogenic factors, thus empowering people to exercise control over lifestyle and behaviours in order to reduce their personal risk of developing cancer. Once empowered with this knowledge, people are then able to make informed choices (within their personal circumstances) regarding risk-reducing sequelae (Wilby, 1998). A conundrum occurs here, as identified by Tones (1997) who positively viewed the need to prevent disease and concentrate on safeguarding the health of the population, but recognized also, that people have a right to exercise choice, but, may not, by virtue of social circumstances, have the opportunity to choose freely.

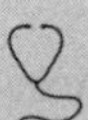

Nursing action points – primary health promotion

Advise patients to

- Avoid unprotected skin exposure to strong sunlight (MacKie, 1992).
- Avoid tobacco smoking and passive inhalation of tobacco smoke (Health Education Authority *et al.*, 1991).
- Drink alcohol socially but do not exceed recognized limits (Hyassala *et al.*, 1992).
- Eat a diet that contains low fat, salt and animal meat content, but is high in fibre (Nicholson, 1996).
- Perform self-examination at regular intervals as appropriate, for example, breast, testicular (MacKie, 1992).
- Abide by health and safety regulations imposed by industrial workplaces (Doll, 1992).

Secondary

This relates to the early detection and treatment of cancers. The earlier a malignant condition is discovered, generally the better the prognosis, in terms of life expectancy (Kelly, 1993). The nurse is in a position to encourage anyone who notices any physiological change to seek medical attention and to advise about investigations that the doctor might requisition.

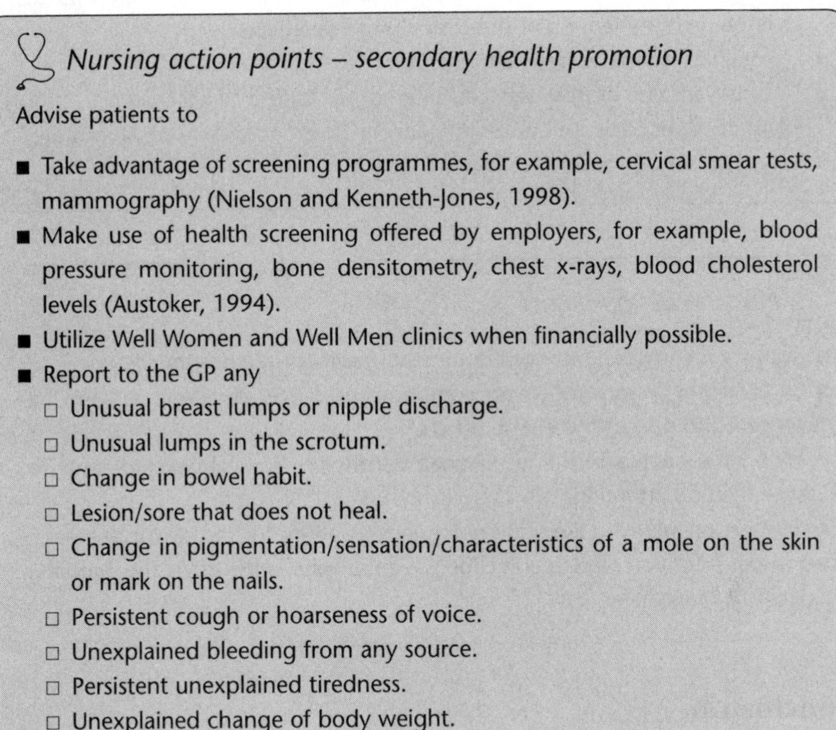

Nursing action points – secondary health promotion

Advise patients to

- Take advantage of screening programmes, for example, cervical smear tests, mammography (Nielson and Kenneth-Jones, 1998).
- Make use of health screening offered by employers, for example, blood pressure monitoring, bone densitometry, chest x-rays, blood cholesterol levels (Austoker, 1994).
- Utilize Well Women and Well Men clinics when financially possible.
- Report to the GP any
  - Unusual breast lumps or nipple discharge.
  - Unusual lumps in the scrotum.
  - Change in bowel habit.
  - Lesion/sore that does not heal.
  - Change in pigmentation/sensation/characteristics of a mole on the skin or mark on the nails.
  - Persistent cough or hoarseness of voice.
  - Unexplained bleeding from any source.
  - Persistent unexplained tiredness.
  - Unexplained change of body weight.

(Marie Curie Cancer Care, 1994)

Tertiary

With increasing knowledge and improved therapeutic interventions, long-term survival rates are lengthening and for many people, cancer may become a chronic illness (Donnelly, 1993). Promotion of well-being is therefore, a focus of nurses who are caring for these patients. Nurses must respect the fact that this group of individuals' knowledge about their own disease trajectory is frequently greater than that of the nurse or doctor, and that particular level of understanding must be the starting point for professionals endeavouring to promote health in their patients.

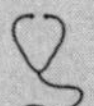

Nursing action points – tertiary health promotion

Advise patients to

- Be positive about control of the malignant disease process.
- Adhere to the treatment programme, asking questions of therapists to promote comprehension of the effects and side effects.
- Maintain as normal a lifestyle as possible.
- Take advantage of the services offered by cancer advice sources, for example, CancerBacup, Cancerlink, Cancer Information Service, Ovacome.
- Access local hospice services where available.

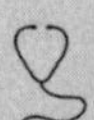

Nursing action points

- Adopt a role model approach in terms of promoting a healthy lifestyle.
- Be aware of factors known to contribute to cancer development and be prepared to discuss these with others.
- Encourage people with unusual anatomical/physiological developments to seek medical attention.
- Support people who are undergoing investigations for malignant disease.
- Promote comfort and dignity for patients living with or in the terminal stages of cancer.

Conclusion

Cancer is a common disease known throughout the world. No age group, gender or culture escapes its development, although there are variations in rates and types of cancer that may be associated with gender, culture, lifestyles and inheritance patterns. Research discoveries over recent decades have added greatly to scientific knowledge regarding cell behaviour and cancer development, with consequent improved detection, treatment and survival rates. It is essential for nurses to keep informed of current findings, so that patients can be offered up to date information about cancer, its predisposing factors, early signs and symptoms and forms of treatment. The overall aim of a cancer patient's care is to maximize the quality of life within the limits imposed by the disease, but in recognition that the patient defines this quality. The multidisciplinary approach to care, including thorough assessment, involving the family (where appropriate) in planning goals with the patient, care interventions and evaluation, is the most effective method of alleviating symptoms associated with cancer and its treatment, and reducing the patient's distress.

Nurses should also be able to communicate empathetically with patients who ask difficult questions, and should demonstrate competence in supporting them psychologically. Quality care for the cancer patient is dependent on effective interdisciplinary collaboration and current knowledge, based on unbiased and rigorously conducted research.

References

Austoker, J. 1994, 'Cancer Prevention in Primary Care'. *British Medical Journal*, 309 (6949), 241–8.

Belcher, A. E. 1992, *Cancer Nursing*. St Louis. Mosby.

Campbell, K. 1999, *Cancer Epidemiology*. London. NT Books.

David, J. 1995, *Cancer Care*. London. Chapman and Hall.

Department of Health (DOH) 1993, *The Health of the Nation*. London. HMSO.

Department of Health (DOH) 1998, *Our Healthier Nation: A Contract for Health*. London. The Stationery Office.

Doll, R. 1992, 'Carcinogenic Risk: Conference Proceedings of the Health and Safety Executive/Europe Against Cancer'. London. HSE.

Doll, R. and Hill, A. 1950, 'Smoking and Cancer of the Lung'. *British Medical Journal*, (ii), 739–48.

Doll, R. and Peto, R. 1976, 'Mortality in Relation to Smoking – 20 years observations on male British doctors'. *British Medical Journal*, (ii), 1525–36.

Doll, R. and Peto, R. 1986, *The Causes of Cancer*. Oxford. Oxford University Press.

Donnelly, G. 1993, 'Chronicity: Concept and Reality', *Holistic Nursing Practice*, 8, 1–7.

Eriksson, J. H. 1990, *Oncologic Nursing*. Massachusetts. Springhouse.

Grieder, C. W. and Blackburn, E. A. 1996, 'Telomeres, Telomeras and Cancer'. *Scientific American*, 2 (2), 96.

Health Education Authority, Health Education Board of Scotland and ASH 1991, *Passive Smoking: Questions and Answers*. London. Health Education Authority.

Hill, J. 1761, *Cautions Against the Immoderate Use of Snuff*. London. Baldwin and Jackson.

Hyassala, L., Rautava, P., Sillanpaa, M. and Tuominen, J. 1992, 'Changes in the Smoking and Drinking Habits of Future Fathers from the Onset of Their Wives Pregnancies'. *Journal of Advanced Nursing*, 17, 849–54.

Imperial Cancer Research Fund (ICRF) – now known as Cancer Research UK – 1998, *Cancer Statistics – Fact Sheet April 1998*. London. ICRF.

Kelly, M. P. 1993, 'The Four Levels of Health Promotion: An Integrated Approach'. *Public Health*, 107 (5), 319–26.

Kennaway, E. L. and Hieger, I. 1930, 'Carcinogenic Substances and Their Fluorescent Spectra'. *British Medical Journal*, (i), 1044–6.

Knudson, A. G. 1986, 'Genetics of Human Cancers: Review'. *Annual Review of Genetics*, 20, 231–51.

MacKie, R. 1992, 'Malignant Melanoma: The Story Unfolds' in *Preventing Cancers*. Heller, T., Bailey, L. and Pattison, S. Milton Keynes. Open University Press. Milton Keynes. Open University Press.

Marie Curie Cancer Care 1994, *Marie Curie Cancer Education Diary*. London. Marie Curie Cancer Care.

McCaffrey, D., Boyle, D. and Engelking, C. 1993, 'Cancer in the Elderly; The Forgotten Priority'. *European Journal of Cancer Care*, 2 (3), 101–7.

Nicholson, A. 1996, 'Diet and the Prevention of Breast Cancer'. *Alternative Therapies*, 2, 32–8.
Nielson, A. and Kenneth-Jones, R. 1998, 'Women's Lay Knowledge of Cervical Cancer/Cervical Screening: Accounting for Non-attendance at Cervical Screening Clinics'. *Journal of Advanced Nursing*, 28 (3), 571–5.
Otto, S. E. 1994, *Oncology Nursing*. St Louis. Mosby.
Pott, P. 1775, *Chirurgical Observations Relative to the Cataract, the Polypus of the Nose, the Cancer of the Scrotum, the Different Kind of Ruptures and Mortification of the Toes and Feet*. London. Hawkes, Clark and Collins.
Prescott, D. M. and Flexer, A. S. 1986, *Cancer: The Misguided Cell*. Sunderland, MA. Sinauer.
Richardson, P. 1995, *Nursing and Cancer*. London. Saunders.
Ruoslahti, E. 1997, in *What you Need to know about Cancer*, Scientific American. New York. 1139–42.
Scientific American 1997, '*What you Need to Know about Cancer*'. Scientific American. New York.
Speechley, V. and Rosenfield, M. 1992, *Cancer Information at your Fingertips*. London. Cass.
Strachan, T. and Read, A. 1996, *Human Molecular Genetics*. Plymouth. BIOS Scientific.
Taylor, M. 1992, 'A Simplified Biology of Cancers' in Heller, T., Bailey, L. and Pattison, S. 1992 (eds) '*Preventing Cancers*'. Milton Keynes. Open University Press.
Tones, K. 1997, 'Health Education as Empowerment' in Siddell, C. and Jones, M. 1997, (eds) *Debates and Dilemmas in Promoting Health*. London. Macmillan.
Wilby, M. 1998, 'Improving the Health Profile: Decreasing Risk for Cancer Through Primary Prevention'. *Holistic Nursing Practice*, 12 (1), 52–61.
Wynden, E. and Goldsmith, R. 1950, 'Tobacco Smoking as a Possible Etiologic Factor in Bronchogenic Carcinoma'. *Journal of the American Medical Association*, 153, 329–36.
Wyke, J. A. 1991, 'Viruses and Cancer' in Franks, L. M. and Teich, N. M. (eds) *Introduction to the Cellular and Molecular Biology of Cancer*. Oxford. Oxford Medical Press.

15 Women's Cancers

SANDRA JOHNSON

When a woman develops symptoms relating to her breasts she may become very anxious and look to a number of sources for support and reassurance. This chapter will address the issue of breast cancer, its development, predisposing factors, investigation procedures and the various treatment options that are currently available to women who develop the disease, plus the effects and side effects of these treatments. Breast cancer screening and nursing interventions for women undergoing therapeutic management will be discussed in order to raise awareness of nurses who will come into contact with breast cancer sufferers in both a professional and personal capacity. The second section of this chapter will adopt a similar approach to cancer of the cervix, as cancer of these two organs is very common and has caused high levels of morbidity and mortality throughout the world.

Contents

Learning Objectives

By the end of the chapter you should be able to demonstrate knowledge of

- The definition of breast cancer.
- How widespread the disease is globally.
- Risk factors associated with breast cancer development.
- Screening programmes to detect the disease.
- How women with breast cancer present their anatomical and physiological signs and symptoms.
- The psychological effect of discovering a breast lump.
- Breast cancer treatments.
- Care of the woman who is receiving therapy for breast cancer.
- Alternative agents who may offer assistance during recovery from treatment.
- Later alternatives.
- Similar aspects relating to cancer of the cervix.

Definition of Breast Cancer

Malignant changes of any of the breast tissues that may occur at any time of life and in any population. These changes, unless treated, will lead to death.

Epidemiology

Breast cancer is not a new disease, it has been recognized throughout the world for centuries but is now the most common malignant condition diagnosed in women in the United Kingdom (UK) and the second most common cancer (Imperial Cancer Research Fund [ICRF] – now known as Cancer Research UK – 1999). A similar situation in the United States of America (USA) is indicated by the American Cancer Society (AMC) (1995), showing that among women in the USA 'breast cancer accounts for one third of all cancers detected, and nearly one fifth of all cancer deaths' (AMC, 1995).

Globally, cancer of the breast is the most common malignancy in women with more than 500 000 diagnoses reported each year, but with variations between developed countries (most common female cancer) and developing countries (second most frequently diagnosed female cancer) (Gail and Benichou, 1994). In Western societies generally, there is an incidence of one in ten females developing breast cancer at some time in their lives, many during their mid-50s with more than two-thirds being post-menopausal, although breast cancer frequency increases with age. It is rare in women under 30 years of age. In the UK in 1997, 34 590 women were recorded as suffering from breast cancer (Cancer Research Campaign [CRC] – now known as Cancer Research UK – 1997) and there is an annual mortality rate of around 14 000. Men are also afflicted with breast cancer but in far fewer numbers, with around 200 diagnoses per year.

Aetiology

A number of factors increase the likelihood of a woman developing breast cancer. These include

- Age
- Nationality
- Exposure to oestrogen
- Family history
- Previous benign breast disease
- Lifestyle

Age

Breast cancer incidence increases with age and doubles with each passing decade, which suggests repeated and accumulated exposure to environmental carcinogens plus other possible factors (McPherson *et al.*, 1995).

Nationality

There is a distinct variation of the incidence of breast cancer between women in different parts of the world with those in Western countries developing the disease in numbers five times greater than women in far Eastern countries. However, studies of Japanese women migrating to Western countries show that, within one or two generations, the migrant population assumes the incidence of the indigenous population, again suggesting a link with environmental factors with possible behavioural factors adding to the statistics (McPherson *et al.*, 1995).

Exposure to Oestrogen

An early menarche (before the age of 11 years) and a late menopause (after 54 years of age) both increase the risk of women developing breast cancer; those who experience the menopause naturally after 55 years of age being twice as likely to develop the disease than those who cease menstruating before the age of 45 years. The hormone connection is the subject of much research and studies have indicated that breast cancer in men is linked to obesity and raised oestrogen levels (Stoppard, 1996). In addition, early (pre-20 years) and frequent pregnancies offer some protection from breast cancer, with women becoming pregnant for the first time over the age of 35 years having an increased risk of developing the disease.

The oral contraceptive pill has been widely studied, but no significant links between it and malignant breast disease have been found. The progesterone only pill presents zero risk, while those compounds containing oestrogen remain of interest to researchers (Faulkner, 1998). Hormone replacement therapy used by pre-and post-menopausal women suggests an increased risk during long-term treatment, of between 1.3 and 2 per cent but there is an associated decreased mortality rate in these instances (Colditz *et al.*, 1995).

Family History

Up to 10 per cent of breast cancer in Western countries is genetically predisposed, and a family history of the disease potentiates all other risk factors. The two known abnormal/mutated genes involved in breast cancer, identified in 1994 (Stoppard, 1996), are BRCA1 that is situated on chromosome 17, and BRCA2 that has been identified on chromosome 13. Many families affected by breast cancer show an excess of other reproductive malignancies and colon cancers, which are attributed to the same, inherited genetic mutation. Breast cancers due to genetic mutation generally occur much earlier in life than non-inherited breast malignancy. In addition, the more relatives a woman has with breast cancer and the younger the age of onset of their disease, the greater her own risk becomes. For example, a woman whose mother developed cancer in both breasts below the age of 35 years has a 25-fold greater risk of breast cancer as against normal risk.

Previous Benign Breast Disease

Women with a history of severe atypical epithelial hyperplasia have an increased risk of four to five times the normal, of developing breast cancer when compared with women with no history of proliferative breast change. When previous benign breast disease co-exists with a first-degree relative with malignant breast disease, then the risk factor is increased nine fold. Women with breast cysts, fibroadenomas, duct papillomas or moderate epithelial hyperplasia have a 1.5 to 2 times increase in risk, but this is not considered to be clinically significant (McPherson *et al.*, 1995).

Lifestyle

Diet

While there is some correlation between the intake of dietary fat and the development of breast tumours in laboratory studies on rats, such evidence cannot be directly applied to humans. Studies of total fat intake have not found that women with breast cancer consume larger amounts than women without; the relationship may reflect total calorie intake rather than fat levels. Breast cancer risk seems to be more influenced by obesity than fat consumption. More recent studies have indicated links between obesity and higher levels of circulating oestrogen, particularly in post-menopausal women who develop fat concentrations around the trunk.

Alcohol

Long-term excesses of alcohol intake interfere with the ability of the liver to metabolize oestrogen, resulting in higher than normal levels of the hormone in the circulation – a predisposing breast cancer factor. However, the studies are inconsistent and moderate alcohol intake is protective against heart disease. It may be wise for a woman with other high-risk factors to be aware of the possibility of the potential for alcohol to further add to the prevailing risks.

Smoking

Smokers tend to have less body fat than non-smokers; hence, less oestrogen is manufactured by the fatty tissues. Smoking appears to be protective against breast cancer since it exerts an anti-oestrogen effect, accelerating the menopause by three to four years and Stoppard (1996) states that women who smoke have higher levels of male sex hormones such as testosterone, which also has an anti-oestrogen effect.

Anatomy and Physiology

The breasts are bilateral rounded protuberances arising from the chest wall between the second and sixth ribs and are mainly glandular in nature. They are fixed to the underlying pectoral muscle by the 'Cooper's ligaments' which also effect an attachment to the overlying skin (see Figure 15.1). The breast size is related more to the amount of fatty (adipose) tissue surrounding the glandular tissue rather than the actual glandular tissue itself; however, breast cancer is most commonly associated with its glandular tissue. There are 15 to 20 lobes (or sections) in each breast which contain a number of smaller sections – lobules – with the lobules composed mainly of glandular cells which, following childbirth, secrete milk. Each of the lobes and lobules are situated in a radial

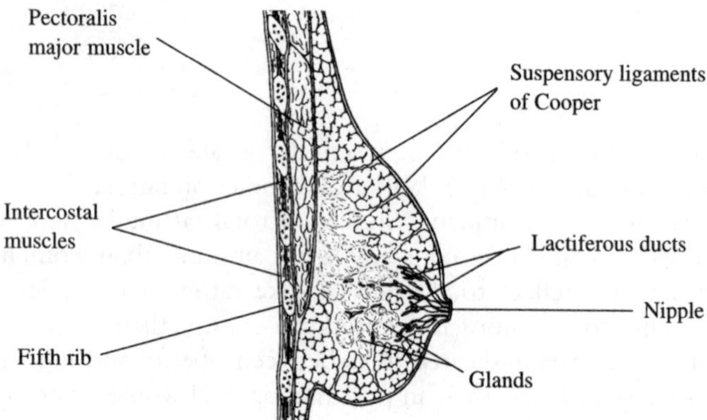

Figure 15.1 Breast, sagittal section

manner, thus giving the breast a conical shape. The glandular cells are clustered together and described as alveoli; these having small drainage ducts that converge towards the nipple – a small protuberance centrally situated which is the site of infant suckling in order to obtain early nutrition. Knowledge of the lymphatic and venous drainage from the breast is important when considering cancer of this organ, as metastatic spread via venous and lymphatic vessels is frequent.

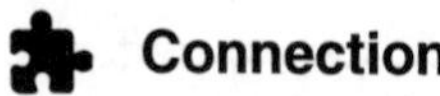

Connection

Chapter 14 (Cancer – an Overview) discusses the aetiology of carcinogenesis.

Pathophysiology

As with all cancers, certain cells that may be genetically or environmentally influenced (or may possess both factors) begin to grow erratically and uncontrollably and to no specific end. In other words, they are not required to replace or repair pre-existent cells. These erratically proliferating cells are abnormal in growth pattern and development and at the end of the cell cycle, vary in many aspects from the parent cell.

Many types of breast cancer exist but the most common histological type is 'infiltrating intraductal carcinoma' which accounts for almost 80 per cent of all breast cancers. Up to 10 per cent of breast cancers in Western countries may be genetically predisposed, but although this is a known fact, it is unknown as yet, as to how many breast cancer genes exist (Kirschbaum, 1999).

Breast cancer presents, in the early stages, as a small, painless lump that is irregular in outline, unilateral and without other symptoms. Many such

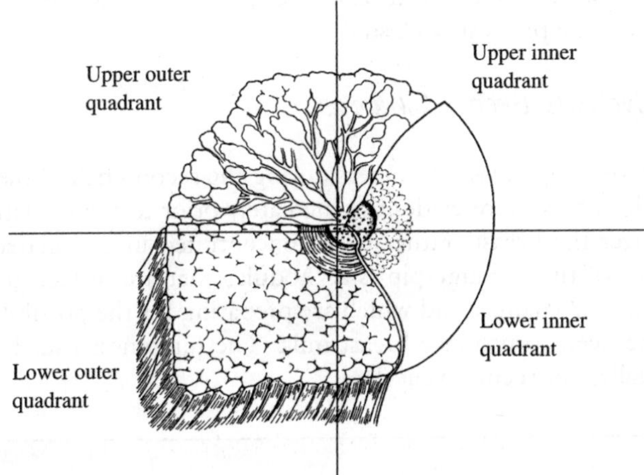

Figure 15.2 Right breast

self-found breast lumps are discovered in the upper, outer breast quadrant and measure about half an inch or one centimetre in size (see Figure 15.2).

Mammography can detect cancerous masses of only one quarter of an inch or half a centimetre in diameter, which obviously improves the prognosis, since treatment can be commenced much earlier, thus reducing the chances of the spread of the cancer.

Clinical Manifestations

Detection of Breast Cancer

Breast Self-examination (BSE)

This is a simple way for a woman to discover the normal size, shape and consistency of her breasts and is a routine that should be commenced in the teenage years and continued on a regular basis throughout life. It involves visual inspection of both breasts in front of a mirror with hands relaxed at the side of the body and again with hands placed at the back of the head. The woman is looking for any change in symmetry, appearance, size or colour of nipples and discharge there from, skin changes or nipple retraction. Then pressing hands on hips, the woman should feel the tension in the chest muscles and repeat the visual observations.

The second part of BSE is for the woman to lie in a relaxed supine position with the right arm behind the head. With the tips of the fingers of the left hand she should palpate the right axilla and along the clavicle for swelling or lumpiness, then repeat the procedure on the right breast. The examination should take the form of gently palpating the breast in a systematic manner (often concentric circles decreasing in size towards the nipple is a chosen pattern).

Nipples should not be squeezed to examine for discharge as this may produce exudate where none previously existed.

Normal Cyclical Breast Changes

Many women develop breast lumpiness during the second half of the menstrual cycle, which becomes more evident immediately prior to menstruation. This is palpable all over the breasts rather than concentrated in an isolated area, and takes the form of tiny 'orange-pip' size nodules that are in fact glands, influenced by hormonal changes and which are preparing for the possibility of pregnancy and the need to produce breast milk. The lumpiness usually disappears post-menstrually, but recurs cyclically.

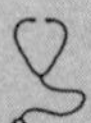

Nursing action points

Ensure that patients are aware that

- Women who have lost a lot of weight may find that due to loss of fat from the breasts, natural lumpiness is more noticeable.
- Tenderness and discomfort or 'heaviness' are extremely common in women's breasts and very rarely is this an indication of breast cancer.
- If tenderness persists, medical opinion should be sought.

Changes Requiring Further Investigation

Observational

- Visible veins become more prominent than usual.
- Changes in colour or texture of breast skin.
- New dimpling or puckering of skin over the breast or nipple, or change in breast outline.
- Discharge or bleeding from nipples.

Palpational

- A new lump that does not vary in size with menstruation.
- It is distinct and not just a thickening of breast tissue.
- It remains unchanged throughout one or two menstrual cycles.
- The lump is unilateral and irregular in outline.
- There is no associated pain.

An early appointment for a medical opinion should be sought and several further investigations will be recommended. Skin dimpling (*peau d'orange*), clear or bloodstained nipple discharge and breast asymmetry may be later signs of breast cancer, but may also be significant symptoms of non-malignant breast disease all of which require further investigation. Lumpiness in the axilla may also be suggestive of breast cancer, but recent events such as inoculations against tetanus or other diseases can cause lymph node swelling in the armpit (Eriksson, 1990). Nipple retraction or ulceration may also be indicative of breast cancer but may be due to other pathological causes and these also require further investigation.

Further Investigations

- Mammography
- Ultrasound
- Fine needle aspiration
- Core biopsy
- Frozen section

Breast Screening via Mammography

The National Health Service (NHS) has established a nationwide programme that offers the opportunity for mammography to all women between the ages of 50 and 64 years at three-yearly intervals, with the aim of reducing deaths by 25 per cent in the screened population. Uptake for the test is about 70 per cent. Women over the age of 64 years (when breast cancer is more frequent) may avail themselves of the test by request to their General Practitioner (GP). In 1999 trials began on screening women from 65 to 69 years of age (ICRF, 1999) to determine the cost-effectiveness of routinely offering the test up to 69 years. Since half of all breast cancer patients are over 65 and this age group accounts for 60 per cent of all breast cancer deaths, extending screening would save an estimated 2000 lives annually (Fletcher *et al.*, 1993). Results of the research have recently encouraged the government to extend the routine screening of women to the age of 69 years. Eligible women receive an invitation to attend a screening centre where a mammogram (type of x-ray) is taken of each breast in two directions. The test is not 100 per cent reliable and does not just detect malignant tumours; for every ten women recalled for further checks, only one will have cancer. Most of the others will be recalled because some form of benign breast disease has been identified (ICRF, 1999).

In women under 50 years of age, breast tissue is more dense and hence the mammogram is more difficult to read and abnormalities more difficult to detect making recall for benign conditions more likely. This could lead to considerable unnecessary anxiety and distress for many women. However, for women with a family history of breast cancer, a mammogram before the age of 50 years might be advisable together with regular clinical examination.

Ultrasound

This investigation produces a picture similar to an x-ray. The patterns are designated by sound wave echoes, which bounce off tissue. The density of the tissue gives pictures that vary in intensity, thus ultrasound is useful for younger women whose breast tissue is generally denser than that of older women. It can detect very small lumps that cannot be felt, particularly tiny cysts, and is very accurate with larger, palpable lumps, being able to distinguish between solid and fluid-filled lumps. The investigation is painless and has no side effects.

Fine Needle Aspiration Cytology

Needle aspiration can differentiate between solid and fluid-filled lumps. The aspiration of solid tumours requires a degree of skill to extract sufficient cells for laboratory analysis.

Core Biopsy

By the use of a specialized cutting needle a small core of tissue can be removed from the lump and sent for laboratory investigation (histology). The result will usually clarify grading and classification of any malignant tumour.

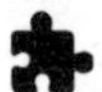 **Connection**

Chapter 14 (Cancer – an Overview) gives details of grading and classification of malignant tumours.

Frozen Section

This investigation is now no longer performed routinely to diagnose breast cancer but may be used to confirm a cytology diagnosis of malignancy prior to proceeding to a more major surgical intervention, to assess excision margins to ensure complete removal of a malignant breast tumour or to assess the involvement of axillary lymph nodes in the cancerous disease, thereby identifying patients who require only a limited dissection.

Screening for Breast Cancer

Screening is 'the practice of investigating apparently healthy individuals with the object of detecting unrecognized disease or people with an exceptionally high risk of developing disease, and intervening in ways that will prevent the occurrence of disease or improve the prognosis when it develops' (Farmer and Miller, 1983).

Cancers are very different in their predisposing factors, development and progress, thus the scope for reducing the ill health and death they cause, varies enormously. Evidence suggests that a large number of deaths from malignant disease might be avoidable, but lack of knowledge leads to some dilemmas regarding cancer prevention.

Primary prevention may mean advising radical possibly unwelcome changes in lifestyle that offer no guarantee of cancer avoidance or ultimate death from the disease. With respect to secondary prevention, which involves screening and early detection, there are doubts as to whether these expensive programmes lead to improved cure rates and not merely longer post-diagnostic survival. Such investigations therefore, have to be carefully appraised for cost-effectiveness financially, politically, physically and psychologically. Screening for breast cancer is not an ideal method of cancer control because to be cost effective and valuable, large numbers of apparently well women have to be subjected to an uncomfortable procedure from which most will gain no obvious benefit, apart from the knowledge that at the time of the examination there was no suggestion of cancer, and some might be physically or psychologically harmed.

In the UK, the Breast Cancer Working Group, which was formally constituted in February 1997 and reported in September of that year, reviewed the relevant interventions for breast cancer. Using the following classification of interventions (Howard *et al.*, 1999), these aimed to

- Improve early detection and treatment of breast cancer.
- Reduce death and complications from breast cancer and its treatments.
- Maintain well-being during and following treatment for breast cancer.

Interventions for Early Detection and Treatment

- Screening of all women in the appropriate age-group
- Limiting the length of use of hormone replacement therapy (HRT)
- Pro-active management of women with a family history of breast cancer

Breast Screening

The aim of breast screening is to detect breast cancer tumours when they are less than 15 mm in diameter. All women between 50 and 64 years are invited for screening every three years using mammography via the NHS breast screening programme. The programme aimed to reduce breast cancer deaths, in the population invited for screening, by at least 25 per cent by the year 2000.

Limiting Hormone Replacement Therapy (HRT)

Use of HRT is valuable in protecting against ischaemic heart disease, osteoporosis and reducing menopausal symptoms in the early and post-menopausal years. These benefits may outweigh the risk of breast cancer developing if HRT use is continued beyond ten years. Its use must be carefully evaluated.

Pro-active Management of Women with a Family History of Breast Cancer

Women with a strong family history of breast cancer may be very fearful of developing the disease and may wish to avail themselves of information offered by specialist breast cancer teams or genetics clinics (Dey and Twelves, 1996).

Main Interventions to Reduce Risk Factors

- Screening all women in the appropriate age group
- Accurate and timely assessment of symptomatic women
- Appropriate treatment of all detected cases
- Appropriate follow-up after treatment

Screening

As above.

Specialist Care

Specialist care from a multidisciplinary team of breast surgeon, breast care nurse(s), pathologist, radiologist and medical or clinical oncologist gives a better five-year survival rate (Clinical Outcomes Group, 1996). Women with symptoms suggestive of breast cancer should be assessed in a specialist breast unit providing clinical examination, mammography or ultrasound, fine needle aspiration, cytology and/or core biopsy (Austoker *et al.*, 1995). Results of tests should be available within five working days to reduce anxiety, with appropriate information, counselling and access to specialist psychological and social care to reduce levels of psychological morbidity (Clinical Outcomes Group, 1996).

Surgery, Chemotherapy, Radiotherapy or Combination Treatments

Depending on the nature and size of the tumour, surgery, chemotherapy or radiotherapy or combinations of these treatments have been shown to reduce the incidence of recurrence of local disease (Veronesi *et al.*, 1995). The use of adjuvant systemic therapies has been shown to be beneficial in terms of life saved that might otherwise have diminished due to metastatic disease (Clinical Outcomes Group, 1996).

Interventions to maintain well-being during and after treatment

- Provision of clear information – verbal and written – at all stages of treatment, with assistance to access sources of social and practical help.
- Effective communication – particularly important here is the breast care nurse who has a key function in facilitating communication and support.
- Access to specialist psychological support – Macmillan nurses are specially trained to offer such a service to patients and their families and the relief of anxiety, depression and physical symptoms from such an intervention helps to improve quality of life (Clinical Outcomes Group, 1996).
- Access to specialist treatment for lymphoedema: this can be a most distressing, irremediable and unpleasant complication of breast cancer (Kirschbaum, 1999). All women who suffer from this condition require specialist support for its treatment.
- Restoration of 'normal' appearance. Reconstructive surgery or prosthetic devices are essential for improving self-esteem, confidence and well-being. These require skilled staff interventions and informed dialogue with the patient as to her individual needs.
- Symptom control, as part of palliative care, should be accessible both in the community, in the patient's own home and in palliative care units for those whose disease is progressing. In conjunction with control of physical symptoms, psychological, social and spiritual support for the patient, relatives and carers is essential (Clinical Outcomes Group, 1996).

Treatment

Advancement of understanding of the nature and progress of breast cancer has meant that many of the extremely radical treatments of three to four decades ago have been superseded by highly individualized, sympathetic therapeutic interventions, conducted in specialized breast care centres. Such specialist centres are managed by a multidisciplinary team of professionals including surgeons, oncologists, trained breast care nurses, radiologists, radiotherapists, pathologists and counsellors, all of whom have education and training within the speciality. This approach ensures rapid attention to women presenting with breast lumps and a streamlined follow-up and follow-through system that is specifically designed to accommodate the individual woman's needs where possible. This means that women who do develop breast cancer are much more likely to find a course of treatment with which they can comply, as opposed to the situation of 20–30 years ago.

Treatment Availabilities

For most women a combination of treatments will be available and therapists will consider clinical and pathological factors that may influence the effectiveness of the treatment options. The classification of the tumour, its grading and staging are significant factors in deciding the most appropriate treatment, but the woman's age, genetic predisposition and general health are also important considerations.

Surgery

The use of surgery locally to eradicate the malignant cells is usually the first choice of treatment but is generally combined with other prophylactic or therapeutic interventions. Surgery may consist of wide local excision, that is, removal of the tumour together with a one centimetre margin of normal tissue, or a quadrantectomy which is a more extensive removal of a quadrant of the breast, but both of these treatment options generally means that the affected breast can be conserved and probably be reconstructed later, if necessary, to match the unaffected breast. For about one-third of patients presenting with breast cancer, breast conservation surgery will not be appropriate and simple mastectomy, which surgically removes the breast tissue and some overlying skin and usually the nipple, would be the most effective surgical intervention. Sainsbury *et al.* (1995) state that 'local recurrence after mastectomy is most common in the first two years and decreases with time,' but that 'local recurrence after breast conservation occurs at a fixed rate each year.' These facts suggest that the follow-up procedure should take account of these differences, in order to detect local recurrence and treat it, or possible spread of cancer to the previously unaffected breast. Mammography, although a very useful diagnostic pre-surgery aid, is less helpful post-operatively, because surgical intervention produces scarring and local distortion in the breast that could lead to misinterpretation of the images.

Radiotherapy

Veronesi *et al.* (1995) argue that all patients should receive breast radiotherapy following wide local excision or quadrantectomy, with individually prescribed doses between three and five weeks. Local boosts of radiotherapy to the excision site or radioactive implants may be useful, but reports to date regarding its beneficial effects are inconclusive.

Side effects of radiotherapy

- Skin reactions
- Hair loss
- Nausea and vomiting
- Dehydration
- Mouth ulceration
- Lethargy
- Mental instability
- Increased susceptibility to infection
- Anaemia

The complications of radiotherapy for breast cancer seen in earlier years have been reduced, mainly due to improved understanding of the dose management, however, skin reactions can still occur in women who are sensitive to therapy and the nurse should be able to offer practical advice and help. This may include the use of baby oil on dry desquamating skin, but not of any application that contains metal such as aluminium (as found in some deodorants or antiperspirants or emollient compounds). Severe skin reactions, although unusual, may require dressings of Flamazine and/or the use of antibiotic sprays to reduce the infection risk. Later skin reactions including telangiectasis, hyperpigmentation and skin necrosis are difficult nursing care problems, but must be approached sympathetically and on an individual basis. The use of applications to reduce itching and hypersensitivity such as anti-inflammatory or antihistamine creams can be helpful and topical antibiotic creams such as metronidazole may be useful in reducing offensive odours produced by fungating wounds.

Most patients who are having radiotherapy around body areas producing hair will experience hair loss. For breast cancer patients, axillary hair may be lost, and if having radiotherapy to the head for metastastic brain deposits, then head hair may be lost together with eyelashes and eyebrows. However, this is usually transient and evidence of regrowth may be seen within six to eight weeks of completion of the treatment. New hair may differ in colour, texture and other features, for example curly or straight, fast or slow growing, lighter or darker, and nurses must be prepared to help women through what can be a most traumatic time of multiple changes in body image. The use of hairpieces or wigs (partially financed by the NHS) can be helpful, but some women may prefer to use head scarves or hats, perceiving their alopecia as other people's problem.

Nausea and vomiting occur because radiotherapy breaks down and kills cells. All of those cells involved will therefore release broken down metabolites into the circulatory system and the excretory systems will remove the toxic products as quickly as they are able to do so, but there will be an inevitable concentration of these toxic metabolites in the circulation that impacts upon the vital centres in the brain. The effect will be varying degrees of nausea, vomiting and associated dehydration with the potential for mouth ulceration, lethargy and mental instability, the latter being compounded given the accumulation of physical and psychological stress factors.

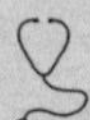

Nursing action points

Nurses should

- Anticipate the distress caused by nausea and vomiting by encouraging the patient to take advantage of prescribed anti-emetic drugs. Sometimes trial and error is needed to find the correct combination of drugs and doses to suit the individual woman in order to achieve control of these very disturbing (and possibly life-threatening) side effects of radiotherapy.
- Have an in-depth knowledge of the physical and psychological effects of dehydration caused by fluctuations in body temperature that can arise in conjunction with radiotherapy and the vomiting itself. The importance of an oral intake of at least three litres of fluid over 24 hours cannot be over-emphasized (David, 1995), to help alleviate the unpleasantness of dehydration, but also for those patients who are feeling nauseated and generally unwell as a result of the physiological accumulation of toxins and the psychological disturbances that the 'cancer' diagnosis can engender, an increased fluid intake is helpful.
- Offer the patient a ready and frequently replenished supply of ice to suck, fizzy soda water or sparkling spring water to sip, taste-bud stimulating citrus-based sugar-free drinks and a comforting hand to hold, or a nurse who is not too busy to just sit with the patient and offer encouragement to partake of a mouthful of fluid, can create an atmosphere whereby even the most depressed woman sees the possibility of a positive outcome. Such interventions by an enlightened and knowledgeable nurse can deepen the resolve of the patient to continue with the treatment and can be a very rewarding experience for both parties.
- Administer mouth care, which is of importance during a period of dehydration as dry oral mucous membranes encourage bacterial and fungal proliferation, the effects of which can seriously compromise a patient's motivation to continue with an increased intake of oral fluids at this crucial time of therapy. Two/four hourly mouth cleansing with a swab moistened with an antiseptic solution can be physically comforting and also act prophylactically against oral thrush and streptococcal invasion.
- Be aware that complementary therapies, such as reflexology, distraction techniques, acupressure and hypnotherapy may all have a place in helping a patient through a difficult therapeutic regime.

Bone marrow depression is a side effect of radiotherapy when large areas of haemopoeitic (blood cell-producing) bone marrow are included in the area of treatment. Haemopoeitic bone marrow produces erythrocytes (red blood cells that carry oxygen), leucocytes and lymphocytes (white cells that protect the body against infective and other potentially damaging proteins and thrombocytes or platelets 'cells' which assist in blood clotting). Therefore, if bone marrow function is depressed, there will be an inevitable reduction in erythrocytes, leading to poor oxygenation of body cells causing lethargy and faintness as brain cells become starved of oxygen and are unable to utilize glucose to form energy and function properly. The reduction in leucocytes and lymphocytes will lead to increased susceptibility to infection and attack by foreign proteins that can be fatal within a very short time.

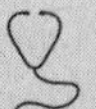

Nursing action points

- Be aware of the early signs of infection for example pyrexia, tachycardia, skin rashes or mucous membrane inflammation, lethargy and general disinterest in local surroundings and activities.
- Report such observations to medical personnel and ensure the best possible outcome for the patient, including the prophylactic assessment of the blood picture every few days.

A decrease in the blood fragment thrombocytes is a further complication, and as these cells diminish in the circulation, local abrasions and wounds, such as those caused by vigorous tooth-brushing or scratching of skin irritations, can lead to a blood loss that cannot be compensated for by normal haemopoeitic bone marrow activity. This compounds the anaemia produced by erythrocyte depletion and causes further feelings of lethargy, breathlessness and disinterest in everyday life activities.

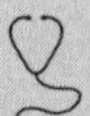

Nursing action points

- Encourage an elevated fluid intake and a diet high in proteins and carbohydrates to help repair and replace damaged and destroyed body cells. Supplementary drinks such as 'Ensure', 'Fortisip' and 'Complan' can be useful if women are physically or psychologically distressed by solid foods during therapy.
- Be aware that other acute problems may be experienced (generally these effects are related to the site of irradiation). For most women who are having radiotherapy for breast cancer, therefore, the difficulties will be mainly related to the chest, axilla, shoulder in proximity to the tumour area and possibly the neck and jaw on the same side, with loosening of teeth and loss of dental fillings being likely.

Chemotherapy

This is the therapeutic use of drugs (chemicals) to assist in the prevention, eradication or control of metastases, or occasionally to reduce the size of a tumour prior to surgery. Once the extent of the primary tumour has been established, and grading, classification and staging are known, further tests such as bone scans or node biopsies will assist the medical team in devising an individual chemotherapy regime for each patient, where such treatment is deemed necessary.

The results of clinical trials (Richards and Smith, 1995) indicate that combinations of drugs are more effective than single drug treatment, and that it is more beneficial to continue the treatment over a period of several months. Drug combinations include cytotoxic (cell poisoning) preparations, for example, fluorouracil, methotrexate and hormonal therapy, for example, tamoxifen. Since some breast cancers are oestrogen/progesterone sensitive and metastatic growth similarly dependent, the choice of chemotherapeutic combinations will necessarily reflect the hormonal status of the woman. Oophorectomy might be an appropriate treatment for some pre-menopausal patients, by depriving breast cancer tumours and metastases of oestrogen, but contemporaneous drug therapies spare the patient from more surgery and its associated morbidity. However, all treatments have positive and negative effects, and the choice depends on relative risk factors such as the age and general health status of the patient, her menopausal status and physical and psychological ability to follow the treatment plan.

Types of Cytotoxic Drugs

Drugs that might be useful in managing/treating human cancers are constantly being researched and introduced into the therapeutic armoury. All cytotoxic drugs affect not just cancer cells, but all cells that are dividing and reproducing, therefore there is likely to be widespread cell damage. But because the blood supply to the tumour (a mass of rapidly dividing cells) is usually much greater than that to normal cells, the tumour cells receive a larger dose of the circulating cytotoxic drugs than normal cells. Improved knowledge of the cell cycle means that research is directed towards attacking rapidly dividing cells when they are at their most vulnerable. The uses of drug combinations are, therefore, crucial to the demise of the tumour and recovery of normal cells. Multiple cytotoxic drug therapy given at intervals, usually over six to nine months allows for increased cancer-cell death as the drugs work in combination and at different times of the cell cycle, and also reduce the development of cancer cell resistance to one drug used in isolation.

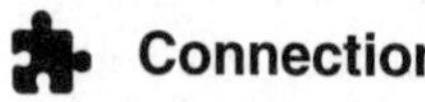

Chapter 14 (Cancer – an Overview) outlines the cell cycle.

Antimetabolites

Antimetabolites act by preventing the formation of constituents needed for cell metabolism, particularly deoxyribonucleic acid (DNA) and ribonucleic acid (RNA), thus the synthesis stage of the cell cycle is severely damaged. For example, 5 fluorouracil, methotrexate mercaptopurine.

Alkylating agents

Alkylating agents work by arresting the separation of DNA strands during cell division so that cell multiplication is inactivated. Many of these drugs have been developed following observations during the First World War, whereby people who were exposed to mustard gas suffered from depleted white blood cells and succumbed to infections that were hitherto not life-threatening. For example, cyclophosphamide, melphalan, carmustine, chlorambucil.

Anti-mitotic Antibiotics

Anti-mitotic antibiotics act at the mitosis stage of the cell cycle and distort the DNA helix, thereby disturbing the capacity of the cell to reproduce. For example, bleomycin, doxorubicin, mitomycin, actinomycin.

Vinca-alkaloids

Vinca-alkaloids work by interfering with protein that assists in nuclear spindle activity. For example, vincristine, vinblastine (derived from the Vinca Rosae or Periwinkle plant).

Miscellaneous

These drugs have either more than one action or are currently known effective anti-cancer drugs, but their mode of action is not thoroughly comprehended. Examples include carboplastin, cisplatin, and mitrozantone.

Other Therapeutic Drug Regimes

Glucocorticoids

These drugs are useful in promoting a feeling of well-being but also inhibit lymphocyte production and reduce the anti-inflammatory response. While women receiving breast cancer treatment might welcome the euphoric state, the symptoms of infection are masked and wound healing delayed.

Hormone Therapy

Any of the earlier surgical interventions, such as bilateral oophorectomy/ adrenalectomy or hypophysectomy which reduce circulating androgens, oestrogens, progesterones and their associated releasing factors, have been superseded by anti-oestrogen drug compounds known as taxanes. These work by arresting the ability of the metastatic cancer cell to divide and reproduce. The most commonly used drug of this group is tamoxifen, which acts by competing with oestrogen and reducing growth stimulation, and its use has been a major contribution to the highest ever recorded UK five-year survival rate of 73.7 per cent (Coombes, 2000). She points out that deaths from breast cancer in the UK have fallen by 30 per cent in the last 20 years, which is the largest recorded reduction worldwide, but this huge reduction may have a number of other contributory factors. Taxotere is mainly used to treat advanced breast cancer when early treatments have been unsuccessful. Currently its use is being tested in earlier stages of breast cancer and in cancer of the ovary. While these drugs are therapeutically effective, they are not without side-effects and alopecia (hair loss), neutropaenia (reduced white cell count), skin rashes, anaemia, nausea and diarrhoea and dependent oedema can all be distressing to the patient.

Many of the chemotherapeutical drugs have similar side effects but some have specific effects that are not shared by other preparations.

Side effects of drugs used to treat breast cancer

- Nausea and vomiting are common with many cytotoxic drugs, as is anorexia and bone marrow depression.
- Some cause alopecia.
- Others are neurotoxic and cause vertigo, due to cerebral oedema, ataxia and a degree of mental confusion, the latter sometimes presenting as aggressive behaviour and personality change (National Cancer Alliance, 1996).
- Nephrotoxicity and cardiotoxicity are properties of some other cytotoxic drugs each interfering with the normal kidney and heart function with corresponding fluid and electrolyte imbalance and cardiac arrhythmias which can be very frightening to the patient.

When involved in the administration of cytotoxic drugs, the nurse needs to be conversant with their specific toxicities and inform the patient of their possible effects so that she is not taken by surprise if they do occur.

Nursing Interventions

- Health education
- Psychological support
- Referral to other agencies
- Tertiary health promotion

Health Education

Information given by nurses is of paramount importance if patients' concerns are to be appropriately addressed and their treatment choices founded on an effective knowledge base. A range of leaflets, audio and videotapes should be available to nurses to enable them to guide patients through the treatment process: a lack of adequate information is one of the most common complaints voiced by recipients of cancer healthcare (National Cancer Alliance, 1996). Nurses must be knowledgeable and continue to improve their knowledge about the pathology of cancer, its treatments, effects and side effects, and thereby be able to encourage their patients to continue with what might be a series of unpleasant and distressing therapeutic interventions. The nurse's self-confidence, personal knowledge and communication skills are obviously paramount in guiding and caring for patients through such times. It is essential that nurses can provide advice regarding the work of various organizations that may be able to offer help in the treatment and post-treatment stages of breast cancer.

Information sources

- Discussion with members of the caring team using terminology that is comprehensible and acceptable to the patient
- Leaflets, journal articles and reference sources available in a variety of languages
- Audio-visual aids such as taped interviews between the patient and the doctor who broke the news of the breast cancer, and of similar interviews between anonymous patients/doctors. Videotapes that explain the disease and treatment options
- Local and national support groups such as CancerBacup
- Counselling services often provided by the NHS or organizations such as Macmillan Cancer Relief. Former cancer patients who are trained by a cancer organization, can liaise with newly diagnosed cancer patients
- Charitable organizations, for example, Marie Curie, The National Cancer Alliance can offer patient-centred services

Psychological Support

An almost universal response to the discovery of a breast lump is shock, which is understandable, because the majority of the population know or have known about the circumstances of a woman with breast cancer. Unfortunately, many women who do find a breast lump postpone or ignore its significance and delay the seeking of appropriate advice due to a preconceived notion that death is inevitable once breast cancer is diagnosed. Surprisingly, Stoppard (1996) indicates that female healthcare workers 'especially nurses' tend to leave reporting their breast lumps until later than the average population, resulting in larger breast lumps and therefore more possibility of distant spread before appropriate treatment had commenced. She also found that women who were studied pre- and post-diagnosis of a benign breast lump suffered from anxiety, coupled with impairment of concentration and rational thought. Additionally, breast loss was only a prime concern in fewer than 13 per cent of women respondents, but the larger majority of almost 60 per cent were most concerned at having cancer. Nurses should be aware of the potential reactions that women may experience if health promotion is to be effective.

Psychologically, women view breast cancer as a very emotive issue, which is natural, particularly as the media portrays health issues, and especially those concerning breast cancer as highly sensational and newsworthy. As a result there is an increase in interest and knowledge among women towards developing an understanding of breast cancer and its trajectory. Nurses are well placed to further increase such understanding.

Sensitivity to the patient's realization that having breast cancer means that she is likely to die (Denton, 1996) must alert nurses to the need for very careful use of communication skills, built upon a sound knowledge-base by which to impart information about the disease, its progress and treatment. Nurses have an important and significant role in recognizing the potential psychological impact that a diagnosis or even a suspicion of breast cancer can engender in women.

Referral to Other Agencies

Mood disturbance is common (Fallowfield, 1991) and if nurses are sensitive to this problem and can assist in the referral of the patient to an appropriate counselling service, further associated sexual problems and depressive illnesses might be avoided.

Vulnerability factors that might alert the caring team to the possibility of psychological morbidity

- Previous psychiatric history
- Lack of support from family and friends
- Pre-existing marital problems
- Visible deformity resulting from cancer and its treatment
- Inability to accept the changes associated with cancer or its therapy
- Youthfulness
- Suppression of negative feelings
- Low expectation of efficacy of treatment

- Low involvement in satisfying activities or occupation
- An intensification of reported physical symptoms regardless of the stage of the cancerous disease
- An adverse familial cancer experience
- Treatment by aggressive chemotherapy

(Watson, 1991)

When nurses observe these features (and observation is a crucial nursing skill) it is imperative that reference to the multidisciplinary team is put into action. While some patients would wish to manage the disease process and its treatment using their own resources, many will undoubtedly appreciate the assistance of helpers aligned to the nursing profession.

Tertiary Health Promotion

Metastatic Breast Cancer

The course of breast cancer is very variable as is the survival rate. The aetiology of the malignancy is significant and patients with hormone-sensitive cancers may live for several years without any intervention other than manipulation of their hormone therapy. Conversely, women with non-hormone sensitive breast cancer have a shorter disease-free interval and shorter survival, which indicates the more aggressive nature of non-hormone dependent disease. While the average post-metastatic disease prognosis is variable, Leonard *et al.* (1995) state that the average period of survival is 18–24 months. Women diagnosed with brain metastases have a median survival time of three months, with liver metastases eight months, lung metastases 15 months, soft tissue metastases 15 months and with bone metastases, the median survival time being 19 months. However, as research progresses and newer therapies become available, survival rates are improving.

Breast Reconstruction

To attempt post-mastectomy symmetry, breast reconstruction may be undertaken on an individual basis, the surgery tailored to the particular needs of the patient. Watson *et al.* (1995) indicate that in those hospitals where breast reconstruction is available, there has been a steady increase in demand with up to 50 per cent of women offered immediate reconstruction availing themselves of the facility. They also argue that there is no evidence that such surgical intervention affects the rate of local or systemic relapse, and the substantial cosmetic and psychological benefits to the woman suggest that this surgery should be made much more widely available. Reconstruction may be via synthetic breast implants, tissue expanders, muscle and subcutaneous tissue implants and combinations of these procedures, in order to give pleasing results to patients where there are no contra-indications.

The Role of the Nurse

Advising the Patient

The nurse's knowledge must be such as to give realistic advice and hope to women who wish to take advantage of reconstruction, as the procedures are not without complications, such as infection, implant fatigue and rupture and tissue necrosis.

Listening to the Patient

If complications occur, the additional stress for a woman who has already undergone mastectomy is not difficult to imagine, and the nurse must be ready to actively listen to the woman's anxieties and understand that the experience of breast cancer is a life-threatening disease with disfiguring treatments that cannot always be redeemed.

Acknowledging Changes in Body Image

Feldman (1989) suggests that body image, sexuality and self-esteem are all closely linked and that poor self-esteem can lead to a negative body image and problems with sexuality. Nurses can establish a rapport with the patient to provide a safe environment in which these problems can be discussed if so wished. The defining of goals, emphasising positive experiences and the identification of new coping strategies, can assist the patient in coming to terms with major life changes.

Leadbeater (2000) explains that it is essential to encourage patients to ask questions that they see as important to them and nurses should be able to respond with accurate answers that are understandable to the woman.

Cervical Cancer

Epidemiology, or the study of the distribution of diseases, can make important contributions to the planning of health services, preventive steps and the evaluation of health care interventions. Cervical cancer is the second most common cancer worldwide (Dey and Woodman, 1996), despite the fact that many developed countries have cervical cytology screening programmes. While these programmes vary in their organization and efficacy, they do aim to reduce mortality from cervical cancer by early detection and treatment of pre-malignant epithelial abnormalities of the cervix. The human papillomavirus (HPV) has consistently been implicated as a sexually transmitted cervical carcinogen

(Reeves *et al.*, 1989; Ley *et al.*, 1991; Dey and Woodman, 1996), and currently much research attention is concentrated on this organism.

Definition of Cervical Cancer

Cervical cancer usually begins at the squamo-columnar junction, or transformation zone of the cervix, and its clinical manifestations vary. It can progress to more widespread local cancer and metastasize distantly.

Epidemiology

Worldwide, cervical cancer is an important cause of morbidity and mortality (Parkin, 1993) with the highest incidence rates being reported in South America and India. The incidence rates in industrialized countries are surpassed by breast, lung and gastrointestinal system malignancies. There are ethnic differences; black Americans have twice the rate of white Americans, and Jewish women record particularly low rates of cervical cancer. In England and Wales, the disease is the fifth most common cancer in women and the second most common gynaecological cancer after ovarian cancer. In 1989 there were 4147 new registrations of cervical cancer (Office of Population, Censuses and Surveys [OPCS], 1989) and it is now the most common cancer in women under 50 years of age. Unlike other gynaecological cancers, its age-specific incidence increases by 40 per cent in women between 20 and 30 years after which it plateaus before a second, but less dramatic increase in the 60–70 year age group. Higher rates are recorded in the north of England, which may reflect the ethnic, socio-economic factors or, differences in uptake of screening. Most certainly, despite regional survival rate variations, it has been shown that the earlier the disease is discovered and the younger the woman, the better the prognosis for all stages of the disease (Meanwell *et al.*, 1988).

There have been steadily decreasing incidence and mortality rates from cancer of the cervix in many developed countries during the last 30 years (Dey and Woodman, 1996), which appear to be related to well organized cervical cytology screening programmes that have achieved high compliance rates. In England and Wales however, the OPCS (1974–89) indicated that there was a 'stand-still' situation that resulted in a national call/recall system being instituted, which appears to have had the effect of lowering mortality (though not incidence) rates.

Aetiology

The majority of cervical cancers are squamous cell, with adenocarcinomas being rare and accounting for less than ten per cent of all those reported. There is a suggestion however (Bjørge *et al.*, 1993) that the rise in incidence of cervical adenocarcinomas in North America and Norway may be due to

- Improved pathological classification
- Improved and earlier detection
- An increased use of oral contraception, which offers less protection than condoms in the transmission of infection

Numerous epidemiological studies consistently indicate an association between sexually related behaviours and squamous cell cervical carcinoma (Brinton, 1992). The relationship between multiple sexual partners and the transmission of any infective organism is obvious (currently 40 per cent of prostitutes in Thailand are HIV positive) (Medical Advisory Services for Travellers Abroad [MASTA], 2000). Additionally, the younger a female begins coitus, the greater number of sexual partners she is likely to encounter, which thus increases her exposure to predisposing risk factors. Women with four or more lifetime sexual partners have a three times greater risk of developing cancer of the cervix compared with women with one or no partners, and there is a two-fold greater risk for women who have sexual intercourse before 16 years of age compared with those who are at least 20 years when intercourse first takes place (Brinton, 1992). Cigarette smoking offers a two to four times increase in the risk of cervical cancer as opposed to non-smokers (Winkelstein, 1990).

Anatomy and Physiology

The essential female reproductive organs comprise the uterus, fallopian tubes and ovaries, and together with the vagina and its supporting structures of muscles and ligaments the female reproductive tract is completed (see Figure 15.3). Breasts are usually described as part of the total system. All of these organs are under the influence of pituitary and ovarian hormones, interacting with the hypothalamus in order to provide the maximum opportunity for the human race to reproduce itself. The cervix is the lower narrower part of the uterus which protrudes downwards into the vagina and is subject to friction from sexual intercourse. The outer covering of the cervix that is exposed to this friction is composed of squamous epithelium which is relatively tough; the cervical canal is lined with columnar epithelium, glandular in origin and secretes sticky mucus that forms a 'plug' in the cervix to protect from ascending pathogens (Clancy and McVicar, 2002; Seeley *et al.*, 1992).

Pathophysiology

Early (pre-malignant) changes in the endo-cervical tissue take place in the 'squamo-columnar junction' or 'transformation zone' (see Figure 15.4). This is the area in the cervix where squamous epithelium, which covers the part of the cervix that protrudes into the vagina, joins with glandular epithelium that

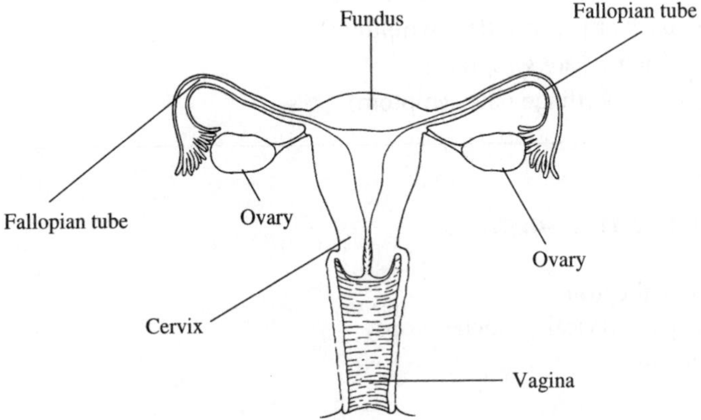

Figure 15.3 Uterus and appendages

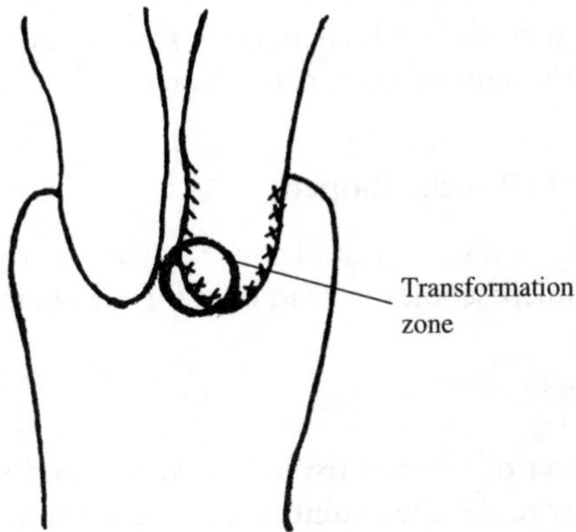

Figure 15.4 Cervix – transformation zone

lines the cervical canal. Hence it is crucial that whenever cervical cytology is undertaken, effective instruments are utilized to enable a suitable sample of transformation zone cells to be secured.

Clinical Manifestations

Symptoms that require attention/investigation

- Thin, watery, blood-stained vaginal discharge
- Post-coital spotting or bleeding
- Metrorrhagia (intermittent, painless, intermenstrual bleeding)
- Menorrhagia (heavy or excessively lengthy menstrual bleeding)

- Ulceration within the vulval/pelvic area
- Pelvic, back or leg pain (late symptoms)
- Ankle oedema (late symptom)
- Vaginal haemorrhage (late symptom)

Diagnostic Investigations

- Endocervical cytology
- Colposcopy/cervical (punch) biopsy
- Cone biopsy

Endocervical Cytology

A small wooden, plastic or brush-like instrument is inserted into the cervix and rotated in order to scrape cells from the 'transformation zone'. These are then affixed to a plastic/glass slide which is then scrutinized in the pathological laboratory for any early signs of malignant change.

Colposcopy/Cervical (Punch) Biopsy

This is a visual scrutiny of the cervix and adnexae with the removal of tiny pieces of tissue that can be microscopically examined for malignant changes.

Cone Biopsy

A 'cone-shaped' section of cervical tissue is removed and sent for histological examination. This may reveal the extent of any pre-malignant or frankly malignant changes in the cervical tissue.

Treatment

When a woman with undiagnosed cervical cancer is pregnant, a conservative approach to assessment is usually the preferred method and treatment delayed until after delivery. If cancer is suspected, a larger, wedge biopsy is necessary, and performed under general anaesthetic (GA) due to the increased risk of haemorrhage from the enhanced blood supply to the reproductive organs during pregnancy.

Surgical interventions to remove a malignant cervix date back to 1892 when Schauta (1902) first performed a successful radical, vaginal hysterectomy. His work was superseded by the German gynaecologist Wertheim who, in 1912, offered reports on a series of over 500 hysterectomies whereby a five year survival rate of 70 per cent had been achieved, but a surgical mortality rate of 19 per cent prevented general acceptance of his intervention at that time. Radiotherapy was, however, gaining greater acceptability in treatment for cervical cancer, but, following the reports of Bonney (1932) and Meigs (1951), which demonstrated better survival rates of around 65 per cent with lower perioperative mortality for surgery, radical hysterectomy became the established treatment for cervix cancer. Burghardt and Holtzer (1977) suggested that minimally invasive cancers could be treated conservatively by local excision (cone biopsy) or simple hysterectomy and more recent recommendations are for treatment by those means.

Treatment varies according to the extent of the disease. The main aim of local conservative treatment is to prevent the spread of cervical cancer to the uterine body or adjacent organs (Anderson, 1993).

Conservative Treatments

- Cryotherapy
- Diathermy
- Laser therapy
- Squamo-columnar junction excision
- Cone biopsy
- Radical excision
- Radiotherapy
- Chemotherapy

Cryotherapy (Cryocautery)

Using probes, fairly large areas of tissue can be destroyed; although Richart *et al.* (1980) argue that this therapy is best reserved for smaller lesions. The intervention can be undertaken without anaesthetic and, provided the depth of the disease does not exceed 4 mm, this process can be considered curative, is cost-effective and does not compromise fertility. Deeper lesions may require further applications and there is a risk that incomplete destruction of the cancer could lead to new epithelial growth covering the remaining cancer cells.

Diathermy

This destroys tissue more effectively than the freezing technique previously described, but has to be performed under local/general anaesthesia. It will destroy tissue up to 1 cm depth, but has the side effect of causing profuse vaginal discharge with scarring of the cervix, but Hammond and Edmonds (1990) stress that this does not appear to affect fertility or normal labour.

Laser (Light Amplification by Stimulated Emission of Radiation) Therapy

The effect of laser therapy used in this situation is heat-producing and the tissue at the focal point of the laser beam is vaporized. The therapy is undertaken via direct vision and thus offers precision and control over the depth of destruction, avoiding damage to sensitive adjacent tissues. Cure rates of 94 per cent of selected patients with adequate tissue destruction have been reported by Jordan *et al.* (1985).

Squamo-columnar Junction (Transformation Zone) Excision

Due to the fact that errors can be made following local destruction techniques (Anderson, 1993) these therapies have been developed as excisional techniques that avoid hysterectomy. Laser and diathermy loop excision are two methods by which deeper local surgery can be undertaken for more invasive cervical cancer, or for where depth of disease is difficult to determine. Laser excision requires a more exacting technique than laser vaporization and takes more time to complete. Diathermy loop excision is probably the treatment of choice for the majority of women with pathological cervical cytology (see Figure 15.5).

It offers good results, and can be undertaken at the first outpatient clinic appointment. It has been shown by Bigrigg *et al.* (1994) to be a quick, easy treatment, relatively free from side-effects and having no detrimental effects on fertility or pregnancy outcomes.

Cone Biopsy

This is performed for either diagnostic or therapeutic requirements. McLaren (1967) reported a success rate of nearly 93 per cent, but with the advent of colposcopy, cone biopsies can be much more specifically structured to each woman's particular lesion, resulting in the removal of smaller amounts of

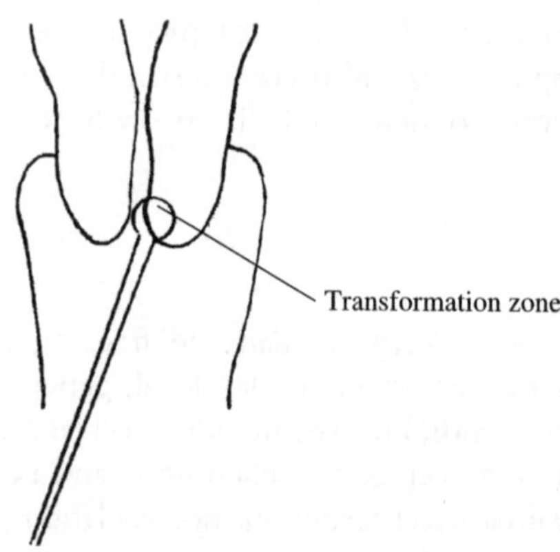

Figure 15.5 Cervix – large loop excision

cervical tissue with subsequently fewer side effects but with equally good, positive outcomes (Jordan, 1989).

Radical Excision

Where early treatment fails then hysterectomy may be necessary, however, as more young women are being screened and diagnosed with cytological abnormalities and treated quickly and effectively by local ablative excisional methods, with cure rates of over 90 per cent (Shafi and Jordan, 1996), hysterectomy is becoming an increasingly rare necessity. The fact that a woman may be diagnosed with cancer of the cervix during pregnancy (though this is a rare occurrence) and proceed to a normal delivery, does not appear to have a poorer prognostic outcome than for the non-pregnant woman. It is the clinical stage at the time of diagnosis that has the main bearing on survival, and treatment, either conservative or radical, is related to the stage of the disease rather than the pregnant condition.

Radiotherapy

This may be used for certain larger cervical lesions in order to reduce pelvic metastases; however there is little evidence to suggest that radiation and hysterectomy need to be combined (Shingleton and Orr, 1995).

Chemotherapy

Cytotoxic drugs will reduce the size of the malignant tumour prior to hysterectomy and improve the amenability of the lesion to surgery; Thomas (1993) suggests that in order to determine whether or not this form of treatment affects recurrence rates or patterns of survival, further study is necessary.

Follow-up

Pelvic examination and Papanicolou smear of the vaginal cuff should be undertaken at three-monthly intervals for the first year post-operatively, then each six months for two years. Other investigations should be arranged according to symptomology (Shingleton and Orr, 1995).

The conditions of invasive cervical cancer and uterine body cancer are outside the scope of this chapter.

Nursing Interventions

Health Promotion

The nurse should be fully aware of the nature and availability of cervical smear tests, and in the UK all women between 20 and 64 years of age are eligible every five years (NHS Screening Programmes, 1999) with some health authorities offering them every three years. The nurse should be able to explain the procedure to women that it is not painful and is usually undertaken by the female practice nurse to avoid embarrassment.

Health Education

- Advice regarding high-risk practices such as smoking and unprotected sexual intercourse should be given in a sensitive and informative manner.
- Encouragement of women to seek medical attention for any unusual vaginal discharge or irregular bleeding must be seen as a prime role of any nurse.

During Investigation and Treatment

Support for the Patient

- Women undergoing treatment for cervical cancer should be allowed time to voice their anxieties and be given appropriate information in accordance with their individual disease status.
- Nursing support for the woman who requires hysterectomy or treatment that will remove wanted fertility is essential, and the offer of advice that the small number of women who encounter side-effects of surgery, such as continence problems or sexual difficulties can usually be assisted by conservative or further surgical intervention. A positive perspective should be maintained.

When caring for women with breast cancer or cancer of the cervix, nurses need to carefully assess the patient's

- Understanding of the reason for hospital admission. Knowledge of malignant disease and its treatment varies and it is essential to establish a mutual focal point from which to progress.
- Historical perspective of her disease process, including onset of symptoms, reporting to the doctor, understanding of the doctor's diagnosis, prescription of investigations and subsequent treatment regimes.
- Psychological perspectives of her disease. Women can under- or overestimate the seriousness of malignancy, which may lead to either denial of the disease and refusal of treatment or even suicide.

Nursing action points

- Be knowledgeable regarding factors likely to increase the risk of breast/cervical cancer and be willing to discuss these with clients/patients.
- Promote the uptake of breast and cervix screening programmes.
- Encourage women with unusual anatomical/physiological developments to seek medical attention.
- Offer physical and psychological care and support for women undergoing investigations and treatment for malignant disease of reproductive tissues.
- Promote comfort and dignity for women living with or in the terminal stages of breast or cervical cancer.

Conclusion

Breast cancer is the most common cancer in women worldwide and is the second leading cause of death from malignant disease (Boring *et al.*, 1994). Many research programmes have assisted in the understanding of this disease, its development, progress and treatment. However, it engenders fear in women who are positively diagnosed and requires a sensitive and holistic approach to medical treatment and nursing care. Treatments, even when tailored to the individual woman's needs, may result in quite devastating side effects that might lead to withdrawal from the therapeutic programme. Nursing interventions should be aimed at educating women about the effects of the disease, choices of treatments and their effects and side effects, and acting as an advocate when a breast cancer sufferer is psychologically unable to indicate a preferred route of therapy. Nurses must always work as part of the multidisciplinary team and consider the effects upon the patient of members of that team. Skills that nurses acquire throughout training, education and practical experience must be employed when helping cancer patients through investigative procedures, treatment regimes and aftercare.

Cancer of the cervix is also a common malignant condition throughout the world. Its incidence varies more widely than breast cancer, although screening and educational programmes regarding the use of condoms during sexual intercourse have assisted in reducing its prevalence in developed countries over the last decade. As with most malignant diseases, cervical cancer, if detected in the early stages, can be completely cured and may cause no problems to the woman who wishes to conceive post-therapy.

Nursing interventions include the education and encouragement of all women to take advantage of cervical cytology and avoid risk factors initially, then to help them accept follow-up treatment if a suspicious or positively diagnosed test is reported, and to advise patients about the effects and side effects of treatments. Nurses have a duty of care to their patients which carries an individual responsibility of maintaining an up to date portfolio of broad nursing knowledge, skills acquisition and appropriate attitudes towards nursing work, together with a more specific, personally designated library of reflection on past experiences and their adaptation to experiences that they will encounter in the future, as new research introduces new ways of thinking and acting towards and with ill people.

References

American Cancer Society (AMC) 1995, *Cancer Facts and Figures*. Atlanta. American Cancer Society.

Anderson, M. C. 1993, 'Invasive carcinoma of the cervix following local destructive radiotherapy for cervical intraepithelial neoplasia'. *British Journal of Obstetrics and Gynaecology*, 100, 657–63.

Austoker, J., Mansel, R., Baum, M., Sainsbury, R. and Hobbs, R. 1995, 'Guidelines for Referral of Patients with Breast Problems'. London. NHS Breast Screening Programme.

Bigrigg, A., Haffenden, D. K. and Sheehan, A. 1994, 'Efficacy and safety of large loop excision of the transformation zone'. *Lancet*, 343, 32.

Bjørge, T., Steinar, O. and Thoreson, G. 1993, 'Incidence, survival and mortality in cancer of the cervix in Norway'. *European Journal of Cancer*, 29A (16), 2291–7.

Bonney, C. 1932, 'Surgical treatment of cancer of the cervix'. *British Medical Journal*, 2, 914.

Boring, C. C., Squires, T. S., Tong, T. and Montgomery, S. 1994, 'Cancer statistics'. *Cancer*, 44, 7–26.

Brinton, L. 1992, 'Epidemiology of cervical cancer – overview' in Munoz, N. and Bosch, F. X. (eds), *The Epidemiology of Human Papillomavirus and Cervical Cancer*. Lyon. 1 ARC.

Burghardt, E. and Holtzer, E. 1977, 'Diagnosis of microinvasive carcinoma of the cervix uteri'. *Obstetrics and Gynaecology*, 49 (6), 641–53.

Cancer Research Campaign (CRC) – now known as Cancer Research UK – 1997, *The Latest Cancer Statistics*. London. CRC.

Clancy, J. and McVicar, A. 2002, *Physiology and Anatomy*. London. Arnold.

Clinical Outcomes Group 1996, *Guidance for Purchasers: Improving Outcomes in Breast Cancer*. Leeds. NHS Executive.

Colditz, J. A., Hankinson, S. E. and Hunter, D. J. 1995, 'The use of estrogens and progestins and the risk of breast cancer in post-menopausal women'. *New England Journal of Medicine*, 332, 1589–93.

Coombes, R. 2000, 'In the pink: breast cancer, down but not out'. *Nursing Times*, 96 (40), 10–11.

David, J. 1995, *Cancer Care*. London. Chapman and Hall.

Denton, S. 1996, *Breast Cancer Nursing*. London. Chapman and Hall.

Dey, M. P. and Woodman, C. B. 1996, 'Epidemiology and pathogenesis of cervical cancer' in Shingleton, H. Fowler, J., Jordan, J. and Lawrence W. 1996 (eds), *Gynaecological Oncology*. London. W. B. Saunders.

Dey, P. and Twelves, E. 1996, 'Breast cancer' in Stevens, A. 1996 (ed.), *Health Care Needs Assessment*. Oxford. Radcliffe Medical.

Eriksson, J. H. 1990, *Oncologic Nursing*. Pennsylvania. Springhouse.

Fallowfield, L. 1991, *Breast Cancer*. London. Routledge.

Farmer, R. and Miller, D. 1983, *Lecture Notes on Epidemiology and Community Medicine*. Oxford. Blackwell Scientific.

Faulkner, A. 1998, *Effective Interaction with Patients*. Edinburgh. Churchill Livingstone.

Feldman, J. E. 1989, 'Ovarian failure and cancer treatment: incidence and interventions for the pre-menopausal woman'. *Oncology Forum*, 16 (5), 651–7.

Fletcher, S., Black, W. and Harris, R. 1993, 'Report on the international workshop on screening for breast cancer'. *Journal of the National Cancer Institute*, 85, 1644–56.

Gail, M. H. and Benichou, D. 1994, 'Epidemiology and biostatistics programme of the National Cancer Institute'. *Journal of the National Cancer Institute*, 86, 573–5.

Hammond, R. H. and Edmonds, D. K. 1990, 'Does treatment for cervical intraepithelial neoplasia affect fertility and pregnancy?' *British Journal of Medicine*, 301, 1344–5.

Howard, R., Goldacre, M., Mason, A., Wilkinson, E. and Arness, M. (eds) 1999, *Health Outcome Indicators: Breast Cancer. Report of a Working Group to the DOH*. Oxford. National Centre for Health Outcomes Development.

International Cancer Research Foundation (ICRF) – now known as Cancer Research UK – 1999, 'Breast Cancer – Spot the Symptoms Early'. London. ICRF 99. MCM. B001.

Jordan, J. A. 1989, *Controversies in Gynaecological Oncology*. London. RCOG.

Jordan, J., Woodman, C. B. and Mylotte, M. J. 1985, 'The treatment of cervical intraepithelial neoplasia by laser vaporisation'. *British Journal of Obstetrics and Gynaecology*, 92, 394–8.

Kirschbaum, M. 1999, *Lymphoedema and Breast Cancer*. London. NT Books. Leadbeater, M. 2000, 'Cancer patients' information needs'. *Nursing Times*, 96(37), 48.

Leonard, R. C., Rodger, A. and Dixon, J. M. 1995, 'Metastatic breast cancer' in Dixon, J. M. (ed.), '*ABC of Breast Disease*'. London. British Medical Journal.

Ley, C., Bauer, H. M. and Reingold, A. 1991, 'Determinants of human papillomavirus infection in young women'. *Journal of the National Cancer Institute*, 83, 997–1003.

Medical Advisory Services for Travellers Abroad (MASTA) 2000, *Travellers Health Brief*. London. Medical Advisory Services for Travellers Abroad.

McLaren, H. C. 1967, 'Conservative management of cervical pre-cancer'. *Journal of Obstetrics and Gynaecology*, 74, 487–92.

McPherson, K., Slee, C. M. and Dixon, J. M. 1995, 'Breast cancer: epidemiology, risk factors and genetics' in Dixon, J. M. (ed.), *ABC of Breast Disease*. London. *British Medical Journal*.

Meanwell, C., Kelly, K. and Wilson, S. 1988, 'Young age as a prognostic factor in cancer of the cervix: analysis of population-based data from 10 022 cases'. *British Medical Journal*, 296, 392–6.

Meigs, J. 1951, 'Radical hysterectomy with bilateral pelvic lymph node dissection'. *American Journal of Obstetricians and Gynaecologists*, 62, 854.

National Cancer Alliance. 1996, *Patient-centred Services; What Patients Say*. Oxford. National Cancer Alliance.

National Health Service (NHS) Cancer Screening Programmes 1999, *Cervical Screening: A Pocket Guide*. Sheffield. NHS Cancer Screening Programmes.

Office of Population Censuses and Surveys (OPCS) 1989, *Cancer Statistics Registrations*. London. OPCS Series MB1. 1974–89.

Parkin, D. M. 1993, 'Estimates of the world-wide incidence of eighteen major cancers in 1985'. *International Journal of Cancer*, 54, 594–606.

Reeves, W., Brinton, L. and Garcia, M. 1989, 'Human papillomavirus infection and cervical cancer in Latin America'. *New England Journal of Medicine*, 320, 1437–41.

Richards, M. and Smith, I. 1995, 'Breast diseases' in Dixon, J. M. (ed.), *ABC of Breast Disease*. London. *British Medical Journal*.

Richart, R. M., Townsend, D. E. and Crisps, W. 1980, 'An analysis of long-term follow-up results in patients with cervical intraepithelial neoplasia treated by cryotherapy.' *American Journal of Obstetricians and Gynaecologists*, 137, 823–6.

Sainsbury, J., Anderson, T. and Morgan, D. A. 1995, in Dixon, J. M. (ed.), *ABC of Breast Disease*. London. *British Medical Journal*.

Schauta, F. 1902, 'Die operation des gebarmutterkrebes mittes des Schuchardt'shen paravaginatschmittes'. *Monatsschrift Geburtshilfe und Gynakologie*, 15, 133.

Seeley, R. R., Stephens, R. D. and Tate, P. 1992, *Anatomy and Physiology*. St. Louis. Mosby.

Shafi, M. I. and Jordan, J. A. 1996, 'Management of pre-invasive lesions of the cervix' in Shingleton, H., Fowler, W., Jordan, J. A. and Lawrence, W. D. (eds), *Gynecologic Oncology*. London. W. B. Saunders.

Shingleton, H. and Orr, J. 1995, *Other Treatments in Cancer of the Cervix*. Philadelphia. J. B. Lippincott.

Stoppard, M. 1996, *The Breast Book*. London. Dorling Kindersley.

Thomas, G. M. 1993, 'Is neoadjuvant chemotherapy a useful strategy for the treatment of stage 1B cervical cancer?' *Journal of Gynaecology*, 2, 62–4.

Veronesi, U., Salvadori, B. and Luinia, A. 1995, 'Breast conservation is a safe method in patients with small cancers of the breast: long-term results of 3 randomized trials on 1973 patients.' *European Journal of Cancer*, 31A, 1574–9.

Watson, M. 1991, *Cancer Patient Care*. Cambridge. British Psychological Society. Cambridge University Press.

Watson, J. D., Sainsbury, J. R. and Dixon, J. M. 1995, 'Metastatic breast cancer' in Dixon, J. M. (ed.), *ABC of Breast Disease*. London. *British Medical Journal*.

Winkelstein, W. 1990, 'Smoking and cervical cancer – current status: a review.' University of Manchester. *American Journal of Epidemiology*.

16

Men's Cancers

SANDRA JOHNSON

The five key areas targeted by the Health of the Nation (Department of Health [DOH], 1992) document, aimed at significant improvement by the year 2000, were: strokes, coronary heart disease, mental illness, sexual health, accidents and cancers. Cervical and breast cancers in women were specifically identified, and have been explored in the previous chapter. However, two common male cancers, testicular and prostatic malignancies received no such interest in the document, despite the fact that testicular cancer is the most common malignant tumour in young men in the United Kingdom (UK), occurring mostly in those aged 15 to 55 years (Imperial Cancer Research Fund [ICRF] – now known as Cancer Research UK – 1999) and prostatic cancer being the second most common in males generally, resulting in around 10 000 deaths annually (Perry, 2000). This chapter examines several issues surrounding these two male cancers, including the reluctance of men to seek help and advice regarding unusual physiological changes. It does not cover palliative care since the two cancers are remarkably susceptible to treatment if discovered early in their course. The intention is for nurses to assist in raising awareness of men to their own anatomy and physiology and to support them in their quest for guidance when deviations from the norm are detected.

Men and women by nature have different healthcare needs, but the question is, 'Are men receiving less sympathetic attention from the DOH than women, given the large amount of literature available for women with gender-specific malignancies and the relatively small amount of information offered to men for two distressing, possibly life-threatening, male-only cancers?' The Royal College of Nursing (RCN) Men's Health Forum (1999) reported that for every one pound spent on men's health, eight pounds is spent on women's health issues. The information within this chapter will attempt to explain this imbalance and, in part, offer nurses the opportunity to influence health promotion and illness prevention in men.

Contents

Learning Objectives

By the end of this chapter you should be able to demonstrate knowledge of

- What is understood by the terms testicular and prostatic cancers.
- The national and international incidence of the disorders.
- Contemporary, evidence-based contributory factors to their development.
- The structure and function of the organs discussed.
- Malignant change affecting the testes and prostate gland.
- The health problems complained about, by men with these diseases.
- Tests that men may have to undergo in order to effect a diagnosis.
- Treatments and nursing care that will assist patients' recovery.

Definition of Testicular Cancer

Testicular cancer is a malignant change of testicular tissue that, if left undetected or untreated, will cause fatality.

Epidemiology

Cancer of the testicle is the most common malignancy in men aged between 15 and 44 years (ICRF, 1999) with Northern Europe having a higher incidence than Southern Europe and with Denmark reporting one of the highest rates in the world. Only 3 per cent of all testicular cancers are diagnosed in males over the age of 70 years (Office for National Statistics [ONS], 1998). Otto (1997) reports a persistent trend of higher incidence in Caucasian Americans than in black Americans and Wardle (1994) observes this difference to be reflected in other non-American populations. A disturbingly rapid increase in the incidence of the disease in England and Wales and many developing countries during the past 20–25 years has been reported by Coleman (1996), who also observed that the risk of testicular cancer is greater in higher socio-economic groups and in unmarried men. It is rare in males of African ancestry and in pre-pubertal males worldwide (Blandy, 1999).

The testicular cancer risk ratio is 1 in 450 males below the age of 50 years in the UK, with just over 1500 new cases diagnosed annually, which represents almost double the figures of 20 years ago (ICRF, 1999). Yet despite these alarming statistics, cancer of the testicle is one of the most curable malignancies with 90 per cent of victims recovering completely, early diagnosis and treatment being the key to a favourable prognosis.

Aetiology

Despite much research being undertaken, it would appear that several factors might be involved in the development of testicular cancer, although none of these would account for the dramatic increase in incidence over recent years.

Predisposing Factors

- Undescended testicle
- Familial tendency
- Antenatal exposure to oestrogen
- Inguinal hernia/hydrocele
- Trauma
- Human immuno-virus disease (HIV)

Undescended Testicle

Males born with an undescended or partially descended testicle are five times more likely to develop testicular cancer than males whose testes lie in the scrotal sac at birth. However, only about 10 per cent of testicular tumours is associated with maldescent and if the condition is surgically corrected before the age of three years, then the risk factor reverts to that of the general population (Blandy, 1999).

Familial Tendency

There appears to be a genetic influence in the development of testicular cancer. A male having a father or brother with the disease is up to five times more likely than the average population, to be similarly affected (Baird, 1988).

Antenatal Exposure to Oestrogen

There is some evidence that the reproductive tissue responds abnormally to high levels of circulating maternal oestrogen in some sensitive fetal males and Blandy (1999) found that rare testicular cancers (Sertoli cell tumours) also cause gynaecomastia (enlarged male breasts) that further supports Baird's (1988) earlier assumption.

Inguinal Hernia/Hydrocele

There is a possible link between these two conditions and testicular cancer, since families prone to the latter appear to report a very high incidence of hernia and hydrocele (Baird, 1988).

Trauma

The testis is easily injured during ordinary working activities. A haematoma (collection of blood) develops in the cavity of the tunica vaginalis (see Figure 16.1) and may enlarge, causing pressure–atrophy of the remainder of the testis. Testicular tumours are well known to occur post-traumatically and, while testicular swellings are relatively commonly presented in general practice, malignant change must be treated as a possibility. Infection of the testes may have a similar effect although evidence so far is inconclusive. The testes may occasionally be the site of metastatic spread from prostate or other malignant tumours.

Human Immuno-Virus Disease (HIV)

There is an association between the development of testicular cancer and HIV, but with this exception, it is unclear whether behavioural patterns contribute to the malignancy (Nichols, 1998).

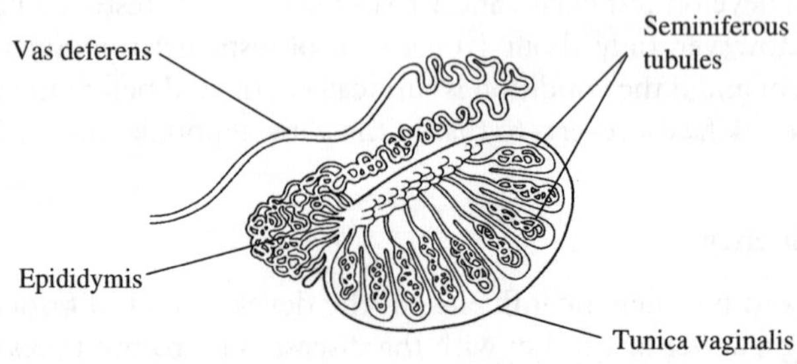

Figure 16.1 Testis

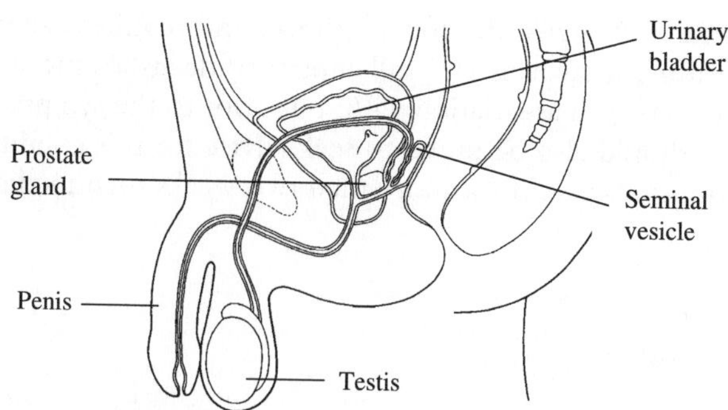

Figure 16.2 Male reproductive tract

Anatomy and Physiology

The male reproductive system comprises the two bilateral testes which lie outside the body in a fold of skin known as the scrotum (Figure 16.2). The testes are the site of spermatozoa manufacture, the sex cells necessary for reproduction, and of the male hormone testosterone. Sperms, manufactured in the seminiferous tubules are stored in a convoluted tube that sits on top of the gland – the epididymis – and are expelled from the male reproductive tract during ejaculation. The prostate gland is essential in the process of sperm motility from their origin to their destination by the secretion of prostatic fluid which lubricates the vas deferens through which they pass. The seminiferous vesicles provide some further lubrication and a fructose-based nutrient to provide the sperms with energy to continue their journey (Marieb, 2001).

Pathophysiology and Clinical Manifestations

Most men with testicular cancer present with a painless lump in the testicle or enlargement of one or both testes. There may be groin or abdominal 'heaviness' or a dull ache in the scrotum; very occasionally testicular cancer may cause acute pain in the early stages. More rarely, patients present with symptoms of metastatic disease for example, severe back pain associated with spinal metastases or breathlessness and coughing of bloodstained sputum, which suggests metastatic disease of the respiratory system.

Approximately 15 per cent of patients show signs of inflammation, which may be mistaken for benign epididymitis or acute orchitis, and a further 15 per cent have a history of fairly recent local injury (Blandy, 1999). All of these may lead to inappropriate early treatment and a delay in diagnosis of cancer and likewise of effective treatment.

Seminal granuloma is an induration in the epididymis which may follow vasectomy; this is an early inflammatory response to extravasated sperms but may resemble the early signs of testicular cancer and requires examination and appropriate treatment, such as anti-inflammatory drugs. Some men will also develop gynaecomastia in association with, but prior to the symptoms of testicular cancer, and should also be urged to seek advice for this condition. Should any of these symptoms persist for more than two weeks then medical attention is imperative.

 **Connection**

Chapter 14 (Cancer – an Overview) discusses the aetiology of carcinogenesis.

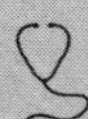 *Nursing action points*

The nurse can play a vital role in primary health care by

- Educating and encouraging men to practice testicular self-examination (TSE) on a regular basis.
- Educating boys that from the time of puberty they should familiarize themselves with their own genital anatomy by regularly examining each testicle with the fingers and thumbs to determine size. It is common to have one testicle larger than the other, in shape and weight. This gives a good foundation by which comparisons can be made in later years. School nurses have a particularly important contribution.

The importance of TSE cannot be overemphasized, since the earlier any malignancy is discovered, the more easily it can be treated with the potential for cure being very high. Unfortunately, only 3 per cent of young men perform this check on a regular basis, mainly through ignorance of its value in health protection (ICRF, 1999) and over 50 per cent of men affected by testicular cancer delay reporting their symptoms to their doctor until the disease has begun to metastasize. Aspects of masculinity clearly play a part in men's decision making with regard to seeking help for physical or mental health problems. Because young men in their teens and early 20s have a feeling of invincibility, they often delay or avoid medical appraisal because they feel it would show them to be vulnerable (Piper, 1997). In recent years, however, there has been a dramatic shift from curative to preventative healthcare, with public health at the forefront of policy initiatives. Schools, workplaces and community settings are identified as key target areas where health improvement programmes can be implemented and nurses can assist in reducing men's unease by providing a relaxed, 'natural' atmosphere in which to address health promoting activities. While these initiatives will not prevent testicular cancer, as the cause remains unknown, they may reduce the time lapse between the discovery of an early tumour and the commencement of treatment.

Investigative Tests

- Ultrasound scan
- Blood tests
- Surgical exploration
- Computerized axial tomography

Ultrasound Scan

Once physical examination confirms the presence of an abnormality, this test, which can be completed in minutes and is painless, should be performed. Results are remarkably reliable (Blandy, 1999).

Blood Tests

Blood is taken for

- Assessment of the enzyme placental alkaline phosphatase (PLAP), which is secreted by gonadocytes
- The hormone human chorionic gonadotrophin (HCG), secreted by the trophoblastic cells
- Alphafetoprotein (AFP), secreted by yolk-sac cells

Surgical Exploration of the Testis/Testes

Under general anaesthetic the scrotum is surgically incised and a malignant testicular tumour can usually be visualized. Verification by frozen section biopsy may be requested, but is not recommended as it can encourage metastatic spread (CancerBacup, 1999).

Computerized Axial Tomography (CT)

A CT scan of the abdomen and chest will identify lymph node involvement and any spread to the lungs (Blandy, 1999).

Once these investigations have been completed and a positive diagnosis reached, treatment will commence and varies according to the classification, grading and staging of the tumour.

Treatment

- Radiotherapy
- Chemotherapy
- Surgical intervention

Staging of Testicular Tumours

- Stage 1 – Tumour confined to testis
- Stage 2 – Lymph node involvement within the abdomen
- Stage 3 – Lymph node involvement above the diaphragm
- Stage 4 – Tumour spread to lungs and liver

There are two main aetiological types of testicular cancer – seminomas and non-seminomas, which are further subdivided according to the cell type from which the tumour originated. Seminomas are the most common and account for around 40 per cent of the total of testicular cancers and are extremely sensitive to radiotherapy thus negating the need for surgical intervention (Dawson and Whitfield, 1997).

For Stage 1 seminomas, a cure rate in excess of 95 per cent has been reported as attributable to radiotherapy (Dawson and Whitfield, 1997); Blandy (1999) claims 100 per cent cure rate with radiotherapy and an identical cure rate obtainable via a single course of the chemotherapeutic agent Carboplastin. For Stage 2, where regional lymph node metastases are present, but smaller than two centimetres in size, a cure rate approaching that of Stage 1 is achievable (Dawson and Whitfield, 1997). For more advanced disease the initial treatment of choice is usually chemotherapy, offering platinum-based drugs and follow-up by computerized tomography scanning to determine the site and size of residual metastases. These may be removed by very careful surgical intervention.

Non-seminomas are more aggressive than seminomas and develop from the more specialized germ cells and, being more aggressive have often spread to the lymph nodes when the patient presents with his symptoms. If the cancer is localized in the testicle then the gland may be removed (orchidectomy) and no further treatment required. However, about 10 per cent of Stage 1 patients have recurrences within two years and will then be treated with adjuvant chemotherapy.

Stage 2 non-seminoma patients who have had orchidectomy and surgical lymph node removal may need no further treatment although some oncologists may offer the patient a short course of combined chemotherapy as prophylaxis against further recurrence. Most Stage 3 non-seminomas can be cured with multi-drug chemotherapy (Nichols, 1998).

Risk of Future Recurrence

Nichols (1998) indicated that the risks for second cancers in later life were significantly higher in men who had previously been positively diagnosed, compared with those having no prior history of testicular malignancy. The risk for subsequent cancer development also increases with time for example 25 years after testicular cancer diagnosis, survivors face a 15.7 per cent risk of a second cancer compared with 9.3 per cent risk for men who had never had a cancer. These facts may be related to the possible carcinogenic properties of the platinum chemotherapeutic drugs, which are retained in the tissues after completion of treatment. However, the research was undertaken on men treated several decades ago and, since chemotherapy treatments now last weeks rather than months or years as they did previously, men treated recently could face considerably lower risks of secondary cancer development in comparison to those treated in the 1970s.

Nursing Interventions

Most people when confronted with the diagnosis of cancer are understandably worried about a range of issues associated with the disease, its progress, treatment and outcome. Young men may feel particularly distressed as they probably belong to social groups where body image, virility and sexuality are seen as very desirable qualities and any threat to these aspects avoided assiduously. They may be embarking on relationships where fathering children is viewed as an essential element of the partnership or, may be at the stage of developing confidence and improved self-esteem after the disturbing changes of puberty. Nurses are in a position to help the patient through a very difficult time whether the treatment is surgery, chemotherapy or radiotherapy.

A model of nursing is usually employed with which to assess the patient's pre-operative health needs with particular reference to breathing, as a general anaesthetic will be necessary, and to appraise nutritional status since anxiety following the diagnosis may have induced loss of appetite, and, if abdominal metastases are present, nausea and vomiting may have compounded weight loss. Maintaining the patient's safety pre-, during, and post-orchidectomy is essential; this includes appropriate preparation for surgery.

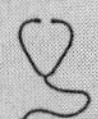

Nursing action points

- Ensure that the patient is clean and comfortable and wearing suitable operating department attire.
- Ensure that the patient has an empty urinary bladder.
- Ensure that the patient is identifiable via a detailed wrist-band.
- Remove any prostheses to suitably labelled containers and store safely.
- Administer prescribed pre-operative medication, at the appropriate time.
- Ensure that the patient has had nothing to eat or drink for four to six hours prior to the anaesthetic.
- Explain all of these measures and the rationale for their implementation to the patient in order to gain his cooperation and allay anxiety.
- Do not hurry this pre-operative period so that the patient can feel confident about asking questions and seeking clarification of any issues that are causing concern.

The Psychological Pre-operative Assessment

This should ascertain the patient's main concerns regarding orchidectomy. One of these is likely to be how the surgery will affect his sexual functioning and reproductive capabilities (Nichols, 1998).

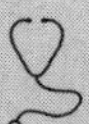

Nursing action points

Explain to the patient that

- The removal of one testicle does not impair fertility or sexual function since the remaining testicle can produce spermatozoa and hormones in adequate amounts for reproduction.
- The removal of retroperitoneal lymph nodes does not affect the ability to have erections or orgasms. It can, however, disrupt the nerve pathways that control ejaculation causing infertility, but newer nerve-sparing techniques have assisted in reducing the incidence of these unwelcome side effects.

Body Image

The patient may also voice fears about body image, expressing feelings of loss or worthlessness as a man. Discussions with the surgeon may result in the implantation of a testicular prosthesis into the scrotal sac during surgery in order to retain normal outward appearance. If the nurse is aware of measures that can be employed to assist the patient in the maintenance of his usual body image then he or she may successfully relieve some of the mental anguish that the patient is experiencing.

Post-operatively

The nurse must maintain the patient's airway, breathing and circulation, monitoring each aspect carefully and regularly.

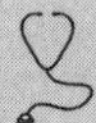

Nursing action points

- Observe the scrotal wound for any haemorrhage, haematoma development or infection.
- Implement measures to resolve these potential problems if they become apparent.
- Ensure a well-balanced diet and oral fluid intake of two to three litres daily, which will assist in post-operative recovery and a return to normal health.

Radiotherapy and/or Chemotherapy

These may be considered as follow-up care after orchidectomy or, in the case of seminoma, the preferred treatment without surgical intervention. No one treatment works for all testicular cancers and the nurse must be aware of, and be able to explain to the patient that seminomas and non-seminomas differ in their tendency to spread, patterns of spread and their response to radiotherapy and chemotherapy. Choice of treatment largely depends upon the type of tumour and the stage of the disease.

Chemotherapy can cause increased risk of infection, nausea and vomiting and hair loss, although not all patients experience these side effects. Some drugs may cause infertility but studies have shown (Henkel, 1996; Nichols, 1998) that the majority of men so treated, recover fertility within 36–40 months.

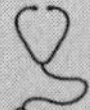

Nursing action points

Following radiotherapy, advise patients that they may

- Become very fatigued.
- Suffer from bone marrow depression and its related problems of susceptibility to infection.
- Suffer from bleeding from mucous membranes.
- Become anaemic.
- Experience an associated temporary infertility.

Nurses must encourage the patient to attend follow-up outpatient clinic appointments and convey an attitude of optimism for him, emphasizing that the cure rate is very high for all types and stages of testicular cancer and many of the more drastic measures taken for Stage 3 and Stage 4 can be avoided if the tumour is discovered and treated in its early stage and compliance with the therapeutic regime is secured.

Conclusion

While this disease is relatively uncommon, it is the most frequently occurring cancer in young men. It responds well to treatment but causes a great deal of mental anguish in those young men who are positively diagnosed. In its early stages, treatment is very effective and has limited side effects, but in later stages treatment has to be more aggressive with correspondingly more severe side effects. Certain factors have been identified as being possibly predisposing to testicular cancer and treatment itself may result in the development of second cancers at a later time in life.

The nurse is in a unique position to help young men identify testicular tumours at an early stage by encouraging regular TSE, a message that might be difficult to convey to the prime risk group, and by sensitive assessment and nursing care throughout treatment, can reduce the physical and psychological trauma associated with the unpleasant therapeutic regime.

Patients who have been treated for testicular cancer also need to be made aware that TSE of the remaining testicle should continue to be performed at monthly intervals and any further abnormalities discovered should be reported immediately to the general practitioner. The nurse should also alert young men to the availability of recently established 24-hour 'Walk-in Clinics' where they can access nursing in an atmosphere of total confidentiality, and where they can be advised of appropriate 'next steps' to take if there is the slightest suspicion of malignant change or doubt about their general health.

Definition of Prostatic Cancer

Malignant change of the prostate gland is rare in young men but very common in older men. It is highly susceptible to therapy, but life-threatening if left untreated.

Epidemiology

Prostatic cancer incidence rates have increased dramatically since 1989, both in the UK and in the United States of America (USA) and this cancer is the second most common malignant disease in British males (lung cancer being the most common). In North American males, cancer of the prostate gland represents the most common malignancy and accounts for 41 per cent of all newly diagnosed male cancers, and, while mortality rates from the disease declined significantly from the mid-1990s, prostatic cancer remains the second leading cause of death from malignant disease in UK and USA males (Otto, 1997).

Worldwide, the pattern of prostatic cancer reveals a high rate in the USA and Northern European countries, particularly amongst Swedish and Danish males, but the lowest incidence rates are recorded in Asia, Eastern Europe and central and South America. However, in a similar historical pattern observed in the behaviour of many cancers, prostatic cancer increases in Asians and others who migrate to the USA, gradually assuming the rates of the indigenous population (Otto, 1997).

Prostatic cancer is associated with the ageing process with around 19 000 men newly diagnosed each year in England and Wales (Munro, 2000) of whom 8500 will die, typically four to five years later. While the disease appears to be increasing in incidence, this may be due to increased interest in the condition, and increase in survival of older men and improved diagnostic procedures. There is a familial link, with men that have a close relative having prostatic cancer having double the risk of developing it themselves. The median age at diagnosis is 72 years with the incidence rate rising every decade after the age of 50 years. Over 80 per cent of all prostate cancer patients are older than 65 years and the disease is nearly twice as common in black males than in white males, with their death rate being nearly three times greater. By the age of 80 years, nearly all of the male population will have a small malignant '*in situ*' prostatic tumour but only 25 per cent of those will prove fatal (Blandy, 1998). While the UK government spends around 4.2 million pounds annually researching prostatic cancer, opinions vary regarding the usefulness of screening methods to detect the disease (Gray, 2000).

Aetiology and Pathophysiology

Typically, the tumour originates in the posterior lobe of the gland near the outer margin and, as it increases in size, causes urinary symptoms. Local invasion occurs as the tumour expands through the prostatic capsule and may spread to the bladder base, and distant spread may involve metastatic deposits in the pelvic, mediastinal and supraclavicular lymph nodes, with lung, liver, kidneys and skeleton being frequent sites of metastatic involvement.

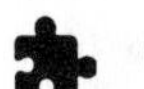

Connection

Chapter 14 (Cancer – an Overview) discusses the aetiology of carcinogenesis.

Anatomy and Physiology

The prostate gland lies at the base of the urinary bladder (see Figure 16.3) and comprises two zones or lobes, which encircle the urethra. Benign hypertrophy, which is extremely common in middle aged and older men, arises usually in the inner lobe whilst malignant changes usually occur in the outer lobe. The bladder and seminal vesicles, vas deferens and ureters lie behind and above the prostate gland. The gland is composed of minute tubules, the contents of which (prostatic fluid) are squeezed out by muscle contraction during ejaculation. This prostatic fluid is thought to lubricate the urethra and enhance the motility of the spermatozoa and possibly provide some form of nourishment to the sex cells.

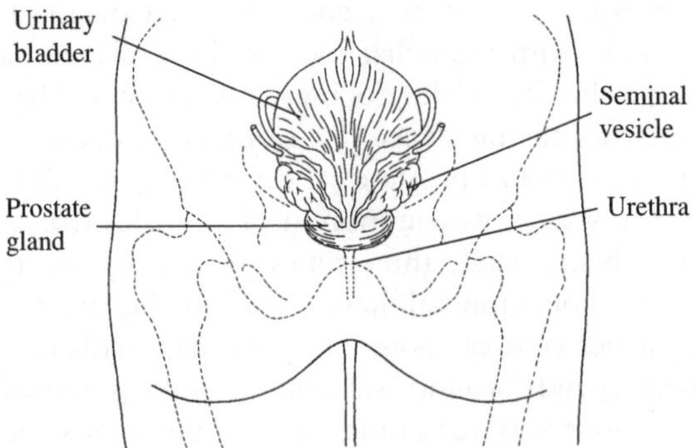

Figure 16.3 Prostate gland in relation to bladder and urethra

Clinical Manifestations

- Poor urinary flow with hesitancy
- Involuntary stopping and starting
- Dribbling at the end of voiding
- Feeling that the bladder is not completely empty following micturition
- Frequency and urgency
- Increasing nocturia
- Haematuria

Typically, the cancer develops slowly and imperceptibly and initially its symptoms and signs are very similar to benign prostatic hypertrophy. As the gland begins to obstruct the urethra, urinary symptoms may start to cause problems such as poor urinary flow with hesitancy, the patient may describe involuntary stopping and starting with dribbling at the end of voiding. He may feel as though the bladder is not completely empty following micturition and bladder instability can occur which may cause frequency and urgency with increasing nocturia. Sometimes haematuria presents when the patient begins to pass urine, but the flow then clears. The patient may relate the symptoms to a minor infection or irritation, but any haematuria should be investigated.

Investigative Tests

Screening for Prostatic Cancer

As with all services provided through the NHS that are designed to assess risks to health, nurses must be able to give current information to men who may be considering screening for prostatic malignancy, and have a degree of knowledge that will justify acting as any patient's advocate. Screening for prostatic cancer raises a number of issues with which nurses must be conversant if they are to act in the patient's best interests (UKCC – now known as the Nursing and Midwifery Council – 1992).

Currently the main screening test is the prostate specific antigen (PSA) which can produce false positive results, but health campaigners are pressing for widespread screening, viewing it as an effective method of reducing prostate cancer deaths. However, the National Screening Committee argues that the belief that mortality rates can be reduced by PSA screening is not founded on hard evidence and in North America, where the test is implemented on a large scale, the evidence does not point to lowered rates of prostatic cancer (Munro, 2000).

While the British government spends around 4.2 million pounds annually on research and favours the test, planning to introduce a national prostate screening programme, Dr Muir Gray of the National Screening Committee condemns the idea and argues that mass screening may do more harm than good, with side effects causing impotence and incontinence (Munro, 2000).

Digital rectal examination may assist in diagnosing prostatic malignancy, but this has low accuracy rates, and any screening programme must be

- Desirable by the target population
- Acceptable in terms of accurate results
- Available to all at risk people and be matched by effective treatment for those showing positive results
- Able to identify early stages of the disease
- Sensitive and specific to the condition

(Austoker, 1994)

Prostatic cancer is not well understood and a large number of men over the age of 70 who die from an unrelated cause harbour foci of potential malignant disease (Kramer *et al.*, 1993), thus it is difficult to distinguish with confidence between innocent and potentially fatal prostatic cancer. In addition, the anxiety and possible further inappropriate invasive investigations and treatment that might be undertaken following false positive testing, could result in greater harm to the patient than if no screening had been implemented initially. Similarly under debate is the issue of trans-rectal ultrasound examination and prostatic biopsy, but Dawson and Whitfield (1997) argue that if, on digital rectal examination, a hard nodule replaces the normal smooth surface of the prostate or it is enlarged, hard and lumpy to the touch, proceeding to ultrasound and biopsy is justifiable. However, they recommend that this should be considered within the context of the individual patient, since biopsy can cause infection and haemorrhage.

Prostatic cancer is found by chance in about 10 per cent of patients who have been offered trans-urethral prostatectomy for an assumed benign hypertrophy of the gland, and the cancer may be detected by a PSA blood test that has been organized as one of a range of tests into general illness. Computerized axial tomography (CT) scan, magnetic resonance imaging and bone scans may be useful in determining the extent of the disease, thus aiding treatment decisions.

Treatment

- Regular monitoring
- Radiotherapy
- Prostatectomy
- Hormone therapy
- Bilateral subcapsular orchidectomy

Localized disease (Stage T1 – where the disease is clinically unapparent) can be initially managed by regular monitoring of the tumour, as few such cancers progress significantly over the following decade. Radiotherapy or radical prostatectomy may be offered at that stage where life expectancy is more than 10 years, but radical prostatectomy is a cause of impotence and/or urinary incontinence in some men. However, this intervention has seen the achievement of a 15-year disease-free survival rate for 85 per cent of men (Dawson and Whitfield, 1997).

Those men whose prostate cancers have advanced beyond the capsule (Stages T3 and T4) will be offered treatment that is designed to contain rather than cure the disease since most of these patients will have undetectable metastatic deposits. Radiotherapy is usually the recommended treatment at these stages although the patient may be offered the choice of radical prostatectomy, particularly if the response to radiotherapy is poor.

With widespread disease, treatment with hormone therapy, based upon the suppression of testosterone secretion or androgen depletion is often implemented. Cyproterone acetate is an anti-androgen whose effect is to reduce prostatic cell growth, it is however hepatotoxic. Goserelin works by antagonizing lutenizing hormone releasing hormone and may be given in conjunction with cyproterone acetate. Bilateral sub-capsular orchidectomy may be performed with a similar effect to treatment with hormone therapy, without the need for regular injections and tablets, but this choice may not appeal to many men (Blandy, 1998).

Where isolated metastases induce pain, local irradiation creates a dramatic palliative response, particularly when these metastases develop in the skeletal system (Otto, 1997) and similar pain relief can be produced by radioactive phosphorus 32, strontium 89 and diphosphonate (Blandy, 1998).

Nursing Interventions

Health Education

Nurses must be familiar with all aspects of this disease if they are to 'safeguard and promote the interests of individual patients and clients' (UKCC, 1992). Therefore, during the early stages when there are altered patterns of urinary elimination related to prostatic enlargement, nurses should advise the patient to seek guidance from the general practitioner who may arrange for further investigations.

If the patient is admitted to hospital for radical prostatectomy, the nurse's role is to help prepare the patient both psychologically and physically for this surgery. The patient needs to be aware of the possible effects of sexual dysfunction post-operatively, but also be informed that prostate cancers are relatively slow-growing typically, and treatable. Anxiety is intensified by poor knowledge of therapeutic procedures and a nurse's fluent and up to date explanations can help to reduce this anxiety (Dearnalay, 1994). It is not unusual for patients and their partners to enter a grieving process once the diagnosis of any cancer is made, so full information of immediate planned treatment and possible follow-up investigations and future therapeutic interventions should be discussed, with a view to giving the patient maximum opportunity for informed consent.

The Nursing Pre-operative Assessment

This involves the identification of potential post-operative physical and psychological problems together with collection of information that will help the nurse to devise an individualized care plan. There may be a pre-operative visit from a member of the operating department staff who can answer questions about the nature of the surgery; from the physiotherapist who will teach the patient breathing and leg exercises in order to reduce respiratory and thrombo-embolic complications.

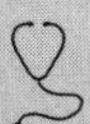

Nursing action points

- The nurse should encourage the patient to practise the exercises prior to surgery and reinforce the teaching of her multidisciplinary team colleagues.
- Bowel preparation may be necessary along with nursing interventions to ensure the patient's safety during his operation.
- The patient should be informed that a urinary catheter will be *in situ* post-operatively and that the urine will be bloodstained for several days.
- The nurse should ensure that the patient has fasted for at least six hours pre-operatively and that any prescribed medication is given appropriately.
- All records of vital signs should be up-to-date, laboratory reports and x-rays available and the consent for operation form signed with the patient's full knowledge of the surgical intervention(s) planned.

Post-operatively

Following surgery, the patient's respiratory function must be closely observed and maintained, his blood pressure and pulse must be carefully monitored and any deviations from the normal range, reported to a senior nurse or doctor. The wound site should be checked regularly for signs of potential haemorrhage and urinary output recorded. Blood clots may occlude the lumen of the urinary catheter therefore it is usual for the bladder to be continuously irrigated to reduce this possibility, and irrigation fluid throughput requires accurate recording.

Pain control must be achieved initially by the nurse administering prescribed strong analgesics and, when the patient is recovered sufficiently, he can be shown how to manage a self-controlled analgesic system in order to maintain a pain-free state. This teaching can take place pre-operatively, but will need to be reinforced following a general anaesthetic as the latter frequently disturbs mental equilibrium for hours or sometimes days following its administration. It is likely that hydration will be via an intravenous infusion for several hours post-operatively, but sips of cold fluids will probably be very welcome. Personal hygiene, including mouth care, should be attended to by the nurse who will also have assessed and continue to assess risk factors for pressure sore development using a recognized scale such as Waterlow (1988) and for deep vein thrombosis potential, for example, Autar (1996).

Bladder spasm is not uncommon following radical prostatectomy and prescribed antispasmodic drugs may need to be administered to relieve this problem.

Stool softeners should be administered as directed, as these will minimize the need to strain to defecate and thus avoid undue abdominal discomfort and pressure on the wound site.

Some patients are discharged with the urinary catheter still in place and the nurse will teach the patient how to manage the closed drainage system and arrange for the community nurse to provide continuity of care for the patient in his own home. Further treatment such as, chemotherapy and/or radiotherapy is generally managed on an outpatient basis with the assistance of the community nursing staff who will administer prescribed intramuscular/intravenous drugs and monitor their effects and side effects and the patient's general health, taking into consideration the effects of the diagnosis and therapeutic regime on the patient's partner.

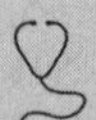

Nursing action points

- The patient and relatives should be given full explanations wherever possible in order to make informed decisions and to reduce anxiety.
- The patient should be prepared physically and psychologically prior to surgery.
- Post-operatively the wound site and urinary output should be monitored for any signs of bleeding or clot formation.
- It is important, post operatively, to reinforce teaching with regard to pain control.
- Hydration, personal hygiene and increased risks due to reduced mobility must be taken into account post-operatively.

- Bladder spasm is not uncommon post-operatively.
- Constipation must be avoided.
- Patients to be discharged with urinary catheter in place will need to be taught how to manage a closed drainage system.

Conclusion

Any person experiencing a diagnosis of cancer is likely to be very distressed at the news due to a variety of reasons. These reasons may involve past experiences of family members or friends having died of the disease, or from caring for people who have suffered badly from the disease or from the effects and side effects of treatments prescribed to control or cure their cancer. The self-concept of patients with cancer may be severely challenged, as 'self' is confronted with a potentially life-threatening situation and a fearfulness of the unknown. Body image is an essential element of self conceptualization, and the fact that this image is viewed by contemporaries as vigorous can be enhancing to that body image and upholding of self-esteem.

When investigations and treatments disturb the body image and self-esteem and possibly leave disturbed bodily functions, it is not surprising that patients feel distressed and find the challenge to self-concept extremely depressing psychologically.

To many people, the mention of cancer is a sentence (death) not just a word, often accompanied by a sense of guilt, failure and futility. Friends and family may avoid the subject (because they don't know what to say), which may deepen the sense of rejection and personal uncertainty for the patient. The side effects from treatment may pose further damaging self-conceptual problems for patients who have limited understanding of cancer, its treatments and outcomes; many patients avoiding treatments due to fear of permanent disfigurement and decreased sexual appeal to partners.

At all stages of care, whether investigatory, receipt of results, beginning, continuation and/or completion of treatment, the nurse has a major role in facilitating self-conceptual adaptation. She or he is often the person present when the patient feels the need for physical and emotional support, thus the nurse must be educationally and practically competent to meet the patient's needs and to assist him to adapt to the new life agenda that is posed. There must be a positive nurse–patient and supportive presence, which must also enable the patient to confront disturbing emotions and enable discussion that can assist the patient to understand realistic outcomes, either positive or negative, according to the specific treatment programme.

While malignant disease is a debilitating and psychologically distressing experience, patients can, and frequently do emerge with a positive self-image and a positive outlook on life. Nurses can play a vital role in this situation, by having confidence in their knowledge, competence in their skills and caring and compassionate attitudes towards their patients.

References

Austoker, J. 1994, 'Screening for ovarian, prostatic and testicular cancers'. *British Medical Journal*, 309, 315–20.
Autar, R. 1996, *Deep Vein Thrombosis – The Silent Killer*. Wiltshire.
Baird, S. B. 1988, *Decision Making in Oncology Nursing*. Oxford. Blackwell Scientific.
Blandy, J. 1998, *Urology*. Oxford. Blackwell Science.
Blandy, J. 1999, *Lecture Notes on Urology*. Oxford. Blackwell Science.
CancerBacup 1999, *Understanding Testicular Cancer*. London. Bacup.
Coleman, M. P. 1996, *Cancer Survival Rates in England and Wales 1971–1995; Deprivation and NHS Regions*. London. Office for National Statistics.
Dawson, C. and Whitfield, H. 1997, *ABC of Urology*. London. British Medical Association. Publishing.
Dearnalay, D. P. 1994, 'Carcinoma of the prostate gland'. *British Medical Journal*, 308, 780–4.
Department of Health (DOH) 1992, *The Health of the Nation*. London. HMSO.
Gray, M. 2000, *The NHS Plan*. London. National Screening Committee.
Henkel, J. 1996, 'Testicular cancer: survival high with early treatment'. *Urology*, 139, 299.
Imperial Cancer Research Fund (ICRF) – now known as Cancer Research UK – 1999, *A Whole New Ball Game*. London. ICRF.
Kramer, B. S., Brown, M. L., Protosky, A. and Gohagan, J. K. 1993, 'Prostate cancer screening; what we know and what we need to know'. *Annals of International Medicine*, 119, 913–14.
Marieb, E. N. 2001, *Human Anatomy and Physiology*. San Francisco. Benjamin Cummings.
Munro, R. 2000, 'Tsar slams prostate screening'. *Nursing Times*, 96 (42), 10–11.
Nichols, C. 1998, *Testicular Cancer*. Indiana. CHSU.
Office for National Statistics (ONS) 1998, 'Cancer Statistics Registration'. *MBI*. 25.
Otto, S. E. 1997, *Oncology Nursing*. St Louis. Mosby.
Perry, M. 2000, 'Dead men walking'. *Nursing Times*, 96 (11), 29–30.
Piper, S. 1997, 'The limitations of well-men clinics for health education'. *Nursing Standard*, 11 (30), 47–9.
Royal College of Nursing (RCN) 1999, *Men's Health – a Public Review*. London. RCN.
UKCC (now known as the Nursing and Midwifery Council) 1992, 'Code of Professional Conduct for Nurses, Midwives and Health Visitors'. London. UKCC.
Wardle, E. 1994, 'Testicular self-examination: attitudes and practices amongst young men in Europe'. *Preventive Medicine*, 23, 206–10.
Waterlow, J. 1988, 'The Waterlow Card for the prevention and management of pressure sores: towards a pocket policy of care'. *Science and Practices*, 1 (6), 8–12.

Index